PLAY THERAPY
WITH CHILDREN AND ADOLESCENTS IN CRISIS

Clinical Practice with Children, Adolescents, and Families

(formerly Social Work Practice with Children and Families)

Nancy Boyd Webb, *Series Editor*

www.guilford.com/CPCAF

This series presents a broad range of topics relevant for today's social workers, psychologists, counselors, and other professionals who work with children, adolescents, and families. Designed for practical use, volumes feature specific discussions of assessment, interventions, therapeutic roadblocks, the therapeutic relationship, and professional and value issues, illuminated by numerous case examples.

Play Therapy with Children and Adolescents in Crisis, Fourth Edition
Nancy Boyd Webb, Editor

Group Work with Adolescents, Third Edition: Principles and Practice
Andrew Malekoff

Social Work Practice with Children, Third Edition
Nancy Boyd Webb

Working with Adolescents: A Guide for Practitioners
Julie Anne Laser and Nicole Nicotera

Child Development, Third Edition: A Practitioner's Guide
Douglas Davies

Helping Bereaved Children, Third Edition:
A Handbook for Practitioners
Nancy Boyd Webb, Editor

Social Work in Schools: Principles and Practice
Linda Openshaw

Working with Traumatized Youth in Child Welfare
Nancy Boyd Webb, Editor

Mass Trauma and Violence: Helping Families and Children Cope
Nancy Boyd Webb, Editor

Culturally Competent Practice
with Immigrant and Refugee Children and Families
Rowena Fong, Editor

Complex Adoption and Assisted Reproductive Technology:
A Developmental Approach to Clinical Practice
Vivian B. Shapiro, Janet R. Shapiro, and Isabel H. Paret

Play Therapy with Children and Adolescents in Crisis

Fourth Edition

Edited by

Nancy Boyd Webb

Foreword by Lenore C. Terr

THE GUILFORD PRESS
New York London

A Division of Guilford Publications, Inc.
370 Seventh Avenue, Suite 1200, New York, NY 10001
www.guilford.com

Paperback edition 2017

Printed in the United States of America

This book is printed on acid-free paper.

Last digit is print number: 9 8 7 6 5 4

The authors have checked with sources believed to be reliable in their efforts to provide information that is complete and generally in accord with the standards of practice that are accepted at the time of publication. However, in view of the possibility of human error or changes in behavioral, mental health, or medical sciences, neither the authors, nor the editors and publisher, nor any other party who has been involved in the preparation or publication of this work warrants that the information contained herein is in every respect accurate or complete, and they are not responsible for any errors or omissions or the results obtained from the use of such information. Readers are encouraged to confirm the information contained in this book with other sources.

Library of Congress Cataloging-in-Publication Data

Play therapy with children and adolescents in crisis / edited by Nancy Boyd Webb ; foreword by Lenore C. Terr.—Fourth edition.
pages cm — (Clinical practice with children, adolescents, and families)
Includes bibliographical references and index.
ISBN 978-1-4625-2221-7 (hardback); ISBN 978-1-4625-3127-1
1. Play therapy—Case studies. 2. Crisis intervention (Mental health services)—Case studies. I. Webb, Nancy Boyd.
RJ505.P6P56 2015
618.92′891653—dc23

2015004736

To the 20 first-grade children and 6 school staff members
who were shot and killed in their elementary school
in Newtown, Connecticut, on December 14, 2012—
and to all the witnesses, survivors, first responders, parents,
and community members who were traumatized
by this tragic event

May this book help mental health practitioners
better understand the terrible aftermath
of such unpredictable and senseless violence,
as they attempt in numerous ways
to help effectively, both in the immediate aftermath
of a tragedy and in ongoing years
when the memories linger.

About the Editor

Nancy Boyd Webb, DSW, LICSW, RPT-S, is a leading authority on play therapy with children who have experienced loss and traumatic bereavement. She is University Distinguished Professor Emerita of Social Work in the Graduate School of Social Service at Fordham University, where she held the endowed James R. Dumpson Chair in Child Welfare Studies and founded the Post-Master's Certificate Program in Child and Adolescent Therapy. Dr. Webb has published numerous books on child therapy, trauma, and bereavement, including *Helping Bereaved Children* and *Social Work Practice with Children* (both now in their third editions). She is an active supervisor, consultant, and trainer who presents frequently at conferences in the United States and internationally. Dr. Webb is a recipient of honors including the Day–Garrett Award from the Smith College School for Social Work, the Clinical Practice Award from the Association for Death Education and Counseling, and the designation of Distinguished Scholar by the National Academies of Practice in Social Work.

Contributors

Jennifer Baggerly, PhD, Department of Counseling and Human Services, University of North Texas at Dallas, Dallas, Texas

David A. Crenshaw, PhD, Children's Home of Poughkeepsie, Poughkeepsie, New York

Esther Deblinger, PhD, Department of Psychiatry and Child Abuse Research Education and Service (CARES) Institute, Rowan University School of Osteopathic Medicine, Stratford, New Jersey

Jana DeCristofaro, LCSW, The Dougy Center: The National Center for Grieving Children and Families, Portland, Oregon

Robin Donath, LCSW, Silver School of Social Work, New York University, New York, New York

Athena A. Drewes, PsyD, RPT-S, Astor Services for Children and Families, Rhinebeck, New York

Valerie L. Dripchak, PhD, LCSW, Department of Social Work, Southern Connecticut State University, New Haven, Connecticut

Pamela Dyson, MA, LPC-S, RPT-S, private practice, Plano, Texas

Ilze Earner, PhD, Lois V. and Samuel J. Silberman School of Social Work, Hunter College, New York, New York

R. Blaine Everson, PhD, LMFT, Department of Counseling, Harold Abel School of Social and Behavioral Sciences, Capella University, Minneapolis, Minnesota

Rowena Fong, EdD, School of Social Work, University of Texas at Austin, Austin, Texas

Allen Garcia, BA, Department of Educational Psychology, University of Nebraska–Lincoln, Lincoln, Nebraska

M. Carlean Gilbert, DSW, LCSW, ACM, School of Social Work, Loyola University Chicago, Chicago, Illinois

Eric J. Green, PhD, Department of Counseling and Human Services, University of North Texas at Dallas, Dallas, Texas

Betsy McAlister Groves, LICSW, Department of Pediatrics, Boston University School of Medicine, Boston, Massachusetts

Craig Haen, PhD, RDT, CGP, LCAT, FAGPA, private practice, White Plains, New York; Drama Therapy Program and Department of Applied Psychology, New York University, New York, New York; Expressive Therapies Doctoral Program, Lesley University, Cambridge, Massachusetts

Joseph R. Herzog, MSW, PhD, Department of Social Work, University of West Florida, Pensacola, Florida

Rana Hong, PhD, LCSW, RPT-S, School of Social Work, Loyola University Chicago, Chicago, Illinois

Tina Maschi, PhD, LCSW, ACSW, Graduate School of Social Service, Fordham University, New York, New York

Joshua Miller, PhD, School for Social Work, Smith College, Northampton, Massachusetts

Kathleen Nader, DSW, private practice, Cedar Park, Texas

Felicia Neubauer, MSW, LCSW, private practice, Medford, New Jersey

Donna L. Schuurman, EdD, The Dougy Center: The National Center for Grieving Children and Families, Portland, Oregon

Heather Schwartz, MA, Department of Educational Psychology, University of Nebraska–Lincoln, Lincoln, Nebraska

Karin Sieger, PhD, Northern Children's Services Philadelphia, Philadelphia, Pennsylvania

Lori Stella, LCSW, Children's Home of Poughkeepsie, Poughkeepsie, New York

Anne L. Stewart, PhD, RPT-S, Department of Graduate Psychology, James Madison University, Harrisonburg, Virginia

Shulamith Lala Ashenberg Straussner, DSW, CAS, Silver School of Social Work, New York University, New York, New York

Susan M. Swearer, PhD, Department of Educational Psychology, University of Nebraska–Lincoln, Lincoln, Nebraska

Jennifer Taylor, LCSW, RPT, Department of Social Work, University of West Florida, Pensacola, Florida

Nancy Boyd Webb, DSW, LICSW, RPT-S, Graduate School of Social Service, Fordham University, New York, New York; private practice, Amesbury, Massachusetts

Maxine L. Weinreb, EdD, Child Witness to Violence Project, Boston Medical Center, Boston, Massachusetts

William F. Whelan, PsyD, Department of Psychology, University of Virginia, Charlottesville, Virginia

Foreword

On a long Sunday afternoon, a professional working with stressed children sometimes wonders, "Why do I do what I do?" We all know that children experiencing horrible luck are not easy to treat. They veer off-subject and speak in code. They run around the office, sometimes trying out light switches or spilling water on the carpet. Once in a while they immerse themselves in an online game or a book they've brought with them. In fact, a number of times one of them sitting in the consulting room claims to be studying for a test or doing a homework assignment. So why do we professionals keep coming back for more? Because children and adolescents, even when they are in crisis, are fun. And what makes them fun is that they almost always give us the opportunity to play.

We play with kids to help solve mysteries—mysteries of betrayal, mysteries of experience, mysteries of meaning, and mysteries of life itself. We use whatever medium the young person likes. Sometimes, in fact, we choose a play medium no one has taught us, or even thought of. Teenagers, for instance, might prefer music, drama, or poetry as a "fun" means of expressing themselves. They might choose design, rather than the superheroes and ice-princesses of younger kids. Whatever their choice, the opportunity for traumatized young people to express themselves and to form meaningful relationships with us very frequently lives and breathes in their play. The chance to enter their worlds of fear and pain exists in our ability to join in. We play right along, sometimes altering the storyline a little, sometimes saying something apt directly to them. Always, we plan as we play. We think almost "sideways." And the wonder of all this: we have fun.

Because children and adolescents exhibit such a pressing need to master overwhelming situations through play, a wonderful variety of playful interventions have been worked out in recent years for mental health professionals. This fourth edition of Nancy Boyd Webb's *Play Therapy with Children and Adolescents in Crisis* gives us a whole new panoply of play modes to read and consider. It offers us new paths to enter the play-worlds of preschoolers as well as adolescents. It includes new ways to play out the tragedies of loss as well as the miseries of failed adoptions, drug-abusing parents, bullying, court appearances, and chronic physical illnesses. As always, with Nancy Boyd Webb as editor, we have an opportunity to enter the mind of the therapist as well as the play-world of the child. Exemplary professionals tell us what they sense as they play, what they think, what they say, what they leave unsaid. In the final chapter, in fact, one of them, Tina Maschi, gives us support in the quest to take care of ourselves as we play out the crises in children's lives.

This fourth edition of Nancy Boyd Webb's book on play therapy represents a separate and very current addition to her earlier editions. Altogether, the four books make up a kind of encyclopedia. I have not discarded my three other books in this collection, nor would I discard this one if Dr. Webb decides to embark on a fifth. Each one informs me on the hows, whys, and whens of play therapy. This fourth edition also gives me information on the whos (from tots to fully developed teens). Reading about play, like play itself, can be fun. And what better activity—on a long Sunday afternoon—might one find?

LENORE C. TERR, MD
Clinical Professor of Psychiatry
University of California, San Francisco

Preface

As I prepare the fourth edition of this book, I am confronted with the 21st-century reality that crises and traumas are inescapable in the everyday lives of all children, adolescents, and their families. No one would describe today's world as peaceful, and it continues to be at least as dangerous as it was in 2007 (when the third edition was published). Mental health practitioners are eager for an overview of the latest treatment methods to help young people and their families who are confronting a wide range of traumatic life events. Trauma may occur as a result of natural disasters, such as tornadoes or wildfires; because of deliberate acts of violence, such as shootings in movie theaters or schools; or because of other unfortunate life events, such as sexual or physical abuse, witnessing abuse of parents or others, bullying, or immigration-related hardships. Regardless of the type of traumatic event, children, teenagers, and their parents often respond with extreme anxiety that requires and benefits from the professional help offered by trained mental health clinicians.

This book aims to provide such professionals and clinicians-in-training with the latest forms of treatment for children and adolescents who have experienced crises and trauma. The various treatment options presented here include approaches that focus on the individual, as well as many that include a parent in conjoint or filial therapy, and others that employ a family treatment model. Numerous newer treatments have been found effective in empirical research studies. From our understanding of child development, we know that young children often cannot express their feelings adequately in words—and, furthermore, that individuals of *all* ages who have been traumatized often avoid remembering and discussing their horrible experiences. This knowledge provides the rationale for using play and expressive therapies, since they encourage the release of feelings through the creative methods of art, puppetry, music, drama, and sandplay. These approaches offer effective ways to deal *symbolically* with frightening experiences that are too upsetting to confront directly and acknowledge as one's own. Many chapters in this book demonstrate the use of a variety of creative methods with young people who have suffered traumatic experiences.

In response to the comments of both academics and practitioners who have used previous editions of this book, this fourth edition adds a focus on traumatized adolescents, in addition to interventions with young children. Because of this inclusion of older youth, the chapter authors in this edition present numerous expressive therapy methods in their work with teenagers who would not want to engage in "play therapy" identified as such. Of course, play therapists also use creative methods such as art, drama, and musical interventions in their treatment of younger children, so the inclusion of expressive therapies in this volume represents more of a semantic shift than a drastic change of intervention approaches. However, the preferred intervention format with adolescents is group rather than individual, as several chapters in this volume demonstrate.

Similarly to the previous editions, this book is divided into five parts, beginning with a theoretical overview that provides the foundations for the use of play and expressive therapies. Part II consists of nine chapters dealing with crises and trauma in family contexts; the three chapters in Part III focus on helping children and teens in school settings. Part IV comprises four chapters on the topic of crises in the larger community and the world, and Part V is devoted to the important topic of professional self-care. Eleven chapters out of the total of 20 are entirely new to this edition, and the other nine have been updated and revised. The topics of the new chapters include growing up with substance-abusing parents, dealing with parental abandonment and divorce, and foster or residential care. The concept of "complex trauma," reflecting the cumulative occurrences of traumatic events in early childhood, is discussed in several chapters; one chapter describes expressive therapies in groups for adolescents who have suffered the negative effects of complex traumas. A cutting-edge topic presented in one chapter is the use of animal-assisted trauma-informed play therapy with children and adolescents who have to testify in court. Another chapter deals with the tragedy of school shootings, such as the one that occurred in Newtown, Connecticut. All the chapters contain case examples, and each chapter concludes with a list of study questions to stimulate class or group discussions about issues raised in that chapter.

The professional backgrounds of the chapter authors are diverse and reflect the range of practitioners who deal with traumatized young people: social workers, psychologists, counselors, drama therapists, and thanatologists. All share a strong commitment to providing the best quality service to the children and adolescents who have been referred to them. I am grateful that they have been willing to share their knowledge and experience for the benefit of other practitioners who will join them in serving traumatized and vulnerable youth in the most difficult circumstances.

Contents

Part IV
CRISES IN THE COMMUNITY AND WORLD

Part V
SUPPORT FOR THERAPISTS

Part I

OVERVIEW AND THEORETICAL FOUNDATIONS

Chapter 1

Family and Community Contexts of Children and Adolescents Facing Crisis or Trauma

NANCY BOYD WEBB

Crises and traumatic events are ubiquitous in modern life and affect people of all ages. Contrary to the myth that the magic years of childhood are a period of guileless innocence and carefree play, the reality of the preteen years, like that of later life, includes experiences that provoke anger, jealousy, fear, and grief as well as joy and pleasure. The teen years have long been considered full of conflict and struggle as young persons grapple to resolve their identity (Erikson, 1968). When children and youth experience crises or traumas, their families and communities inevitably also are involved. Sometimes adults actually are the instigators of the victimization of children and teens, as in cases of abuse or family violence. In other situations (such as natural disasters), no one person is responsible, and the entire affected community must deal together with the shared traumatic experience.

This revised volume focuses on adolescents as well as young children who are struggling to respond to crises and/or traumatic events. The book presents the use of play and expressive therapies to help these young people cope with and resolve their difficulties. The book begins with a focus on the family and community environment in which youth live because of the critical importance of this social context to the nature of young people's reactions in crises or traumatic situations. We know that young children depend on the adults around them for security and protection, and the younger they are, the more this is the case. Adolescents may attempt to respond either independently or with the help of peers, but these efforts may fail in the face of extreme trauma. Evidence in the professional literature increasingly attests to the influence of adults' responses to crises or traumas on the subsequent nature of children's reactions (Arroyo & Eth, 1996; Pfefferbaum, 1997; Rustemi & Karanei, 1996; Swenson et al., 1996). Because children watch and take their cues from adults, when their caregivers feel and act terrified, children become even more panicked—since they know that they themselves are helpless and powerless. Adolescents may try to act "cool" in tumultuous situations, but they can be deeply affected and traumatized nevertheless, even though they may not show immediate symptoms (Appleyard, Egeland, van Dulmen, & Stroufe, 2005).

This book recognizes and discusses the vast range of stressful and traumatic events that may impair everyday functioning and cause emotional pain to children and adolescents. The specifics of an *individual* child's or adolescent's responses, and the challenge of making a differential diagnosis, are presented by Nader in Chapter 2. The present chapter discusses the role of family and community factors in a youth's surrounding social environment that have the potential to ameliorate or worsen his or her response to a crisis or trauma. The nature of the crisis or traumatic event is also considered, since this can have differing effects on the type of support the young person receives. I have previously diagrammed the three groups of interacting factors affecting a

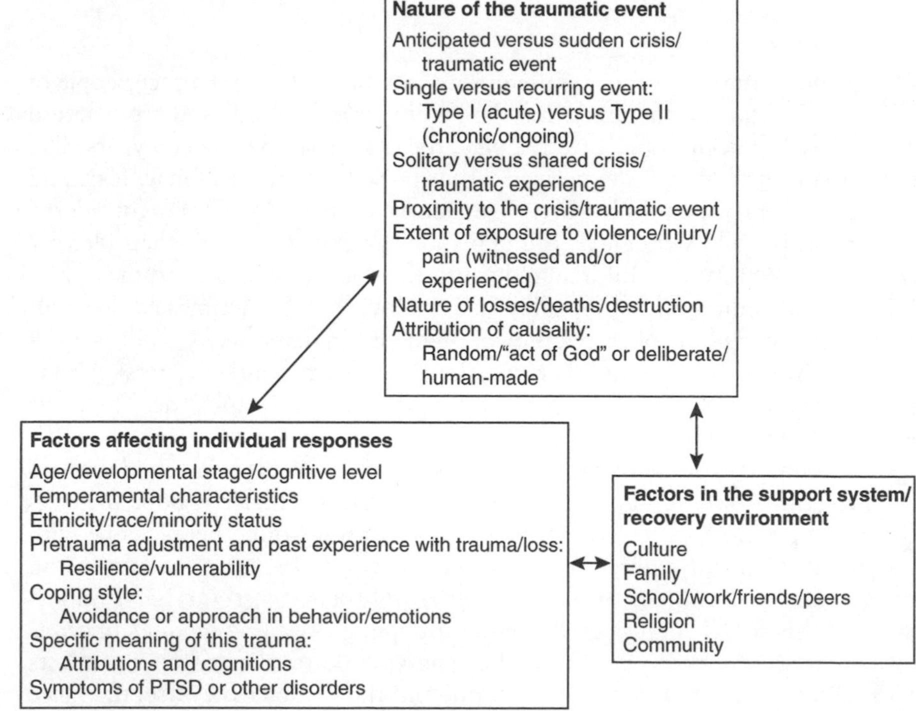

FIGURE 1.1. Interactive components of the tripartite assessment of a child's responses to a crisis/traumatic event. From Webb (2004a). Copyright 2004 by The Guilford Press. Adapted by permission.

child's responses to crisis or trauma, and have labeled the process of assessing these factors a "tripartite assessment" (Webb, 1993, 1999, 2004a, 2006, 2010, 2011; see Figure 1.1). Because this conceptualization is not age-specific, it can apply to adolescents as well as young children.

The next section presents an overview of the concepts of "stress," "crisis," and "trauma" as preliminary to examining the role of environmental risk and protective elements in buffering or escalating a young person's response to a crisis or traumatic event.

STRESS, CRISIS, AND TRAUMA

The conditions of stress, crisis, and trauma involve distinct but overlapping concepts. Whereas the "average" person (adult or child) carries out his or her life with the ability to withstand most of the ups and downs of a typical day, some people are less resilient to stress because their temperaments or their personal histories make them vulnerable. For example, an 11-year-old girl may wake up 20 minutes late and have to skip breakfast to avoid being late for school. The child in this situation feels some stress, but her stress level soon diminishes once she decides to omit her breakfast and to grab something to drink or eat on the way to school, thereby allowing her to arrive on time. In contrast, another girl in a similar situation may not see any alternative to being late; she becomes hysterical and decides not to go to school at all because she is afraid of being reprimanded for being late. Furthermore, she fears that the school will report her absence to her working mother, who will respond punitively. If we speculate that this second girl has a history of being harshly treated by her mother, we can see that the same circumstance—waking late—creates stress for both girls, but precipitates a crisis for the second girl, who may already be functioning on a marginal level because of her history of abuse. Figure 1.2 depicts the interaction and progression among the concepts of stress, crisis, and trauma.

Stress

Everyone knows how it feels to be under stress in situations that are challenging or threatening. Responses to stress may take one of three different forms: (1) attempting to get away from the uncomfortable circumstances ("flight"); (2) aggressively confronting the cause of the problem ("fight"); or (3) constricting/inhibiting one's emotional and behavioral responses ("freeze"). Selye (1978) coined the expression "fight or flight," to which "freeze" has been added by those studying behavioral reactions to dangerous situations (Blaustein & Kinniburgh, 2010).

The body under stressful circumstances actually undergoes physiological changes due to the outpouring of steroid hormones from the adrenal glands; these hormones cause increased heart and breathing rate, blood pressure,

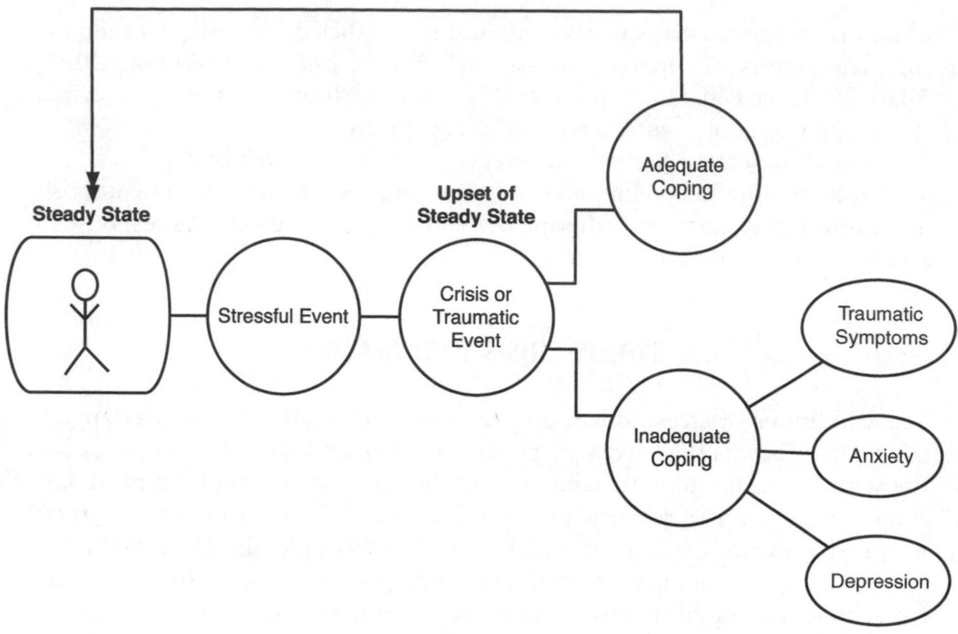

FIGURE 1.2 The interaction of stress, crisis, and trauma.

metabolic rate, and blood flow to the muscles (Benson, 2000; Selye, 1978). Although Selye maintained that stress in itself is not harmful, he pointed out that it may precipitate a state of crisis if the anxiety that accompanies it exceeds the individual's ability to function adequately.

In other words, people have different levels of stress tolerance, as well as different ways of responding to stress. Young children are particularly vulnerable to stress because of their youth, immature defenses, and lack of life experience. They often require assistance from adults to obtain relief from their anxiety and to learn new coping methods. Some adolescents under stress may rely on alcohol and drugs, and/or engage in other risky behaviors to help them cope, and these methods may actually place them at increased risk of danger (Blaustein & Kinniburgh, 2010).

Crisis

The term "crisis" refers to a situation that appears to exceed an individual's coping ability, and results in psychological disequilibrium, malfunctioning of emotions, cognition, and behavior (James & Gilliland, 2004; Roberts, 2005). The person perceives and believes that the event or situation is an intolerable difficulty that exceeds his or her resources and ability to cope. This emphasis on the *perception* of the event, rather than on the event itself, appropriately draws attention to the unique underlying meaning of the situation to each individual. As demonstrated in the case of the two girls who wake late for school, different people experience the same situation differently, and idiosyncratic factors determine their separate perceptions of a crisis.

Another example of distinctive responses to the same stressful situation involved a group of third-grade children, following the news of the sudden death of one of their classmates in an automobile accident. All the children in the victim's class displayed some degree of shock, concern, and curiosity about the death, but individual reactions varied greatly. One child told his teacher the next day (falsely) that his father had died suddenly the previous evening. Another child complained of headaches and stomachaches for a week with no physical cause, and a third child, who was a close friend of the dead child, had frightening nightmares for several weeks about being chased by a monster. However, most of the children in the class did not develop symptoms and did not appear to be traumatized by the death (in the opinions of the teachers and the school social worker), although the child with the nightmares did benefit from six play therapy sessions, which helped reduce her anxiety. See Webb (2002) for a full discussion of this situation.

Anna Freud (1965, p. 139) stated that "traumatic events should not be taken at their face value, but should be translated into their specific meaning for the given child." I believe that the same is true of crisis events more generally. We know that different people who are present at the same event will have different responses: Not only will their experiences differ, but the individual characteristics they bring to bear upon the psychological processing are different, and *this processing takes place in differing recovery environments*. For a child or teen in crisis, the "recovery environment" holds particular significance because of the young person's dependence on family members, peers, and others to provide support and guidance. Thus the tripartite assessment of the young person in crisis includes an analysis of (1) individual factors interacting with (2) the resources of the family and the social support network, in the face of (3) a specific crisis situation.

An underlying principle of crisis intervention theory is that crises can and do happen to everyone (James & Gilliland, 2004; Parad & Parad, 1990; Webb, 1999). No previous pathology should be assumed when, for example, a child becomes withdrawn and apathetic after the child's mother is hospitalized for surgery. Although individual differences influence personal vulnerability to breakdown and the form and timing of the disturbance, no one is immune from the possibility of becoming overwhelmed in the aftermath of a crisis.

Therefore, the phrase "stress overload" seems very relevant to crisis situations, and it explains the progression from stress to a state of crisis, as depicted in Figure 1.2. The overload causes the individual to feel disorganized, confused, and panicked. When these feelings continue without relief, anxiety, depression, and/or at least some symptoms of posttraumatic stress disorder (PTSD) may develop. In fact, some theorists believe that "the degree of distress caused by an event is the major factor determining the probability of the onset of psychiatric disorder" (McFarlane, 1990, p. 70). Therefore, a crisis intervention approach that aims to lessen the anxiety of the people involved in a crisis and to bolster their coping strategies has the potential for the primary prevention of psychiatric disorders. As we will see in many cases presented in this book, crisis intervention services are frequently short term because most crises by their very nature are time-limited. "A minimum of therapeutic intervention during the brief crisis period can often produce a maximum therapeutic effect through the use of supportive social resources and focused treatment techniques" (Parad & Parad, 1990, p. 9).

Trauma

In contrast to the possibility of brief and successful treatment of anxious individuals following crisis events, therapy for *traumatized* persons may take considerably longer. The word "trauma" comes from the Greek, meaning "wound." In the fifth edition of the *Diagnostic and Statistical Manual of Mental Disorders* (DSM-5), the American Psychiatric Association (2013) defines a traumatic event as one in which a person was exposed to threatened or actual death, grave injury, or sexual violence in any of four different circumstances: direct experience of a traumatic event; personally witnessing an event as it happened to others; learning that a traumatic event happened to a close relative or close friend; or repeated experience of exposure to painful details of a traumatic event. As mentioned previously, children often become terrified through witnessing adults in states of panic, high arousal, or frozen shock during traumatic events. The challenge of assessing a young person who has been exposed to a crisis or a traumatic event is discussed by Nader in Chapter 2.

THE NATURE OF THE CRISIS OR TRAUMATIC EVENT AND ITS IMPACT ON CONTEXTUAL SUPPORT

The tripartite assessment covers seven components that influence the nature of a crisis or traumatic situation. The present discussion focuses on how these factors may affect not only the individual, but also the type of support (or lack thereof) provided by the family and social environment. These specific components include the following:

- Anticipated versus sudden crisis/traumatic event
- Single versus recurring event: Type I (acute) versus Type II (chronic/ongoing) crisis/trauma
- Solitary versus shared crisis/traumatic experience
- Proximity to the crisis/traumatic event
- Extent of exposure to violence/injury/pain (witnessed and/or experienced)
- Nature of losses/deaths/destruction
- Attribution of causality: Random/"act of God" or deliberate/human-made

Anticipated versus Sudden Crisis/Traumatic Event

The Scout motto, "Be prepared," implies by contrast the undesirability of being caught off guard. Some events that lead to crises or traumas are by their nature unpredictable. Examples include natural disasters with no preliminary warning, the sudden death of a parent who was previously well, and the killing and injury of innocent bystanders in a wanton shooting episode. These contrast with other situations that gradually build up to a crisis or trauma. Examples of anticipated crises include a family's move to another community, the departure of the father from the home as the beginning of a marital separation, and the terminal illness of a family member. Stressful events that develop toward predictable outcomes present the opportunity for gradual comprehension and assimilation of the impending transition or loss.

However, many well-meaning adults deliberately try to shield young people from worry, and they avoid exposing them until the last minute to situations they believe will prove upsetting. For instance, they do not talk about a father's impending overseas military deployment until the day of his departure. This prevents the youth from "getting ready" psychologically, asking questions, and bracing themselves for the upcoming stressful loss. Often adults do not know how to talk with young people about future stressful matters, especially when they themselves are afraid and anxious.

The crisis techniques of "role rehearsal" and "anticipatory guidance" (Parad & Parad, 1990) aim to help individuals prepare in advance for future difficult situations. For example, a child who has advance knowledge, through pictures and explanations, about surgical masks and medical procedures shows less anxiety when confronted with these in a hospital. This mastery in advance through reflection or fantasy provides a form of psychological preparedness that ideally will lead to enhanced coping in future stressful situations. A folk saying claims that "a job well dreaded is more than half done." Even though the dreading is unpleasant, it permits anticipatory problem solving and emotional preparation. Parents, teachers, and community members who have contact with children and teens should be encouraged not to shield them, but to help prepare them for possible future stressful life experiences, and to assist them in talking about and dealing with their current worries as well.

Single versus Recurring Crisis/Trauma Events: Type I versus Type II Trauma and the Diagnosis of Complex Trauma

The notion of the "straw that breaks the camel's back" suggests that accumulated stress may weigh so heavily on a person that not even one minor additional stress can be tolerated. Thus the precipitating factor in a crisis may not be as significant as the events that have preceded it and created a "vulnerable state" for the individual. For example, a child who has suffered repeated physical abuse may respond aggressively after a relatively minor occurrence, such as a reprimand from a teacher, because of the child's preexisting vulnerable state.

Terr (1991) has proposed the concepts of "Type I" trauma, which occurs following *one* sudden shock, and of "Type II" trauma, which is "precipitated by a *series* of external blows" (p. 19; emphasis added). Responses to Type I traumas may include detailed memories and misperceptions about what happened, whereas reactions to Type II traumas often involve denial, numbing, dissociation, and rage. Sometimes the two types of traumas coexist. When untreated, either type can lead to serious disorders in both children and adults, but this is particularly true of Type II. For example, common sense suggests that the witnessing of a teacher's murder may have very different repercussions for a young person whose development is proceeding normally and whose parents offer appropriate comfort and support, as compared with a teen who lives in a dangerous neighborhood where guns and violence are commonplace and whose older siblings talk about needing a gun for self-protection. In most circumstances, Type I traumas do not lead to long-term symptoms, and recovery occurs in more than three-quarters of cases, even after very tragic experiences (Cohen, 2004; McFarlane, 1990). Type II traumas take much longer to resolve, however, and may require long-term treatment.

The term "complex trauma" refers to multiple, chronic, relational traumas such as abuse, neglect, violence, and parental misattunement, which begin in early childhood and which are usually ongoing and interpersonal (Herman, 1992; Kliethermes & Wamser, 2012; Shelby, Aranda, Asbill, & Gallagher, 2015). Because about one-fifth of youth in the United States have been exposed to more than one type of victimization (Grasso, Greene, & Ford, 2013), and the initial exposure typically occurs at about 5 years of age, this may mean that complex trauma is a relatively common condition in youth (Shelby et al., 2015). The symptoms may include various forms of emotional dysregulation, somatatization, and aggressive behavior (Saxe, MacDonald, & Ellis, 2007). Although this condition has been studied primarily in adults (Nader, 2008), there is growing attention to the assessment and treatment of this condition in children and adolescents (Kliethermes & Wamser, 2012). In Chapter 12 of this book, Haen discusses group treatment for adolescents who have been diagnosed with complex trauma.

Solitary versus Shared Crisis/Traumatic Experience

If "misery loves company," then we would expect the sharing of a crisis or traumatic experience to offer a degree of comfort and support that is absent when an individual undergoes such a stressful crisis alone. Certainly the dynamic of guilt ("What did *I* do that caused this?") and issues of personal responsibility ("What *should* I have done?") are irrelevant or greatly reduced in shared situations. Although every crisis or traumatic event is experienced ultimately on a personal level, the knowledge that others are enduring similar turmoil may reduce the stigma of victimization. For example, a child victim of incest may gain extraordinary benefits from participation in a support group of similarly victimized children.

However, the commonality of a shared crisis or traumatic event does not automatically lead to bonding among the individuals involved. Terr (1979), reporting on the aftermath of the kidnapping of a school bus of summer school students, found that the traumatized youngsters avoided contact with one another after the horrible experience was over. As if to escape the memories of their ordeal, these children tried to blend into the community and to stay away from the students who had shared the trauma and who reminded them of the frightening experience. This type of avoidance was also noted by many group therapists who unsuccessfully attempted to convene bereavement support groups soon after the New York World Trade Center terrorist attacks of September 11, 2001 (Hartley, 2004). Avoidance is one of the characteristics of PTSD, as discussed below.

Age is a crucial factor in determining the extent to which the sharing of a crisis or traumatic situation helps children. Whereas peer support may be very crucial for adolescents, the influence of peers is not strong until the middle years of elementary school. Preschool children rely on their familiar adult caregivers, rather than on peers, to provide them comfort and security when they are upset. Unfortunately, parents and teachers often minimize children's anxious responses (La Greca & Prinstein, 2002) thereby increasing the likelihood that children in distress will not receive timely treatment.

Proximity to the Crisis/Traumatic Event

A research study in California following a sniper attack in a school playground (Pynoos & Nader, 1989) found that children who were in closer physical proximity to the shooting developed more symptoms of PTSD than children who were on the periphery or not on the playground when the attack occurred. Proximity to the shooting resulted in more severe responses, both soon after the event and 14 months later (Nader, Pynoos, Fairbanks, & Frederick, 1990). These findings, which seem intuitively valid, confirm that proximity to a crisis or traumatic event results in intense sensory responses together with a heightened sense of life threat, all of which can contribute to symptom formation.

However, as I have written previously (Webb, 2004b, p. 8), "proximity can be viewed as emotional, as well as geographic." Many employees who worked in the New York World Trade Center lived some distance from ground zero. Their family members who watched the disastrous events of 9/11 on television were clearly in close "emotional proximity" to the traumatic events. In fact, in this age of high media exposure, even very young children may watch horrific events such as the World Trade Center's destruction, and see such things as the clouds of smoke and people jumping from buildings to escape. Research after both the Oklahoma City bombing of 1995 and the 9/11 attacks showed an association between televised coverage of the terrorist events and children's adverse psychological outcomes (Pfefferbaum et al., 2004). These exposure experiences may qualify as "vicarious traumatization" (McCann & Pearlman, 1990), since they involve auditory and visual scenes of horror. Unfortunately, many families did not protect their children from watching repeated media replays of these traumatic events, and some children became very confused and troubled by seeing them. In these instances, "proximity to the event" occurred within their own living rooms!

Extent of Exposure to Violence/Injury/Pain (Witnessed and/or Experienced)

As the preceding discussion suggests, we live in a violent world that does not shield children from graphic exposure to conflict in all forms and locales, including the family, school, and community. American society seems to have a high baseline tolerance for violence, which within the family takes the form of child abuse, spouse or partner abuse, incest, and other assault episodes. Pynoos and Eth (1985, p. 19) believe that "children who witness extreme acts of violence represent a population at significant risk of developing anxiety, depressive, phobic, conduct, and posttraumatic stress disorders." (This risk, of course, is even higher when children are themselves the victims of such violent acts.) Indeed, the presence of severe threat to human life in which the individual's response involves intense fear, helplessness, and horror constitutes the precondition for a traumatic experience in the DSM-5 diagnosis of PTSD, as I have noted earlier and as discussed by Nader in Chapter 2.

Child witnesses typically experience a sense of helplessness and confusion when confronted with human-induced acts of violence. Especially when these traumatic events occur in their own families, children become flooded with feelings of anger, vulnerability, and fear because they realize that the very people who are supposed to love and protect them are instead deliberately hurting them or other family members. This usually interferes with the development of a secure attachment relationship (Davies, 2004, 2011).

When violence results in deaths—as, for example, in the school shootings of 20 children in Newtown, Connecticut—the community and newspapers may sensationalize the event, and the people involved may feel overwhelmed by an emotional battery of reactions, including anger, hatred, and guilt (see Miller, Chapter 14, this volume). Although a family can help a child survivor by ensuring his or her safety and protection after the traumatic situation is over, the pupils who witnessed the deaths of their classmates and feared for their own lives will not easily forget this, and many will need specialized treatment to help them deal with their traumatic memories (Rivera, 2013). Fortunately, schools have become more attuned to the wisdom of providing some form of psychological debriefing or first aid to students following a school-based crisis or trauma such as the Newtown event, but often witnesses will still require individual treatment. In Chapter 14, Miller discusses appropriate school interventions following violent and traumatic events.

Nature of Losses/Deaths/Destruction

Losses play a major role in many crises and traumatic situations, and the associated reactions of confusion, anger, and desperation may be understood as mourning responses associated with the losses. When the losses include death of or separation from family members, grief and mourning are appropriate responses. Less obvious losses occur in situations such as moving or school promotion, which require giving up a familiar location or status and developing new relationships. Teachers can attest to the high level of anxiety in September until children become comfortable with the expectations and people in their new grade. This anxiety usually does not cause a state of crisis for most youth, but it can put them into a vulnerable state in which their ability to cope is reduced temporarily. Even adolescents may be uncomfortable in a new grade until they become accustomed to their schedules and their different teachers.

The converse of loss is attachment. If no positive bonding existed, no mourning would be necessary. Bowlby's (1969) seminal work on attachment highlighted the biological source of the need for proximity in human relationships, with the prototype of attachment being the mother–infant relationship. Although object constancy permits the mental retention of loved persons in the memory, nonetheless a child whose parents separate and/or divorce is deprived of daily contact with one of his or her attachment figures, and thus suffers the loss both of this person and that of the intact nuclear family. Other losses following divorce often include a change of residence, school, and lifestyle. But it is the loss of contact with an attachment object (the nonresident parent) that results in the most serious deprivation for children. Multiple losses cause multiple stressors, adding to the potential for crisis.

Illness, although a common occurrence in growing up, may involve a number of temporary or permanent restrictions on a young person's life, which he or she may experience as losses. A youth with a terminal illness, for example, must adapt to bodily changes, environmental restrictions, changed expectations for the future, and changed relationships. These all constitute losses. Physical injury or pain constitutes a serious threat to a youth's basic sense of body integrity, compounding the other stresses associated with medical treatment. The family has an important role in helping the child cope with a serious medical crisis. (See Gilbert & Hong, Chapter 15, this volume, for further discussion.)

Losses constitute a significant component of a crisis or traumatic event. Both losses that are "vague," such as the loss of a sense of predictability about the environment (e.g., following a tsunami or terrorist attack), and more evident or specific losses, such as the death of a pet, can create stress and anxiety. In addition, memories of past experiences of loss and bereavement often become reawakened in current loss situations, thereby complicating the individual's responses.

Attribution of Causality: Random/"Act of God" or Deliberate/Human-Made

People often seek to attach blame after something "bad" happens. For example, because preschool children are naturally egocentric, such a child may believe that something he or she did or did not do caused a parent's death. As children grow, their understanding becomes more mature and sometimes reveals their search for logical reasons for tragic events. This was illustrated by an 8-year-old boy who asked in disbelief following the 9/11 attacks, "Why did they do it, when *we* taught them to fly?" (Webb, 2004b, p. 10). The child's black-and-white sense of right and wrong was shattered, and this may have led to erosion of this boy's faith in human nature. An older child usually has more understanding about the complexity of human behavior and motivation, including the reality of deliberate malevolent actions. This awareness may lead to disillusionment about other people and increased anxiety about the safety of the world. Of course, sensitive caregivers can buffer children and teens' anxiety by reassuring them that the current experience is not typical of *all* people, and that goodness exceeds evil in the world.

As compared with a terrorist or other human-made act, when a crisis/traumatic event occurs as the result of a seemingly random occurrence or "act of God," the element of blame is often less intense. Many adults respond with a kind of fatalistic attitude that there is nothing anyone could have done to prevent this type of crisis. This acceptance makes the resulting grief less complicated. However, blaming still may occur with regard to the management of disaster relief efforts. For example, in the aftermath of Hurricane Katrina in 2005, many people complained about inadequate government intervention to alleviate their suffering, and thousands of families were subjected to both physical and emotional pain as a result of the massive dislocation and destruction they witnessed and experienced after the disaster.

CONTEXTUAL ELEMENTS THAT HELP OR HINDER YOUTH IN CRISIS AND TRAUMATIC SITUATIONS

A crisis happens to a specific individual within the context of his or her social and physical environment. I now consider some of the features of this contextual surround that may either help or hinder a child or adolescent in crisis. The nature of the support system is particularly important for children in crisis/traumatic situations because their youth and dependence make them especially reliant on others to assist them (Pfefferbaum et al., 2004).

Culture and Religion

The term "culture" encompasses the beliefs, values, morals, customs, and world views that are held in common by a group and to which its members are expected to conform (Webb, 2001). Cultural values pervade all aspects of life and are often shaped by specific religious practices and beliefs. For example, the responses of many Buddhists following the December 2004 tsunami in the Far East reflected their fatalistic belief in karma, with the acceptance of such events as part of the cycle of life. In striking contrast, many fundamentalist Christians in south Florida after Hurricane Hugo in 1989 attributed the storm to God's intent to "teach them a lesson." These different perceptions demonstrate how culture and religion constitute the lenses through which people view their worlds.

Whereas all people experience stress, their culture determines whether and in what manner they acknowledge this distress. For example, Fang and Chen (2004) reported the case of Chinese parents living in New York after the 9/11 World Trade Center bombing who were unable to understand their daughter's traumatic nightmares and school failure as part of the girl's anxiety reaction. They did not want her to consult the school psychologist about her poor grades and difficulty concentrating because the parents considered that this would reveal the girl's "weakness" and therefore "shame" the family. Psychological problems are considered disgraceful in some cultures, and the challenge for counselors and therapists is to find a way to frame these difficulties in terms of "normal" responses in difficult situations (Nader, Dubrow, & Stamm, 1999). The cultural and religious backgrounds of different groups influence both the way a crisis or traumatic event is perceived and the nature of the response (McGoldrick, Giordano, & Garcia-Preto, 2005). McGoldrick (1982, p. 6) states categorically that "the language and customs of a culture will influence whether or not a symptom is labeled a problem . . . [and that] problems can be neither diagnosed nor treated without understanding the frame of reference of the person seeking help as well as that of the helper."

Thus it is imperative for a therapist to identify and weigh the significance of cultural and religious factors in trying to understand a family's reaction to a crisis or traumatic situation. In the previous example, had the school social worker telephoned the Chinese parents and suggested that they seek a mental health evaluation for their daughter, the parents would have felt disgraced and angry, and they probably would have declined the suggestion and blamed their daughter for speaking about her problem to outsiders. However, had the social worker stated that she was sending *all* parents some information about the typical reactions of children and youth after disasters, and then pointed out that it was important to help children so that their schoolwork did not suffer, the chances of parental cooperation would have been far greater.

Nuclear and Extended Family

Most people seek out their close family members at times of crisis, either directly or via telephone or electronic communication. Proximity seeking is a hallmark of attachment. Young children are no exception, and in stressful situations they cry for their mothers (or other primary caregivers) and cling to them for comfort. The nature of the mothers' responses, in turn, has a strong influence on how the children will react—even during the stresses of wartime. Freud and Burlingham (1943) reported that children who remained with their mothers in London during the Blitz of World War II fared better than those who were evacuated to the countryside, where they lived more safely but with strangers. When parents remain calm, their children tend to follow suit. However, this places a great burden on parents who themselves may be traumatized. Even in a noncrisis situation, parents may be preoccupied with financial worries, professional concerns, or other matters that can significantly diminish their availablity to their children.

A "genogram" is the starting point for identifying all family members who potentially can provide support to a child in crisis. In the process of creating a three-generation genogram with the family, the crisis therapist learns not only the names of family members, but also their geographic location, their frequency of contact with one another, and something about the quality of their various relationships. It is helpful to ask parents in completing the genogram, "Of all these various family members, which ones do you consider most important to your children?" The response sometimes reveals the influence of an aunt or uncle, which might not otherwise be known.

The family members' demographic characteristics (e.g., age, socioeconomic status, level of education), in addition to their cultural characteristics, often affect the particular ways they respond to a crisis or trauma. In particular, we must recognize that children growing up in impoverished families frequently lack support from their parents, who may be under financial stress and suffer more depression and psychological distress than do more affluent parents (Huston, 1995). Therefore, children who most need adult protection, due to dangerous inner-city neighborhoods with very high levels of interpersonal violence, may not have this resource (Fick, Osofsky, & Lewis, 1994). The ideal of a safe, nurturing, supportive environment is far from the reality of many young people in poverty.

School, Friends, and Community Supports

An "eco-map" (Hartman, 1978) provides a diagrammatic tool for illustrating the available types of support surrounding a family or household. The eco-map provides an excellent means of analyzing potential resources in a young person's network of friends, church, school, health care, and other institutions.

The Beatles sang about getting by "with a little help from my friends," and this continues to be true for those fortunate enough to have caring friends who can help. It is not surprising that more supportive environments tend to be associated with a better adjustment to stressful situations.

Beyond the family circle, the school can serve as either a refuge or a source of dread for a young person, depending on the degree to which he or she feels comfortable in the classroom setting and especially in the peer environment. School-age children and teens typically seek out friends who are similar to themselves. This friendship group broadens a young person's sphere of contacts outside the family, and sometimes provides an important source of support at times when the youth's own family members may be caught up in their own conflicts, such as separation and divorce (Davies, 2011). On the other hand, a young person who does not fit in at school may suffer the effects of negative peer contacts, which can cause him or her to dread going to school for fear of ostracism or bullying. In Chapter 13 of this book, Swearer, Schwartz, and Garcia deal with this situation more fully.

Community problems can affect children to varying degrees, depending on their scope and meaning to the child. For example, a youngster living in a run-down tenement building surrounded by gang warfare will probably react more strongly if he or she witnesses a shooting than will a child the same age who lives in a safe neighborhood. The first child realizes (probably not for the first time) that his or her neighborhood is not safe, and therefore this child may experience an increased sense of vulnerability. Children in this situation may benefit greatly from community programs in which they can participate in sports, recreation, or church activities under the careful supervision of coaches, teachers, or religious leaders, who serve as both protectors and positive role models. Unfortunately, all too frequently communities in poor neighborhoods lack the kind of after-school activities that could assist underprivileged youth to grow up with positive views about themselves and their world.

CONCLUDING COMMENTS

The term "resilient" has been used to describe individuals who demonstrate successful adaptation despite high-risk status, chronic stress, or prolonged or severe trauma (Egeland, Carlson, & Stroufe, 1993; Garmezy, 1993; Masten, Best, & Garmezy, 1990). "Resilience" is defined as "the ability to recover readily from illness, depression, adversity, or the like" (*Webster's College Dictionary*, 1968, p. 1146). If we consider resilience to be an *internal* capacity, we must also acknowledge that this ability inevitably interacts with *external* factors, which may be either nurturing and supportive or difficult and depriving (or some combination of the two). Thus resilience is a transactional *process* that "develops over time in the context of environmental support" (Egeland et al., 1993, p. 518).

However, the existence of risk factors such as poverty, parental divorce, parental substance misuse, or parental mental illness by no means sentences a young person to negative life outcomes, according to Rak and Patterson (1996). These authors optimistically report that protective factors, such as individual temperament and unexpected sources of support in the family and community, can buffer a youngster who is at high risk and help him or her succeed in life. See Davies (2011) for a full discussion of the intricacies and interrelationship among risk and protective factors in the child, the family, and the community.

Clearly, multiple factors affect each child and adolescent in each situation—factors that the tripartite assessment summarizes. Consideration of the numerous elements that help or hinder a young person's unique adaptation in different crisis situations constitutes the heart of understanding. And, ideally, such understanding will lead to appropriate assessment and treatment, as we will see in the following chapters.

STUDY QUESTIONS

1. What are some options a counselor can employ to help a young person from an abusive family who lives in a poor and violence-prone community?
2. Discuss the impact on a child of living in a deeply religious family that does not approve of after-school activities such as participating in sports and social events. Can you suggest some ways to convince the parents that these activities might be beneficial for their child?
3. How can a counselor/social worker help family members deal with negative behavior toward them and their children based on racial prejudice?
4. List some methods to help influence a child not to join a gang or participate in antisocial activities.

REFERENCES

American Psychiatric Association. (2013). *Diagnostic and statistical manual of mental disorders* (5th ed.). Arlington, VA: Author.

Appleyard, K., Egeland, B., van Dulmen, M., & Stroufe, A. (2005). When more is not better. The role of cumulative risk in child behavior outcomes. *Journal of Child Psychology and Psychiatry, 46*(3), 235–245.

Arroyo, W., & Eth, S. (1996). Post-traumatic stress disorder and other stress reactions. In R. J. Apfel & B. Simon (Eds.), *Minefields in their hearts: The mental health of children in war and communal violence* (pp. 52–74). New Haven, CT: Yale University Press.

Benson, H. (2000). *The relaxation response.* New York: HarperCollins.

Blaustein, M. E., & Kinniburgh, K. M (2010). *Treating traumatic stress in children and adolescents: How to foster resiliency through attachment, self-regulation, and competency.* New York: Guilford Press.

Bowlby, J. (1969). *Attachment and loss: Vol. 1. Attachment.* London: Hogarth Press.

Cohen, J. A. (2004). Early mental health interventions for trauma and traumatic loss in children and adolescents. In B. T. Litz (Ed.), *Early intervention for trauma and traumatic loss* (pp. 131–146). New York: Guilford Press.

Davies, D. (2004). *Child development: A practitioner's guide* (2nd ed.). New York: Guilford Press.

Davies, D. (2011). *Child development: A practitioner's guide* (3rd ed.). New York: Guilford Press.

Egeland, B., Carlson, E., & Sroufe, L. A. (1993). *Resilience as Process. Development and Psychopathology, 5*, 517–528.

Erikson, E. H. (1968). *Identity: Youth and crisis.* New York: Norton.

Eth, S., & Pynoos, R. S. (1985). Interaction of trauma and grief in childhood. In S. Eth & R. S. Pynoos (Eds.), *Post-traumatic stress disorder in children* (pp. 171–186). Washington, DC: American Psychiatric Press.

Fang, L., & Chen, T. (2004). Community outreach and education to deal with cultural resistance to mental health services. In N. B. Webb (Ed.), *Mass trauma and violence: Helping families and children cope* (pp. 234–255). New York: Guilford Press.

Fick, A. C., Osofsky, J. D., & Lewis, M. L. (1994). Perceptions of violence: Children, parents, and police officers. In R. S. Pynoos (Ed.), *Posttraumatic stress disorder: A clinical review* (pp. 261–276). Lutherville, MD: Sidran Press.

Freud, A. (1965). *Normality and pathology in childhood.* New York: International Universities Press.

Freud, A., & Burlingham, D. T. (1943). *War and children.* London: Medical War Books.

Garmezy, N. (1993). Stress-resistant children: The search for protective factors. In J. E. Stevenson (Ed.), *Recent research in developmental psychopathology* (pp. 213–233). Oxford, UK: Pergamon Press.

Grasso, D., Greene, C., & Ford, J. D. (2013). Cumulative trauma in childhood. In J. D. Ford & C. A. Courtois (Eds.), *Treating complex traumatic stress disorders in children and adolescents* (pp.79–99). New York: Guilford Press.

Hartley, B. (2004). Bereavement groups soon after traumatic death. In N. B. Webb (Ed.), *Mass trauma and violence: Helping children and families cope* (pp. 167–190). New York: Guilford Press.

Hartman, A. (1978). Diagrammatic assessment of family relationships. *Social Casework, 59*, 465–476.

Herman, J. L. (1992). Complex PTSD: A syndrome in survivors of prolonged and repeated trauma. *Journal of Traumatic Stress*, 5, 377–391.

Huston, A. C. (1995, August). *Children in poverty and public policy.* Presidential address presented at the meeting of Division 7 (Developmental Psychology) of the American Psychological Association, New York.

James, R. K., & Gilliland, B. E. (2004). *Crisis intervention strategies* (4th ed.). Pacific Grove, CA: Brooks/Cole.

Kliethermes, M., & Wamser, R. (2012). Adolescents with complex trauma. In J. A. Cohen, A. P. Mannarino, & E. Deblinger (Eds.), *Trauma-focused CBT for children and adolescents: Treatment applications* (pp. 175–196). New York: Guilford Press.

La Greca, A. M., & Prinstein, M. J. (2002). Hurricanes and earthquakes. In A. M. La Greca, W. K. Silverman, & M. C. Roberts (Eds.), *Helping children cope with disasters and terrorism* (pp. 107–138). Washington, DC: American Psychological Association.

Masten, A. S., Best, K. M., & Garmezy, N. (1990). Resilience and development:

Contributions from the study of children who overcome adversity. *Development and Psychopathology*, *2*, 425–444.

McCann, L. I., & Pearlman, L. (1990). Vicarious traumatization: A framework for understanding the psychological effects of working with victims. *Journal of Traumatic Stress*, *3*(1), 131–149.

McFarlane, A. C. (1990). Post-traumatic stress syndrome revisited. In H. J. Parad & L. G. Parad (Eds.), *Crisis intervention book 2: The practitioner's sourcebook for brief therapy* (pp. 69–92). Milwaukee, WI: Family Service America.

McGoldrick, M. (1982). Ethnicity and family therapy: An overview. In M. McGoldrick, J. K. Pearce, & J. Giordano (Eds.), *Ethnicity and family therapy* (pp. 3–30). New York: Guilford Press.

McGoldrick, M., Giordano, J., & Garcia-Preto, N. (Eds.). (2005). *Ethnicity and family therapy* (3rd ed.). New York: Guilford Press.

Nader, K. (2008). *Understanding and assessing trauma in children and adolescents: Measures, methods and youth in context*. New York: Routledge.

Nader, K., Dubrow, N., & Stamm, B. H. (Eds.). (1999). *Honoring differences: Cultural issues in the treatment of trauma and loss*. Philadelphia: Brunner/Mazel.

Nader, K., Pynoos, R. S., Fairbanks, L., & Frederick, C. (1990). Children's PTSD reactions one year after a sniper attack at their school. *American Journal of Psychiatry*, *147*, 1526–1530.

Parad, H. J., & Parad, L. G. (Eds.). (1990). *Crisis intervention book 2: The practitioner's sourcebook for brief therapy*. Milwaukee, WI: Family Service America.

Pfefferbaum, B. J. (1997). Posttraumtatic stress disorder in children: A review of the past 10 years. *Journal of the American Academy of Child and Adolescent Psychiatry*, 36(11), 1503–1509.

Pfefferbaum, B. J., De Voe, E. R., Stuber, J., Schiff, M., Klein, T. P., & Fairbrother, G. (2004). Psychological impact of terrorism on children and families in the United States. *Journal of Aggression, Maltreatment and Trauma*, *9*(3–4), 305–317.

Pynoos, R. S., & Eth, S. (1985). Children traumatized by witnessing acts of personal violence. In S. Eth & R. S. Pynoos (Eds.), *Post-traumatic stress disorder in children* (pp. 19–43). Washington, DC: American Psychiatric Press.

Pynoos, R. S., & Nader, K. (1989). Children's memory and proximity to violence. *Journal of the American Academy of Child and Adolescent Psychiatry*, *28*, 236–241.

Rak, C. F., & Patterson, L. E. (1996). Promoting resilience in at-risk children. *Journal of Counseling and Development*, *74*, 368–373.

Rivera, R. (2013, January 29). Reliving horror and faint hope at massacre site. *New York Times*, p. A1.

Roberts, A. R. (Ed.). (2005). *Crisis intervention handbook: Assessment, treatment, and research* (3rd ed.). New York: Oxford University Press.

Rustemi, A., & Karanei, A. N. (1996). Distress reactions and earthquake-related cognitions of parents and their adolescent children in a victimized population. *Journal of Social Behavior and Personality*, *11*, 767–780.

Saxe, G. N., MacDonald, H. Z., & Ellis, B. H. (2007). Psychosocial approaches for children with PTSD. In M. J. Friedman, T. M. Keane, & P. A. Resnick (Eds.). *Handbook of PTSD: Science and practice* (pp. 359–375). New York: Guilford Press.

Selye, H. (1978). *The stress of life*. New York: McGraw-Hill.

Shelby, J., Aranda, B., Asbill, L., & Gallagher, J. (2015). Simple interventions for complex trauma: Play-based safety and affect regulation strategies for child survivors. In E. J. Green & A. C. Myrick (Eds.), *Play therapy with vulnerable populations: No child forgotten* (pp. 61–92). Lanham, MD: Rowman & Littlefield.

Swenson, C. C., Saylor, C. F., Powell, M. P., Stokes, S. J., Foster, K. Y., & Belter, R. W. (1996). Impact of a natural disaster on preschool children: Adjustment 14 months after a hurricane. *American Journal of Orthopsychiatry, 66*, 122–130.

Terr, L. C. (1979). Children of Chowchilla. *Psychoanalytic Study of the Child, 34*, 547–623.

Terr, L. C. (1991). Childhood traumas: An outline and overview. *American Journal of Psychiatry, 148*(1), 10–20.

Webb, N. B. (Ed.). (1993). *Helping bereaved children: A handbook for practitioners.* New York: Guilford Press.

Webb, N. B. (Ed.). (1999). *Play therapy with children in crisis: Individual, group, and family treatment* (2nd ed.). New York: Guilford Press.

Webb, N. B. (Ed.). (2001). *Culturally diverse parent–child and family relationships: A guide for social workers and other practitioners.* New York: Columbia University Press.

Webb, N. B. (2002). Traumatic death of a friend/peer: Case of Susan, age 9. In N. B. Webb (Ed.), *Helping bereaved children: A handbook for practitioners* (2nd ed., pp. 167–193). New York: Guilford Press.

Webb, N. B. (2004a). A developmental–transactional framework for assessment of children and families following mass trauma. In N. B. Webb (Ed.), *Mass trauma and violence: Helping families and children cope* (pp. 23–49). New York: Guilford Press.

Webb, N. B. (2004b). The impact of traumatic stress and loss on children and families. In N. B. Webb (Ed.), *Mass trauma and violence: Helping families and children cope* (pp. 3–22). New York: Guilford Press.

Webb, N. B. (Ed.). (2006). *Working with traumatized youth in child welfare.* New York: Guilford Press.

Webb, N. B. (Ed.). (2010). *Helping bereaved children: A handbook for practitioners* (3rd ed.). New York: Guilford Press.

Webb, N. B. (2011). *Social work practice with children* (3rd ed.). New York: Guilford Press.

Webster's College Dictionary. (1968). New York: Random House.

Chapter 2

Differential Diagnosis in the Assessment of Children and Adolescents after Crises and Traumatic Events

KATHLEEN NADER

Accurate diagnosis is important to providing successful interventions for both youth and adults. Following traumatic events, youth are often assessed for possible posttraumatic stress disorder (PTSD), and may be examined for acute stress disorder (ASD) or more complicated forms of posttraumatic reactions (e.g., complicated trauma or complicated grief) as well. The fifth edition of the *Diagnostic and Statistical Manual of Mental Disorders* (DSM-5; American Psychiatric Association [APA], 2013) has added attachment disorders to trauma- and stressor-related disorders (TSRD), now a separate category from anxiety disorders as defined in DSM-IV (APA, 1994). Importantly, youth may respond to their traumatic experiences with disorders, symptoms, and patterns of thought and behavior (that affect their quality of life and functioning) other than those described in the diagnostic criteria for TSRD (Nader, 2008). A number of factors, including genetic factors, influence whether children exposed to traumas develop behavioral and emotional difficulties or, conversely, evidence resilience and better functioning (Kim-Cohen et al., 2006; Nader & Fletcher, 2014). Trauma is associated with a number of disorders. In fact, without a trigger such as trauma or other adversity, the probability of gene-related dysfunction or specific disorder is reduced (Lau & Pine, 2008).

For disorders in DSM-5, much co-occurrence and symptom overlap exist (see Table 2.1). Studies often focus on one disorder, without taking into account the frequent comorbidity of disorders and the effects of disorder combinations on the nature of response and recovery (Kessler, 2000). PTSD presents with high rates of comorbidity. Evidence suggests that treatments for simple PTSD may not be applicable to complex trauma or to PTSD with comorbid disorders

TABLE 2.1. PTSD Symptoms and the Other Disorders with Which They May Be Associated

Symptom	Other disorders that may have the symptom
Distressing memories	CBD; MDD; OCD
Distressing dreams	N; ND; N-REM; SAD
Dissociative reactions	AW; CvD; DID; PsyD (e.g., Sch, schizoaffective disorder); SUD
Recurrent psychological distress	Ag; anxiety disorders; CBD; OCD; Pan; SPh; SAD
Physiological reactions	CvD; D/DD; FD; Pan; SAD; Sch; SSD
Avoidance or efforts to avoid memories, thoughts, or feelings	CBD; OCD
Avoidance or efforts to avoid people, places, conversations, activities, objects, or situations	ADHD; Ag; APD; CBD; OCD; SPh; SoAD
Amnesias	CvD; DA; DID; HD; N
Persistent negative beliefs about self or the world	AN; APD; BDD; BPsD; CBD; CD; GAD; PDD; PPD; PrDD; Sch
Blame of self or others	CBD (self); OCD (self); ODD (others)
Persistent negative emotional states (e.g., fear, horror, anger, guilt, shame)	AN; BPD-MDE; CBD; CW; CanW; D; D/DD; MDD; PrDD; RAD; SAD; Sch; SPh; SUD (W); TBI
Diminished interest or participation in activities	AN; BPD-MDE; CBD; MDD; PrDD; PsyD (e.g., schizoaffective disorder); ScPD; SPh
Detachment or estrangement from others or socially withdrawn behavior	AN; APD; BDD; BPsD; CBD; ExD; N-REM; OCD; PsyD (e.g., schizoaffective disorder); RAD; SAD; ScPD; SchPD; SCD; SoAD; SUD
Inability to experience positive emotions	BPD-MDE; CBD; CW; MDD; PsyD (e.g., Sch); RAD; SAD; ScPD; SUD
Irritability and angry outbursts	ADHD; AN; CanW; CD; D; DMDD; GAD; ID; IED; MDD; ODD; PrDD; RAD; Sch; SUD; TBI
Recklessness or self-destructive behavior	CD; DA; DID; PsyD
Hypervigilance, increased startle, excessive fear or anxiety, or frozen watchfulness	Ag; AI; anxiety disorders; APD; ASD; CanW; D; OCD; Pan; PsyD (e.g., schizoaffective disorder); SAD; SPh; SUD
Poor concentration	ADHD; AI; BPD-ME; BPD-MDE; CW; D; GAD; ID; MDD; PDD; PrDD; SAD; SUD

(continued)

TABLE 2.1. *(continued)*

Symptom	Other disorders that may have the symptom
Sleep disturbance	Anxiety and mood disorders; AN; AW; BPD-MDE; CI; CanW; D; GAD; HD; ID; MDD; PDD; PrDD; Sch; SUD; SWD; TBI
Derealization or depersonalization	CvD; D/DD; Pan; Sch; SUD
Dissociative amnesia	CvD; DA; DID; HD; Med; N; SUD; TBI
Increased suicide risk	ADHD; AI; AN; BDD; BN; BPD; BPsD; DA; Dep; DID; DMDD; MDD; ND; OCD; ODD; Pan; PsyD (e.g., Sch, schizoaffective disorder); SAD; SPh; SSD; SUD

Note. Copyright 2006, 2014 by Kathleen Nader. AD, Asperger's disorder; ADHD, attention-deficit/hyperactivity disorder; Ag, agoraphobia; AI/W, alcohol intoxication or withdrawal; AmD, amnestic disorders; AN, anorexia nervosa; APD, avoidant personality disorder; ASD, autism spectrum disorder; BDD, body dysmorphic disorder; BN, bulimia nervosa; BPD, bipolar disorders; BPsD, borderline personality disorder; CanW, cannabis withdrawal; CBD, persistent complex bereavement disorder; CD, conduct disorder; CI/W, caffeine intoxication or withdrawal; CvD, conversion disorder; D, delirium; DA, dissociative amnesia; Dep, depressive disorders; D/DD, depersonalization/derealization disorder; DID, dissociative identity disorder; DMDD, disruptive mood dysregulation disorder; ExD, excoriation disorder; FD, factitious disorder; GAD, generalized anxiety disorder; HD, hypersomnolence disorder; ID, insomnia disorder; MDD, major depressive disorder; MDE, major depressive episode; ME, manic episode; Med, medical disorders; N, narcolepsy; ND, nightmare disorder; N-REM, non-rapid eye movement sleep arousal disorders; OCD, obsessive–compulsive disorder; ODD, oppositional defiant disorder; P, paranoid schizophrenia; Pan, panic disorder or panic attack specifier; PDD, persistent depressive disorder; PPD, paranoid personality disorder; PnD, pain disorder; PsyD, schizophrenia spectrum and other psychotic disorders; PrDD, premenstrual dysphoric disorder; RAD, reactive attachment disorder; SAD, separation anxiety disorder; SCD, social communication disorder; Sch, schizophrenia; SoAD, social anxiety disorder; SPh, specific phobia; ScPD, schizoid personality disorder; SWD, sleep–wake disorders; SSD, somatic symptom disorder; SUD, stimulant or other substance use disorder or withdrawal; TBI, traumatic brain injury.

(Ford, Courtois, Steele, van der Hart, & Nijenhuis, 2005; van der Kolk, Roth, Pelcovitz, Sunday, & Spinazzola, 2005).

CHILDHOOD ADVERSITIES AND ADULT DISORDERS

Adversities have been stronger predictors of early-onset than of later-onset disorders. Trauma exposure and PTSD in childhood are linked to a variety of negative outcomes in childhood and adulthood—for example, PTSD (Kulkarni, Graham-Bermann, Rauch, & Seng, 2011), bulimia nervosa (Wonderlich et al., 2007), and depressive disorders (Dennis et al., 2009)—as well as other symptoms such as hypo- or hypercortisolism (see Nader & Weems, 2011) and hostility (Dennis et al., 2009). Although most posttrauma studies examine specific disorders such as PTSD, Kessler, Davis, and Kendler (1997) found that the effects of particular adverse events are not confined to any one class of disorders. When studies control for lifetime comorbidities, the effects of a variety of adversities—whether or not they meet DSM Criterion A for PTSD or ASD—are distinguished more by their similarities than by their differences. Kessler and colleagues found that adults' recollections of one-time natural or human-made disasters were related to mood, anxiety (then including PTSD), and maladaptive coping (addiction) disorders, but not to conduct disorder (CD) or adult antisocial behavior. A history of multiple trauma exposures is common among adult women with disorders such as PTSD and major depressive disorder (MDD) (Dennis et al., 2009). Psychotic symptoms or experience in childhood increase the likelihood of adult-onset psychosis (Laurens, Hodgins, West, & Murray, 2007; van Os, Hanssen, Bijl, & Vollebergh, 2001). Although many individuals with psychosis have no history of trauma, psychosis-like symptoms or experiences may follow traumas.

As Webb (2004 and Chapter 1, this volume) points out in her discussion of tripartite assessment (see also Nader, 2008; Shaw, 2000), a youth's traumatic reactions are shaped by aspects of the youth (e.g., genetics, traits, previous experiences, neurobiology) and the youth's background (e.g., socioeconomic status, culture, subculture); the nature of the event (e.g., chronicity, intensity, individual experience, personal meaning); and the pre- and posttrauma environments. Cultural issues, for example, influence coping strategies (Pole, Best, Metzler, & Marmar, 2005), support systems (Danieli & Nader, 2006; Nader & Danieli, 2005), and sanctioned reactions to trauma (Nader, 2008). This chapter examines aspects of a child or adolescent that influence traumatic response, the range of a youth's reactions, and differential diagnosis.

CHILD FACTORS THAT INFLUENCE RESPONSE

Not all youth exposed to adversity develop problems or psychopathology (Yates, Egeland, & Sroufe, 2003). Some youth with little apparent life difficulty do develop problems. Risk and protective factors are not universally predictive of outcomes for youth (Sonderegger, Barrett, & Creed, 2004); they may be mediated by other influences. Nevertheless, aspects of youth's personalities, genetics, self-views, and other personal strengths and weaknesses often influence their characteristic reactions to stress (Davies, 2011; Nader, 2008; Nader & Fletcher, 2014). Risk and vulnerability may interact or operate in concert. For example, evidence suggests that specific genetic qualities (e.g., short-allele serotonin polymorphism, specific dopamine polymorphisms, and the Met allele carriers of the brain-derived neurotrophic factor [BDNF] gene) are associated with increased sensitivity to positive and negative environmental conditions. Such genetic factors have shown increased reactivity to stressful environments and higher responsiveness to positive environmental changes in studies of animals and of human children and adults (Del Giudice, Ellis, & Shirtcliff, 2011; Drury et al., 2012; Nader & Fletcher, 2014). For example, children with negative emotionality/difficult temperament (associated with short-allele serotonin polymorphism; see Nader & Fletcher, 2014) who were followed from 1 month to 4.5 years of age (Pleuss & Belsky, 2009) appeared to be both more negatively and more positively affected by the quality of care they experienced than other young children. That is, they exhibited more behavior problems when faced with low-quality care, and fewer behavior problems when experiencing high-quality care. Similar environmental by genetic effects have been reported for older children (e.g., ages 7 and 9; Belsky, Bakermans-Kranenburg, & van IJzendoorn, 2007).

Risk Factors

"Risk factors" are variables that are empirically associated with a disorder and predict the *increased probability* of the disorder's occurring (Ingram & Price, 2001; Nader, 2008). "Vulnerabilities" are a subset of risk factors that may exist in any of a youth's physiological, cognitive, affective, or social/behavioral systems. In addition to the risks created by such environmental conditions as experiences of premature birth, poverty, parental mental illness, divorce, war, and maltreatment, risk has been associated with individual traits such as negative emotionality and introversion, antisocial behavior or other conduct disturbances, poor responses to challenges, fewer or lower cognitive skills, external locus of control, and low self-esteem (Caspi, 1998; Luthar, 2003; Nader, 2008; Rothbart & Bates, 1998; Yates et al., 2003). Genes may influence traits and mental health outcomes (Nader, 2015; Nader & Fletcher, 2014). As noted, the short-allele variant of the serotonin transporter gene and particular dopamine polymorphisms have been associated with increased susceptibility to the negative impacts of stress. The absence or diminishment of resilience factors may add to risk.

Resilience Factors

"Resilience" suggests reduced vulnerability and the presence of protective factors. Studies have identified a number of variables that may serve as resilience factors or, when absent, may add to risk (Nader, 2008). Protective factors include personal qualities (such as intelligence, the ability to trust, a sense of self-worth, self-confidence, a realistic assessment of one's control, the ability to function well in relationships, and the capacity for appropriate self-regulation), as well as environmental conditions (such as access to needed resources, a good support system, secure caregiver–child attachments, effective parenting, and socioeconomic advantages) (Fergusson & Horwood, 2003; Masten & Powell, 2003; Nader, 2008).

Environmental and child intrinsic factors interact. A child's personality and biochemical tendencies may elicit or repel responsive care, for example (Yates et al., 2003). Supportive, responsive, structured, and affectively stimulating environments contribute to children's self-worth, social competence, empathic involvement with others, self-confidence, curiosity, and positive affective expression. Secure attachments and the consequent youth competencies foster the development of flexible problem-solving skills, effective emotion regulation, and an expectation of success in the face of adversity (Nader, 2008, 2014). Children with the long variant of the serotonin transporter (5HTT) gene have appeared to be protected against, for example, the adverse effects of institutionalized care (Bakermans-Kranenburg, Dobrova-Krol, & van IJzendoorn, 2011).

Stages of Response

Individuals exposed to the same event will have different timetables for processing aspects of the event—specific traumatic episodes and reactions such as anxiety, grief, and rage. Following traumas and across the course of treatment, a child or adolescent may emerge from varying degrees or stages of numbing. In order to cope, the youth may unintentionally intersperse periods of numbing and avoidance between phases of intrusion and arousal, or between attempts to face aspects of his or her experience and response. The youth's periodic need for avoidance of traumatic memories and thoughts can be honored across the course of his or her response while the youth is gently assisted therapeutically (Nader, 1997, 2004). When an event is perceived to be over rather than ongoing (such as the end of a war vs. ongoing conflict), or when the numbing wears off, there may be a reassessment of the experience or an aspect of it, its results, and one's role in it; of beliefs and expectations; and of the meaning of events and interactions.

THE RANGE OF CHILD REACTIONS FOLLOWING CRISIS AND TRAUMA

Traumas can have immediate and long-term effects as well as cascading effects in a young child's life (Nader, 2008). Childhood traumatic experiences have been associated with childhood and adult psychiatric disorders; physical problems and disorders; academic or job-related difficulties; emotional and behavioral problems; relationship difficulties; and suicidal ideation and attempts (Boney-McCoy & Finkelhor, 1995; Kessler, 2000; Nader, 2008; van der Kolk, 2003). In addition to formally defined disorders, traumatic experiences may result in persistent changes that dynamically influence actions and reactions in all important arenas of life. Faulty information processing, for example, may include patterns of thinking that foster violent behavioral patterns, problematic script-like or reenactment behaviors, and/or a distorted sense of self (Crick & Dodge, 1996; Dodge, Bates, Pettit, & Valente, 1995; Nader, 2008; Schippell, Vasey, Cravens-Brown, & Bretveld, 2003). Especially after multiple types of trauma exposure—and especially when traumas include chronic or severe interpersonal traumas—traumatic reactions may be more complex than the diagnosis of PTSD (Herman, 1992; van der Kolk et al.,

2005). Although complex trauma is not included in DSM-5 (van der Kolk & Courtois, 2005), a number of the symptoms proposed for complicated PTSD are now among PTSD symptoms. As noted, treatment methods for PTSD may result in inadequate treatment for more complex forms of trauma, such as proposed complicated PTSD or PTSD with comorbid disorders (Ford et al., 2005; van der Kolk & Courtois, 2005).

Trauma- and Stressor-Related Disorders

In DSM-5 (APA, 2013), the TSRD category includes reactive attachment disorder (RAD), disinhibited social engagement disorder (DSED), PTSD, ASD, adjustment disorders, and other specific TSRD. Dissociation is a risk factor for PTSD. Although often found in the aftermath of trauma, dissociative disorders are not included as a part of TSRD. Additionally, although some changes were made in DSM-5, and a new category was added for children under age 6, not all concerns about the applicability of DSM PTSD to children were addressed in the final revision (see Nader & Fletcher, 2014). Moreover, to greater and lesser extents, all types of childhood trauma may result in developmental disruptions, in more complex forms of trauma, and in other or comorbid disorders. These disorders may occur immediately after or at length after traumatic experiences. PTSD with delayed expression (APA, 2013) can be persistent and debilitating (Nader & Fletcher, 2014).

Reactive Attachment Disorder

In response to social or emotional neglect or deprivation, or repeated changes in primary caregiver, a child may develop RAD, before the age of 5 (APA, 2013). Both RAD and a disinhibited disorder have been found in previously institutionalized children (Gleason et al., 2011). RAD is indicated when a young child—whose behavior is not explained by autism, intellectual disability, or clinical depression—demonstrates consistent inhibition and emotional withdrawal with caregivers (i.e., rarely seeks or responds to comfort when distressed) and shows limited social or emotional responses to others, little positive affect, and unexplained negative moods (irritability, sadness, or fearfulness). RAD has been associated with attachment security problems, reduced cognitive abilities, and depressive symptoms (Gleason et al., 2011; Smyke et al., 2012). Signs of RAD have improved with placement in foster care (Smyke et al., 2012).

Disinhibited Social Engagement Disorder

When a child experiences extremes of insufficient care (i.e., social neglect or deprivation, repeated changes of primary caregiver, or limited opportunities for selective attachment such as in institutional care), the child may be diagnosed with DSED (after the age of 9 months). The disorder is characterized by little or no reluctance to approach or interact with unfamiliar adults, by excessively familiar behavior, by little or no checking back with caregiver, and/or by willingness to leave with an unfamiliar adult, as well as by socially disinhibited behavior. Like RAD, the disorder may occur with developmental delays and other signs of severe neglect (APA, 2013). DSED may persist through adolescence with some variations in patterns of behavior (see Scheeringa, 2014). Although social impulsivity is also characteristic of attention-deficit/hyperactivity disorder (ADHD), children with DSED do not show attention difficulties or hyperactivity. Nevertheless, indicators of DSED have been associated with signs of activity/impulsivity and of ADHD (although distinct from ADHD) and modestly associated with inhibitory control difficulties (Gleason et al., 2011). Such children have shown reduced cognitive abilities and have shown less resolution of symptoms with placement in foster care than children diagnosed with RAD have (Smyke et al., 2012).

Posttraumatic Stress Disorder

For children over age 6, PTSD requires exposure to threatened or actual death, grave injury, or sexual violence through either direct experience, witnessing in person, or learning of a violent or accidental trauma to a close friend or relative (APA, 2013). The algorithm for a PTSD diagnosis requires one intrusion symptom (PTSD Criterion B), one or both avoidance symptoms (Criterion C), two or more negative alterations in cognitions or mood (Criterion D), and two or more marked alterations in arousal or reactivity (Criterion E) plus functional impairment. For PTSD in children ages 6 and under, the symptom list is somewhat different: It requires one intrusive symptom, one symptom of avoidance or negative alteration in cognitions, and two arousal symptoms, plus dysfunction (APA, 2013). PTSD commonly occurs with comorbid disorders such as separation anxiety disorder (SAD) or oppositional defiant disorder (ODD) in young children.

When there is a traumatic stressor that meets PTSD Criterion A, other diagnoses may be excluded or comorbid (APA, 2013). For example, panic disorder is excluded when panic occurs after traumatic reminders; obsessive–compulsive disorder (OCD) is ruled out if symptoms relate specifically to the trauma (e.g., obsessive thoughts relate to the trauma and compulsions are absent). However, if symptoms are severe enough, they may warrant a separate diagnosis. For example, rather than PTSD with dissociative symptoms, PTSD and a dissociative disorder may be diagnosed. Somatic symptoms that occur with PTSD can be distinguished from conversion disorder, and PTSD flashbacks can be distinguished from psychotic disorders. If symptoms do not persist longer than 1 month after a trauma, ASD is appropriate.

Acute Stress Disorder

Following traumatic experiences, ASD lasts a minimum of 3 days and a maximum of 1 month. DSM-5 lists the PTSD and other symptoms ASD comprises (APA, 2013, pp. 280–281).

Adjustment Disorders

When stressor-related symptoms are clinically significant but do not meet full diagnostic criteria for PTSD, adjustment disorder can be used with specification of its nature (i.e., with depressed mood, anxiety, mixed anxiety and depressed mood, conduct disturbance, mixed conduct and emotional disturbance, or unspecified disturbance). Children with subsyndromal PTSD have demonstrated clinically significant impairment (Carrion, Weems, Ray, & Reiss, 2002; Davis et al., 2000; Nader, 2008; Nader & Fletcher, 2014; Vila, Porsche, & Mouren-Simeoni, 1999).

Complex Trauma

Complex PTSD or developmental trauma disorder (DTD) in children is still undergoing testing and can occur without full PTSD. Although complicated traumatic reactions have been documented more frequently for stressors that are interpersonal, early, extreme, or prolonged stressors (APA, 1994, 2000; Pearlman, 2001; Terr, 1991; van der Kolk & Courtois, 2005; van der Kolk et al., 2005), complex trauma has also occurred after later and single-incident traumas such as natural disasters (Nader, 1997; van der Kolk et al., 2005). The symptoms of complex trauma have been organized in more than one way (APA, 1994, 2000; Herman, 1992; Pearlman, 2001; van der Kolk, 2003; Williams & Sommer, 2002; Wilson, 2004). Evidence suggests that many of the symptoms described for complicated traumatic reactions are significantly explained by polyvictimization (Finkelhor, Shattuck, Turner, & Ormrod, 2014; Nader & Fletcher, 2014). DTD can be understood as representing failures in emotional and behavioral self-regulation (Ford, 2011). The symptoms of altered self-capacities have been linked with symptoms of suicidality, impulse control problems, substance abuse, and other tension reduction behaviors (e.g., self-injury; Briere & Spinazzola, 2005). Youth with multiple exposures and complicated reactions have benefited from treatments designed to improve their ability to regulate emotions and impulsivity (Cloitre et al., 2010; Ford, Wasser, & Connor, 2011; Ford et al., 2013; Taylor & Harvey, 2010). As noted, some of DTD's identified symptoms are now part of PTSD as defined in DSM-5.

Other Specified Trauma- and Stressor-Related Disorders

When symptoms produce clinically significant distress, but do not meet criteria for the types of TSRD described earlier, a child (or adult) may be diagnosed with other specified TSRD. This grouping includes cultural disorders; delayed-onset or prolonged-duration adjustment-like disorders; and persistent complex bereavement disorder (PCBD) (APA, 2013, p. 289). I discuss the last of these, and various other syndromes that can be defined as "complicated grief," below.

COMPLICATED GRIEF

Grieving is normal following a significant loss. It may be complicated (intensified and prolonged) by a number of factors, including depression (Corruble, Chouinard, Letierce, Gorwood, & Chouinard, 2009; Zisook et al., 2010), posthumous disillusionment (Stalfa, 2010), attachment issues (prolonged grief disorder; Boelen, van den Hout, & van den Bout, 2006; Prigerson et al., 2009), conduct or other pronounced disturbances (Pearlman, Schwalbe, & Cloitre, 2010), and/or traumatic experience (Melhem, Moritz, Walker, & Shearer, 2007; Nader & Salloum, 2011). Young children may experience the loss of a parent as traumatic (APA, 2013). Although it appears that prolonged grief disorder is likely to be included in the 11th revision of the *International Classification of Diseases* (ICD-11) (Maercker et al., 2013), PCBD (309.89) is listed in DSM-5 under "Conditions for Further Study" (APA, 2013, pp. 789–790), pending additional research on the types and nature of complicated grief (see Nader & Salloum, 2011, for discussion of types). In children, symptoms may be manifested in play and behavior, anxiety, or regression (APA, 2013). PCBD may co-occur with PTSD or occur without PTSD—for example, when the loss is experienced as personally devastating (Jacobs, 1999). It is distinguished from SAD in that the anxiety focuses on the deceased rather than on a living attachment figure (APA, 2013).

Other Trauma-Linked Disorders

Comorbid disorders are common for traumatized individuals (Nader, 2008), and trauma can be found to be significant in the histories of individuals with a number of disorders (Nader & Fletcher, 2014). Adults with a history of trauma have demonstrated dissociative, depressive, substance use, anxiety, personality, psychotic, and medical disorders (Gold, 2004; Kimerling, Prins, Westrup, & Lee, 2004; Krug, 1996). Disorders found in association with PTSD for youth are ADHD, CD, depressive disorders (e.g., MDD or depressive disorder not otherwise specified), ODD, phobic disorders (i.e., social phobia [social anxiety disorder] or specific phobia), and other anxiety disorders (e.g., SAD, panic disorder) (Carrion et al., 2002; Cicchetti, 2003; Ford, 2002; Greenwald, 2002; Udwin, Boyle, Yule, Bolton, & O'Ryan, 2000; van der Kolk et al., 2005; Weinstein, Staffelbach, & Biaggio, 2000). For both youth and adults, substance use and eating disorders have been associated with childhood traumas (Pasquini, Liotti, Mazzotti, Fassone, & Picardi, 2002). The relationship between PTSD and other disorders can be bidirectional. For instance, depression is both a possible result of trauma and a risk factor for the development of PTSD (Kimerling et al., 2004).

Trauma or adversity is prominent in the expression of genetic vulnerabilities (Nader & Fletcher, 2014). As noted earlier, the likelihood of gene-related mental health dysfunction is reduced without a trigger such as trauma or other adversity (Lau & Pine, 2008). Although some of them occur without traumas, the following disorders have been statistically significantly associated with psychological traumas: alexithymia (Frewen, Dozois, Neufeld, & Lanius, 2012), bipolar disorders (Savitz, van der Merwe, Stein, Solms, & Ramesar, 2007), childhood CD (McReynolds & Wasserman, 2011), depression (Gatt et al., 2009), and psychosis (van Winkel, Stefanis, & Myin-Germeys, 2008). A strong relationship between depression and stressful life events appears to be moderated by genetic vulnerability (Gatt et al., 2009). PTSD may result in increased stress sensitivity, and genetically linked stress sensitivity may increase vulnerability to PTSD (Nader & Fletcher, 2014).

Alterations in Information Processing

Trauma may alter categorization and interpretation of experience, including attention, expectations, and enactments toward self and others, as well as patterns of cognitive associations (Mash & Dozois, 2003; Nader, 2008; van der Kolk, 2003; Yee, Pierce, Ptacek, & Modzelesky, 2003). For example, depressed youth may engage in negative self-evaluations, set unrealistic and perfectionistic goals, believe that efforts to achieve goals are futile, or feel hopeless or pessimistic about the future (Hammen & Rudolph, 2003). Actions based on faulty information processing may result in reactions from others that confirm the faulty processing (Caspi, 1998; Nader, 2008).

Aggression

The commission of violence has been indirectly and directly linked to exposure to violent and other traumas such as natural disasters (see Buchanan, 1998; Kohly, 1994; Nader, 1997, 2015; Simmons & Johnson, 1998). In addition to its association with trauma, aggression has been correlated with traits, information-processing tendencies, neurochemistry, experience, and aspects of parenting and socialization (Aber, Brown, & Jones, 2003; Barry, Frick, & Killian, 2003; Dodge et al., 1995; Laird, Jordan, Dodge, Pettit, & Bates, 2001; Nader, 2008). Temperamental characteristics and early experiences may set up anticipatory attitudes that affect behaviors and relationships (Caspi, 1998). Abused youth, for example, may perceive, interpret, and make decisions about social interactions that increase the likelihood of their aggressive acts (Crick & Dodge, 1996; Dodge et al., 1995). Overtly aggressive youth tend to make more hostile attributions, generate more aggressive responses, and more frequently expect rewards from aggressive problem solving (Crick, 1995).

Script-Like Reenactments

Intense traumatic impressions become etched into a youth's memory following traumatic experiences (Terr, 1991). Multiple intensely registered impressions include, for example, the experience of an immobilized onlooker, a person in flight from danger, or a defender; horrible images, sounds, and physical sensations; and strong desires or compulsions to act—to intervene, rescue, fight back, attack the source of danger, or take other action (see Nader, 2008). These impressions influence a traumatized youth's behavior toward and thinking about self and others. Consequently, in addition to the thoughts and images that may repeatedly intrude after traumatic events, traumatic impressions may replay behaviorally in repeated enactments of trauma-related roles or trauma-engendered scripts (Nader, 2008). The attributional biases related to these scripts may include altered expectations of protection and of the trustworthiness and personal value of self and others (Thomas, 2005). These script-like reenactments may play out across the lifespan in the roles of persecutor, rescuer, victim, immobilized witness, and comforter, among others (Ford, 2002; Liotti, 2004; Nader, 2008; Nader & Mello, 2001).

Neurobiological Changes

Research has documented reductions in brain volume and neurochemical changes following traumatic experiences (Bremner, 2003; De Bellis et al., 1999; Sapolsky, 2000). Such changes as a result of severe or prolonged trauma may have profound, compounding, and long-term effects on a child's life and development (Nader, 2008; Nader & Fletcher, 2014). These neurobiological changes can affect cognitive, behavioral, and emotional functioning—"the way youths greet the world, function in it, interact with others, cope with adversity, and respond to life's challenges" (Nader, 2008, p. 57; see also Nader & Fletcher, 2014).

DIFFERENTIAL DIAGNOSIS: DISTINGUISHING PTSD AND ASD FROM OTHER CLINICAL DIAGNOSES

Overlapping symptoms among disorders (Table 2.1) may make differential diagnosis difficult. The descriptions of Jake (Box 2.1) and Billy (Box 2.2) demonstrate the overlap in symptoms and the difficulty in determining a diagnosis (see Table 2.2). Exposure to an actual traumatic experience often helps to distinguish the anxieties of other disorders from those of simple or complex PTSD or ASD. For DSM disorders, a PTSD diagnosis, if possible, supersedes other diagnoses when symptoms are directly related to a DSM PTSD Criterion A experience.

Anxiety and Related Disorders

Prior to DSM-5, PTSD was classified as an anxiety disorder, and it shares several symptoms with anxiety disorders (and OCD, which was likewise formerly classified as an anxiety disorder). Abnormalities found in functional neuroimaging studies that are common to PTSD have also been reported for other anxiety-related disorders (e.g., OCD; Francati, Vermetten, & Bremner, 2007;

BOX 2.1. Excerpts from the Case of Jake

History

Symptoms

Jake has a history of aggression toward his family and sometimes toward his peers. He does not seem to have empathy for others. His parents describe him as stubborn, defiant, and uncommunicative. He sometimes angrily refuses to obey his parents. In contrast, after his sister goes to bed, he becomes a calm, likeable boy in the nurturing presence of his parents. He is fearful of being alone and fearful in general.

When something triggers stress, he hyperventilates or has a stomachache. . . . His excellent intelligence can be interrupted by stress or an inability to concentrate or keep focus. He has frequent angry outbursts. He is cautious or angry toward others. . . .

Jake currently engages in poor self-care (e.g., does not want to brush his teeth). He is afraid of all health care practitioners and refuses to cooperate with them. . . . Jake cannot sleep at night unless the covers are tightly wrapped around him.

Jake's symptoms are exacerbated by noise or commotion. Rhythmic motion and music soothe him. . . .

Family History

Jake's parents are intelligent and caring caregivers. Both of his parents have a history of depression and anxiety. Jakes younger sister is charming and has a comfortable relationship with both parents. Although sometimes comfortable in dyads under nurturing circumstances, Jake's relationship with his family has been frequently strained. . . . When Jake was 2, his father was treated successfully for cancer. His mother was often absent from home during his treatment.

Presentation in Interviews

Jake is an intelligent, attractive 10 year-old boy. . . . Jake appears to be very cautious with other people.

He looks warily at individuals who enter his proximity. He is on alert when being approached. He often does not respond to greetings or to questions from others. . . . He tenses when approached and looks ready to fight or protect himself. . . . Jake sometimes behaves defiantly or with intense resistance. He exits when a situation no longer holds interest or reward for him. . . . He reports negative expectations of the future. . . .

Diagnosis

Jake's diagnosis before referral was sensory integration dysfunction. He responded well to occupational therapy that included methods of rhythmic activity and techniques that soothe or gather focus. . . .

Tests ordered: EEG, neurochemical tests

Rule out: ADHD, ODD, disruptive mood dysregulation disorder, PTSD, low-cortisol aggression, serotonin polymorphism, anxiety disorder

BOX 2.2. Excerpts from the Case of Billy

History

Symptoms

Billy's mother reports a history of aggression. He lashes out if anyone grabs an arm or a shoulder. Sometimes he just wants to fight someone. He has nightmares at night and falls asleep during the day. Billy was formerly a good student and a happy boy. Now he is in a special class because of his disruptive behavior and inability to concentrate or remember. He cannot eat in the school cafeteria because the smells of some foods make him nauseated. He is always aware of his surroundings and seems to need to know whether there is possible danger. . . . Teachers describe him as defiant now. . . .

Event

On a hockey day, Billy was in his hockey shirt like the other players. When he was walking down the hall, a boy came up to him, grabbed his arm, and yelled something like "You think you're so great, big hockey player!" Later Billy was in the cafeteria eating with the other players when the same boy came in with a gun and started shooting at the players. A few of the players had made fun of this boy on more than one occasion. Billy saw the first bullets hit his fellow players and saw the blood and tissue flying across the table. Billy saw the bullets coming toward him, almost as if in slow motion. He sat frozen at first and was jarred into action by the impact of the first bullet. He dove under the table. . . .

Diagnostic Interviews

Billy is 12 years old. . . . Billy calmly stated that he did not "need to see a shrink." He was quiet and resisted cooperating, at first. Then he seemed to relax and provided thorough information in response to questions. He said that he could not stand to think about the shootings. He just wanted to sleep. He said that he didn't feel anything most of the time, but must be angry because he just wanted to punch someone. He wanted to fight. . . . Billy is highly reactive in response to reminders of the event. When someone grabs his arm or shoulder the way the shooter grabbed him, he just swings at him or her. He doesn't think about it first: "It just happens." . . . "After the shooting, people were screaming and running and throwing up. I just can't go back in there without feeling sick to my stomach." . . .

Diagnosis

Inaccurate diagnosis: CD. Accurate diagnosis: PTSD.

TABLE 2.2. Differential Diagnosis

Symptom	Jake (age 10)	Billy (age 12)
Distressing memories	Memories of interactions with other youth	Memories of a shooter, of people who were shot, of bullets coming toward him, of screaming . . .
Distressing dreams	Nightmares about being in danger	Nightmares of being shot at or being in other danger
Dissociative reactions	Occasional daydreams	Automatic aggressive reactions in response to reminders of event
Intense psychological distress	Anxious in general; hyperventilates when stressed	Avoids or erupts
Physiological reactions	Stomachaches when stressed	Nausea in response to specific food odors
Avoidance of thoughts and feelings	Will not talk about distress; just does not answer questions	Sometimes just doesn't feel anything; goes to sleep when cannot avoid reminders of experience
Avoidances of activities, people, and places	Avoidance of all health care professionals	Refusal to go into the cafeteria at school
Inability to remember an aspect of experience	(None reported)	(Vivid memories)
Negative beliefs about self and others	Very sensitive about others' view of him; has negative expectations about people and experiences	Expects danger; sits with back to wall in public places; thinks he will not live to be 21
Blames self or others	Blames others when he feels embarrassed, or gets angry over own poor performance	Feels rage toward shooter; disparages shooter and contradicts labels of shooter that make him sound skilled
Diminished interest in activities	Has continued interest in activities; leaves or erupts in anger if performs poorly in activity; avoid activities in which he fears he might be embarrassed	Has continued interest in activities; avoids some activities that serve as reminders of his experience; engages in risk-taking activities
Negative emotional states	Often in a bad mood; angers easily; embarrasses easily	Often depressed or angry; occasionally appears unemotional
Feelings of detachment or estrangement	Won't speak about it, but feels unlikeable	Feels separate and different from others; trust issues make him cautious; feels that others do not or would not fully understand

(continued)

TABLE 2.2. *(continued)*

Symptom	Jake (age 10)	Billy (age 12)
Inability to experience positive emotions	Is often depressed or anxious; shows little joy; shows satisfaction and some happiness over building things or doing something well	Often feels depressed; shows no joy or satisfaction; seems more dependent than loving to trusted others
Irritability or outbursts of anger	Frequent angry outbursts; constant irritability; aggressive behavior to family and peers	Impulsive reactivity; angry outbursts
Reckless or self-destructive behavior	Cautious	Places self in danger with risk taking
Hypervigilance	Excessive fear; wariness toward others; cautious about being approached	Always watching to see if there is danger in his vicinity
Exaggerated startle response		
Poor concentration	Concentration can be interrupted by anxieties	Finds it impossible to concentrate for any length of time
Sleep disturbance	Must have covers tightly around him in order to sleep	Excessive sleep in the day; interrupted by nightmares at night
Impaired functioning: academic, social, other	Social functioning is problematic; will not cooperate with medical practitioners of any kind	Impaired academic functioning; associates only with aggressive youth; does not have the concentration to work
Diagnosis	Disruptive mood dysregulation disorder (with anxiety and depressive symptoms) (Short-allele serotonin polymorphism)	PTSD Complex trauma with antisocial and self-destructive behaviors

Nakao et al., 2005). Nevertheless, PTSD can be distinguished from anxiety and related disorders in various ways. Some of the symptoms of PTSD may mimic those of panic disorder, but PTSD symptoms are linked to the trauma. The risk of OCD is increased after trauma (Gross & Hen, 2004; Lafleur et al., 2011), and OCD may be comorbid with PTSD (Spinazzolla, Blaustein, & van der Kolk, 2005). Like PTSD, the anxiety associated with OCD includes intrusive, recurrent urges, thoughts, or images, and/or repetitive behaviors or mental acts that the person feels compelled to perform (APA, 2013). However, preoccupations or intrusive thoughts related to PTSD are related to "real-life concerns" (i.e., to the traumatic experience), whereas OCD obsessions do not usually relate to "real-life concerns" and may appear odd, irrational, or magical in nature. In OCD, repetitive mental acts and/or actions that constitute compulsions are engaged to counteract recurrent thoughts, actions, images, or impulses (obsessions) (McNally, 2001). By contrast, posttraumatic cognitive, behavioral, or physiological repetitions reproduce aspects of the traumatic experience, are a part of the intrusions of the trauma, and may include attempts to process or master aspects of the experience (Horowitz, 1975). In addition, they may be less ritualized than with OCD (Jung & Steil, 2011).

SAD—excessive and developmentally inappropriate fear or anxiety about separation from an attachment figure—may follow traumatic exposure and may accompany PTSD or ASD (APA, 2013; Nader & Pynoos, 1993). When they occur posttraumatically, such fears may reflect regression, fear about a recurrence of the trauma, and/or ongoing concerns about personal safety (Pynoos & Nader, 1988; Shaw, 2000). Such anxieties may relate to intrusion and avoidance of traumatic memories, rather than concerns about the well-being of attachment figures or separation from them (APA, 2013).

Traumatic events can precede the onset of specific phobia. When things feared or avoided are directly linked to the trauma, a diagnosis of specific phobia is only assigned if all criteria for PTSD are not met (APA, 2013). Fear of possible humiliation is prominent in social phobia (now called social anxiety disorder; APA, 2013), but in PTSD or ASD, fear of humiliation and other social anxieties are related to the traumatic experience or engendered by it through altered information processing. Following traumatic experiences, youth may avoid social situations for a number of reasons: for example, because (1) stimuli (e.g., noise, motion, emotion) become overwhelming; (2) the youth feel unsafe in crowds or away from caregivers; (3) people remind the youth of the traumatic experience and thus cause distress; (4) the youth feel humiliated or embarrassed because of having been victimized or because of traumatic injuries; (5) trust or self-esteem has been damaged; or (6) irritability or anger makes relationships difficult.

Somatic Symptom and Related Disorders

Somatic symptom and related disorders include pronounced somatic symptoms linked with significant impairment and distress (APA, 2013). Depression, anxiety, somatic complaints, and psychotic-like behaviors (for dissociative or disorganized youth) may occur in combination among traumatized youth (Cohen & Mannarino, 2004). In addition, pain symptoms are common to depressive, anxiety, and psychotic disorders (APA, 1994, 2000). In contrast to the specific diagnosis of somatic symptom disorder, the physical complaints associated with trauma occur within the context of the trauma and are among other anxieties and symptoms (with some cultural exceptions). Members of some cultures (e.g., Asian or Hispanic cultures) may present with somatic complaints rather than other symptoms of trauma (Kinzie, Boehnlein,

& Sack, 1998; Pole et al., 2005; Shiang, 2000). In all cases, actual medical disorders must be ruled out in the process of diagnosis. The neurobiology of extreme stress can inhibit immune functioning (Sapolsky, 1998). Medical disorders are among long-term consequences of trauma (see Nader & Fletcher, 2014).

Dissociative Disorders

As noted, dissociative symptoms may accompany PTSD and are possible in complex trauma. Dissociative disorders may occur with or without exposure to traumatic events and with or without PTSD (APA, 2013). When full PTSD can be diagnosed, the subtype PTSD with dissociative symptoms should be considered. Dissociative symptoms and disorders such as amnesia may occur as a result of medical disorders, substance use, seizure disorders, or brain injury. Dissociative identity disorder (DID) has often been linked to severe and repeated traumas (Silberg, 1998). For DID, it may be necessary to distinguish between the existence of separate identities and auditory hallucinations (e.g., in schizophrenia) or the shift between cyclical mood states (e.g., in bipolar disorders).

Psychotic Disorders

Under particular conditions, severely traumatized youth may display transient psychotic symptoms (Cohen & Mannarino, 2004). Severely abused or incarcerated and tortured youth, for example, may display psychotic symptoms when frightened by being restrained on an inpatient psychiatric unit. Dissociative symptoms such as disorganized behavior, flat affect, and social withdrawal may have a presentation similar to symptoms of psychotic disorders. In addition, adverse life events have been associated with increased levels of psychotic symptoms in at-risk individuals (van Winkel et al., 2008). Whereas trauma has been significant in the histories of a subgroup of psychotics, many others have no history of trauma (Zelst, 2008; see Nader & Fletcher, 2014, for a summary).

ADHD and Disruptive, Impulse-Control, and Conduct Disorders

Problems in self-control of emotions and behaviors may occur after traumas. The impulsiveness common to ADHD, ODD, CD, and PTSD may reflect neurochemical commonalities. A diagnosis of ADHD or ODD may be a misdiagnosis of PTSD (Greenwald, 2002). Traumatization may also include concentration difficulties, fidgeting, impatience, difficulty delaying responses, and disruptive behaviors. Fidgetiness and difficulty sitting still may reflect posttraumatic jumpiness, nervousness, and hypervigilance. In addition, both PTSD and ADHD may include disturbed sleep patterns. Difficulties with impulse control and intermittent explosive behaviors (as in intermittent explosive disorder) may occur following traumas. Impulse-control disorders are not diagnosed when the impaired impulse control is an aspect of PTSD (APA, 2013).

Youth with CD violate the rights of others or major societal age-appropriate rules or norms (APA, 2013). Several studies suggest an association of traumatization with CD and ODD (Ford, 2002). The two disorders have symptoms in common with PTSD. Like youth with CD, previously well-behaved youth who have been traumatized may exhibit bullying or threatening behaviors, initiate fights, engage in other aggression, and otherwise violate rules and norms. Like youth with ODD—which involves anger/irritability, argumentativeness/defiance with adults, blaming others, and vindictiveness (APA, 2013)—traumatized youth may exhibit defiance, easy loss of temper, quick annoyance, anger, irritability, resentfulness, and argumentativeness. Ford (2002) points out that posttraumatic oppositional refusal to follow rules or engage in particular activities may reflect the persistent posttraumatic avoidance of reminders of the trauma.

Sleep–Wake Disorders

Sleep disturbances occur as associated symptoms of several disorders, such as depressive, bipolar, or anxiety disorders (APA, 2013). If the sleep disturbance associated with PTSD becomes severe enough, it may be included as a separate diagnosis. Sleep disturbances may contribute to other symptoms, such as deficits in concentration, memory, energy, feelings of well-being, motivation, and mood, as well as increases in clumsiness, fatigue, and malaise (APA, 1994, 2000; Nader, 2008). A diagnosis of nightmare disorder is not applied separately if nightmares occur as symptoms of PTSD or bereavement. Adults have experienced a reduction of other trauma symptoms after treatment for nightmares (Krakow, Hollifield, et al., 2001). Similar treatment of a small group of adolescents reduced nightmares but did not diminish concurrent symptoms (Krakow, Sandoval, et al., 2001).

Personality Disorders

A personality disorder (PD) is a durable pattern of behavior and internal experience that deviates notably from the norms of the individual's culture, is inflexible and pervading, and results in impairment or distress (APA, 2013). Although most PDs are not apparent before adolescence or young adulthood, paranoid PD (pervading suspicion and distrust of others) and schizotypal PD (distorted perceptions and eccentric behavior, plus discomfort in and restricted capacity for relationships) may be apparent in childhood. Recognition of the early signs and symptoms of PDs may assist preventive interventions. Care must be taken in interpreting behaviors, however, because (1) a dimensional, rather than a categorical, perspective suggests that PDs represent maladaptive variations of personality traits; (2) some of the behaviors of PDs are common for particular age groups (e.g., dependent behaviors for young children, narcissistic behaviors for adolescents); and (3) symptoms otherwise associated with PDs are reasonably expectable following exposure to traumatic events. The distrust and suspiciousness of paranoid PD; the social detachment and restricted range of affect common to schizoid PD; the impulsivity and instability of affect, self-image, and relationships associated with borderline PD; the hypersensitivity to negative evaluation, feelings of inadequacy, rigidity, and social inhibition linked to avoidant PD; the clinging and submissiveness of dependent PD; and the obsessive thoughts and need for control associated with obsessive–compulsive PD can all occur following exposure to traumatic events (APA, 2013; Ingram & Price, 2001). Because of the overlap in symptoms, DSM-IV and DSM-IV-TR (APA, 1994, 2000) advised caution in using PD diagnoses during an episode of a mood or anxiety disorder (which then included PTSD).

CONCLUSIONS

PTSD captures only a part of posttraumatic psychopathology in youth. A number of comorbid disorders, symptoms, and patterns of thought and behavior other than those described in the diagnostic criteria of PTSD occur for youth and may increasingly disrupt life across time. A number of risk and resilience factors may affect youth's traumatic reactions. Aspects of a youth as an individual, the youth's background and environment, his or her individual traumatic experience and history, and the manner of assessment may interact or transact in determining the youth's reactions to adversity. There is a great deal of overlap in symptoms for youth disorders. PTSD and ASD are distinguished from other disorders by exposure to a Criterion A stressor event and by symptoms that relate directly to or are colored by the event. Assessors of youth must examine multiple factors and symptoms in addition to PTSD.

STUDY QUESTIONS

1. What are the differences between DSM-5 PTSD and complex PTSD? Why are they important?
2. Do you think that Billy (Box 2.2) has complex trauma? Why or why not?
3. What are risk and resilience factors? Name commonly recognized ones.
4. Which symptoms of PTSD overlap with other disorders? Why doesn't Jake (Box 2.1) receive a diagnosis of PTSD?

REFERENCES

Aber, J. L., Brown, J. L., & Jones, S. M. (2003). Developmental trajectories toward violence in middle childhood: Course, demographic differences, and response to school-based intervention. *Developmental Psychology, 39*(2), 324–348.

American Psychiatric Association (APA). (1994). *Diagnostic and statistical manual of mental disorders* (4th ed.). Washington, DC: Author.

American Psychiatric Association (APA). (2000). *Diagnostic and statistical manual of mental disorders* (4th ed., text rev.). Washington, DC: Author.

American Psychiatric Association (APA). (2013). *Diagnostic and statistical manual of mental disorders* (5th ed.). Arlington, VA: Author.

Bakermans-Kranenburg, M., Dobrova-Krol, N., & van IJzendoorn, M. (2011). Impact of institutional care on attachment disorganization and insecurity of Ukrainian preschoolers: Protective effect of the long variant of the serotonin transporter gene (5HTT). *International Journal of Behavioral Development, 36*(1), 1–8.

Barry, C. T., Frick, P. J., & Killian, A. L. (2003). The relation of narcissism and self-esteem to conduct problems in children: A preliminary investigation. *Journal of Clinical Child and Adolescent Psychology, 32*(1), 139–152.

Belsky, J., Bakermans-Kranenburg, M. J., & van IJzendoorn, M. H. (2007). For better and for worse: Differential susceptibility to environmental influences. *Current Directions in Psychological Science, 16*, 300–304.

Boelen, P., van den Hout, M., & van den Bout, J. (2006). A cognitive-behavioral conceptualization of complicated grief. *Clinical Psychology Science and Practice, 13*, 109–128.

Boney-McCoy, S., & Finkelhor, D. (1995). Psychosocial sequelae of violent victimization in a national youth sample. *Journal of Consulting and Clinical Psychology, 63*, 726–736.

Bremner, J. D. (2003). The effects of stress on the brain. *Psychiatric Times, 20*(7), 18–22.

Briere, J., & Spinnazzola, J. (2005). Phenomenology and psychological assessment of complex posttraumatic states. *Journal of Traumatic Stress, 18*(5), 401–412.

Buchanan, A. (1998). Intergenerational child maltreatment. In Y. Danieli (Ed.), *International handbook of multigenerational legacies of trauma* (pp. 535–552). New York: Plenum Press.

Carrion, V. G., Weems, C. F., Ray, R. D., & Reiss, A. L. (2002). Toward an empirical definition of pediatric PTSD: The phenomenology of PTSD symptoms in youth. *Journal of the American Academy of Child and Adolescent Psychiatry, 41*(2), 166–173.

Caspi, A. (1998). Personality development across the life course. In W. Damon (Series Ed.) & N. Eisenberg (Vol. Ed.), *Handbook of child psychology: Vol. 3. Social, emotional, and personality development* (5th ed., pp. 311–388). New York: Wiley.

Cicchetti, D. V. (2003). Neuroendocrine functioning in maltreated children. In D. Cicchetti & E. Walker (Eds.), *Neurodevelopmental mechanisms in psychopathology* (pp. 345–365). Cambridge, UK: Cambridge University Press.

Cloitre, M., Stovall-McClough, K., Nooner, K., Zorbas, P., Cherry, S., Jackson, C., et al. (2010). Treatment for PTSD related to childhood abuse: A randomized controlled trial. *American Journal of Psychiatry, 167*, 915–924.

Cohen, J., & Mannarino, A. (2004). Posttraumatic stress disorder. In T. Ollendick & J. March (Eds.), *Phobic and anxiety disorders in children and adolescents: A clinician's guide to effective psychosocial and pharmacological interventions* (pp. 405–432). New York: Oxford University Press.

Corruble, E., Chouinard, V., Letierce, A., Gorwood, P., & Chouinard, G. (2009). Is DSM-IV bereavement exclusion for major depressive episode relevant to severity and pattern of symptoms?: A case–control, cross-sectional study. *Journal of Clinical Psychiatry, 70*, 1091–1097.

Crick, N. R. (1995). Relational aggression: The role of intent attributions, feelings of distress, and provocation type. *Development and Psychopathology, 7*, 313–322.

Crick, N. R., & Dodge, K. A. (1996). Social information-processing mechanisms in reactive and proactive aggression. *Child Development, 67*(3), 993–1002.

Danieli, Y., & Nader, K. (2006). Respecting cultural, religious and ethnic differences in the prevention and treatment of psychological sequelae. In L. Schein, G. Spitz, H. Burlingame, & P. Muskin (Eds.), *Psychological effects of catastrophic disasters: Group approaches to treatment* (pp. 203–234). New York: Haworth Press.

Davies, D. (2011). *Child development: A practitioner's guide* (3rd ed.). New York: Guilford Press.

Davis, W. B., Mooney, D., Racusin, R., Ford, J. D., Fleischer, A., & McHugo, G. J. (2000). Predicting posttraumatic stress after hospitalization for pediatric injury. *Journal of American Academy of Child and Adolescent Psychiatry, 59*(5), 576–583.

De Bellis, M., Keshavan, M., Clark, D., Casey, B., Giedd, H., Boring, A., et al. (1999). Developmental traumatology: Part II. Brain development. *Biological Psychiatry, 45*, 1271–1284.

Del Giudice, M., Ellis, B. & Shirtcliff, E. (2011). The adaptive calibration model of stress responsivity. *Neuroscience and Biobehavioral Reviews. 35*, 1562–1592.

Dennis, M., Flood, A., Reynolds, V., Araujo, G., Clancy, C., Barefoot, J., et al. (2009). Evaluation of lifetime trauma exposure and physical health in women with posttraumatic stress disorder or major depressive disorder. *Violence against Women, 15*, 618–627.

Dodge, K. A., Bates, J. E., Pettit, G. S., & Valente, E. (1995). Social information-processing patterns partially mediate the effect of early physical abuse on later conduct problems. *Journal of Abnormal Psychology, 104*(4), 632–643.

Drury, S., Gleason, M., Theall, K., Smyke, A., Nelson, C., Fox, N., et al. (2012). Genetic sensitivity to the caregiving context: The influence of 5HTTLPR and BDNF Val66Met on indiscriminate social behavior. *Physiology and Behavior, 106*, 728–735.

Fergusson, D. M., & Horwood, L. J. (2003). Resilience to childhood adversity: Results of a 21-year study. In S. S. Luthar (Ed.), *Resilience and vulnerability: Adaptation in the context of childhood adversities* (pp. 130–155). New York: Cambridge University Press.

Finkelhor, D., Shattuck, A., Turner, H., & Ormrod, R. (2014). Poly-victimization in developmental context. In K. Nader (Ed.), *Assessment of trauma in youths: Understanding issues of age, complexity, and associated variables* (pp. 132–141). New York: Routledge.

Ford, J. D. (2002). Traumatic victimization in childhood and persistent problems with oppositional-defiance. *Journal of Aggression, Maltreatment and Trauma, 6*(1), 25–58.

Ford, J. D. (2011). Assessing child and adolescent complex traumatic reactions. *Journal of Child and Adolescent Trauma, 4*(3), 217–232.

Ford, J. D., Courtois, C. A., Steele, K., van der Hart, O., & Nijenhuis, E. R. S. (2005). Treatment of complex posttraumatic self-dysregulation. *Journal of Traumatic Stress, 18*(5), 437–447.

Ford, J. D., Grasso, D., Greene, C., Levine, J., Spinazzola, J., & van der Kolk, B. (2013). Clinical significance of a proposed developmental trauma disorder diagnosis: Results of an international survey of clinicians. *Journal of Clinical Psychiatry, 74*(8), 841–849.

Ford, J. D., Wasser, T., & Connor, D. (2011). Identifying and determining the symptom severity associated with polyvictimization among psychiatrically impaired children in the outpatient setting. *Child Maltreatment, 16*, 216–226.

Francati, V., Vermetten, E., & Bremner, J. (2007). Functional neuroimaging studies in posttraumatic stress disorder: Review of current methods and findings. *Depression and Anxiety, 24*, 202–218.

Frewen, P., Dozois, D., Neufeld, R., & Lanius, R. (2012). Disturbances of emotional awareness and expression in posttraumatic stress disorder: Meta-mood, emotion regulation, mindfulness, and interference of emotional expressiveness. *Psychological Trauma: Theory, Research, Practice, and Policy, 4*, 152–161.

Gatt, J., Nemeroff, C., Dobson-Stone, C., Paul, R., Bryant, R., Schofield, P., et al. (2009). Interactions between BDNF Val66Met polymorphism and early life stress predict brain and arousal pathways to syndromal depression and anxiety. *Molecular Psychiatry, 14*, 681–695.

Gleason, M., Fox, N., Drury, S., Smyke, A., Egger, H., Nelson, C., III, et al. (2011). Reactive attachment disorder: Indiscriminately social/disinhibited and emotionally withdrawn/inhibited types. *Journal of the American Academy of Child and Adolescent Psychiatry, 50*(3), 216–231.

Gold, S. N. (2004). Trauma resolution and integration program. *Psychotherapy: Theory, Research, Practice, Training, 41*(4), 363–373.

Greenwald, R. (Ed.). (2002). *Trauma and juvenile delinquency: Theory, research, and interventions*. New York: Haworth Press.

Gross, C., & Hen, R. (2004). The developmental origins of anxiety. *Neuroscience, 5*, 545–552.

Hammen, C., & Rudolph, K. D. (2003). Childhood mood disorders. In E. J. Mash & R. A. Barkley (Eds.), *Child psychopathology* (2nd ed., pp. 233–278). New York: Guilford Press.

Herman, J. (1992). *Trauma and recovery*. New York: Basic Books.

Horowitz, M. J. (1975). Intrusive and repetitive thoughts after experimental stress. *Archives of General Psychiatry, 32*, 1457–1463.

Ingram, R. E., & Price, J. M. (Eds.). (2001). *Vulnerability to psychopathology: Risk across the lifespan*. New York: Guilford Press.

Jacobs, S. (1999). *Traumatic grief: Diagnosis, treatment, and prevention*. Philadelphia: Brunner/Mazel.

Jung, K., & Steil, R. (2011). The feeling of being contaminated in adult survivors of childhood sexual abuse and its treatment via a two-session program of cognitive restructuring and imagery modification: A case study. *Behavior Modification, 36*(1), 67–86.

Kessler, R. C. (2000). Posttraumatic stress disorder: The burden to the individual and to society. *Journal of Clinical Psychiatry, 61*(5), 4–14.

Kessler, R. C., Davis, C., & Kendler, K. (1997). Childhood adversity and adult psychiatric disorder in the US National Comorbidity Survey. *Psychological Medicine, 27,* 1101–1119.

Kim-Cohen, J., Caspi, A., Taylor, A., Williams, B., Newcombe, R., Craig, I., et al. (2006). MAOA, maltreatment, and gene–environment interaction predicting children's mental health: New evidence and a meta-analysis. *Molecular Psychiatry, 11,* 903–913.

Kimerling, R., Prins, A., Westrup, D., & Lee, T. (2004). Gender issues in the assessment of PTSD. In J. P. Wilson & T. M. Keane (Eds.), *Assessing psychological trauma and PTSD* (2nd ed., pp. 565–599). New York: Guilford Press.

Kinzie, J. D., Boehnlein, J., & Sack, W. H. (1998). The effects of massive trauma on Cambodian parents and children. In Y. Danieli (Ed.), *International handbook of multigenerational legacies of trauma* (pp. 211–221). New York: Plenum Press.

Kohly, M. (1994). *Reported child abuse and neglect victims during the flood months of 1993.* Jefferson City: Missouri Department of Social Services, Division of Family Services, Research and Development Unit.

Krakow, B., Hollifield, M., Johnston, L., Koss, M., Schrader, R., Warner, T. D., et al. (2001). Imagery rehearsal therapy for chronic nightmares in sexual assault survivors with posttraumatic stress disorder [Electronic version]. *Journal of the American Medical Association, 286*(5). Retrieved from *jama.ama-assn.org/issues/v286n5/abs/joc10245.html*

Krakow, B., Sandoval, D., Schrader, R., Keuhne, B., McBride, L., Yau, C. L., et al. (2001). Treatment of chronic nightmares in adjudicated adolescent girls in a residential facility. *Journal of Adolescent Health, 29*(2), 94–100.

Krug, R. (1996). Psychological effects of manmade disasters. *Journal—Oklahoma Dental Association, 86*(4), 40–44.

Kulkarni, M., Graham-Bermann, S., Rauch, S., & Seng, J. (2011). Witnessing versus experiencing direct violence in childhood as correlates of adulthood PTSD. *Journal of Interpersonal Violence, 26,* 1264–1281.

Lafleur, D., Petty, C., Mancuso, E., McCarthy, K., Biederman, J., Faro, A., et al. (2011). Traumatic events and obsessive compulsive disorder in children and adolescents: Is there a link? *Journal of Anxiety Disorders, 25*(4), 513–519.

Laird, R. D., Jordan, K. Y., Dodge, K. A., Pettit, G. S., & Bates, J. E. (2001). Peer rejection in childhood, involvement with antisocial peers in early adolescence, and the development of externalizing behavior problems. *Development and Psychopathology, 13,* 337–354.

Lau, J., & Pine, D. (2008). Elucidating risk mechanisms of gene–environment interactions on pediatric anxiety: Integrating findings from neuroscience. *European Archives of Psychiatry and Clinical Neuroscience, 258,* 97–106.

Laurens, K., Hodgins, S., West, S., & Murray, R. (2007). Prevalence and correlates of psychotic-like experiences and other developmental antecedents of schizophrenia in children aged 9–12 years. *Schizophrenia Bulletin, 33,* 239.

Liotti, G. (2004). Trauma, dissociation, and disorganized attachment: Three strands of a single braid. *Psychotherapy: Theory, Research, Practice, Training, 41*(4), 472–486.

Luthar, S. S. (Ed.). (2003). *Resilience and vulnerability: Adaptation in the context of childhood adversities.* New York: Cambridge University Press.

Maercker, A., Brewin, C., Bryant, R., Cloitre, M., Reed, G., van Ommeren, M., et al. (2013). Proposals for mental disorders specifically associated with stress in the ICD-11. *Lancet, 381,* 1683–1685.

Mash, E. J., & Dozois, D. (2003). Child psychopathology: A developmental systems perspective. In E. J. Mash & R. A. Barkley (Eds.), *Child psychopathology* (2nd ed., pp. 3–71). New York: Guilford Press.

Masten, A. S., & Powell, J. L. (2003). A resilience framework for research, policy and practice. In S. S. Luthar (Ed.), *Resilience and vulnerability: Adaptation in the context of childhood adversities* (pp. 1–25). New York: Cambridge University Press.

McNally, R. J. (2001). Vulnerability to anxiety disorders in adulthood. In R. E. Ingram & J. M. Price (Eds.), *Vulnerability to psychopathology: Risk across the lifespan* (pp. 304–321). New York: Guilford Press.

McReynolds, L., & Wasserman, G. (2011). Self-injury in incarcerated juvenile females: Contributions of mental health and traumatic experiences. *Journal of Traumatic Stress, 24*, 752–755.

Melhem, N., Moritz, G., Walker, M., & Shear, K. (2007). Phenomenology and correlates of complicated grief in children and adolescents. *Journal of the American Academy of Child and Adolescent Psychiatry, 46*(4), 493–499.

Nader, K. (1997). Childhood traumatic loss: The interaction of trauma and grief. In C. R. Figley, B. E. Bride, & N. Mazza (Eds.), *Death and trauma: The traumatology of grieving* (pp. 17–41). London: Taylor & Francis.

Nader, K. (2004). Treating traumatized children and adolescents: Treatment issues, modalities, timing, and methods. In N. B. Webb (Ed.), *Mass trauma and violence: Helping families and children cope* (pp. 50–74). New York: Guilford Press.

Nader, K. (2008). *Understanding and assessing trauma in children and adolescents: Measures, methods, and youth in context.* New York: Routledge.

Nader, K. (Ed.). (2014). *Assessment of trauma in youths: Understanding issues of age, complexity, and associated variables.* New York: Routledge.

Nader, K. (2015). Assessing childhood traumatic reactions: The variables that influence reactions and methods of assessment. In P. Clements & S. Seedat (Eds.), *Mental health issues of child maltreatment* (pp. 455–501) St. Louis, MO: STM Learning.

Nader, K., & Danieli, Y. (2005). Culture and terrorism. In Y. Danieli, D. Brom, & J. Waizer (Eds.), *The trauma of terror: Sharing knowledge and shared care* (pp. 399–410). New York: Haworth Press.

Nader, K., & Fletcher, K. (2014). Childhood posttraumatic stress disorder. In E. J. Mash & R. A. Barkley (Eds.), *Child psychopathology* (3rd ed., pp. 476–528). New York: Guilford Press.

Nader, K., & Mello, C. (2001). Interactive trauma/grief focused therapy. In P. Lehmann & N. F. Coady (Eds.), *Theoretical perspectives for direct social work practice: A generalist–eclectic approach* (pp. 382–401). New York: Springer.

Nader, K., & Pynoos, R. (1993). School disaster: Planning and initial interventions. *Journal of Social Behavior and Personality, 8*(5), 299–320.

Nader, K., & Salloum, A. (2011). Complicated grief reactions in children and adolescents. *Journal of Child and Adolescent Trauma, 4*, 233–257.

Nader, K., & Weems, C. (2011). Understanding and assessing cortisol levels in children and adolescents. *Journal of Child and Adolescent Trauma, 4*(4), 318–338.

Nakao, T., Nakagawa, A., Yoshiura, T., Nakatani, E., Nabeyama, M., Yoshizato, C., et al. (2005). A functional MRI comparison of patients with obsessive–compulsive disorder and normal controls during a Chinese character Stroop task. *Psychiatry Resident, 139*, 101–114.

Pasquini, P., Liotti, G., Mazzotti, E., Fassone, G., & Picardi, A. (2002). Risk factors in the early family life of patients suffering from dissociative disorders. *Acta Psychiatrica Scandinavica, 105*, 110–116.

Pearlman, L. A. (2001). Treatment of persons with complex PTSD and other trauma-related disruptions of the self. In J. P. Wilson, M. Friedman, & J. Lindy (Eds.), *Treating psychological trauma and PTSD* (pp. 205–236). New York: Guilford Press.

Pearlman, M., Schwalbe, K., & Cloitre, M. (2010). *Grief in childhood: Fundamentals of treatment in clinical practice.* Washington, DC: American Psychological Association.

Pleuss, M., & Belsky, J. (2009). Differential susceptibility to rearing experience: The case of childcare. *Journal of Child Psychology and Psychiatry, 50*(4), 396–404.

Pole, N., Best, S. R., Metzler, T., & Marmar, C. R. (2005). Why are Hispanics at greater risk for PTSD? *Cultural Diversity and Ethnic Minority Psychology, 11*(2), 144–161.

Prigerson, H., Horowitz, M., Jacobs, S., Parks, C. M., Aslan, M., Goodkin, K., et al. (2009). Prolonged grief disorder: Psychometric validation of criteria proposed for DSM-V and ICD11. *PLoS Medicine, 6*(8), e1000121.

Pynoos, R., & Nader, K. (1988). Psychological first aid and treatment approach for children exposed to community violence: Research implications. *Journal of Traumatic Stress, 1*(4), 445–473.

Rothbart, M. K., & Bates, J. E. (1998). Temperament. In W. Damon (Series Ed.) & N. Eisenberg (Vol. Ed.), *Handbook of child psychology: Vol. 3. Social, emotional, and personality development* (5th ed., pp. 105–176). New York: Wiley.

Sapolsky, R. M. (1998). *Biology and human behavior: The neurological origins of individuality* [Videotape series]. Chantilly, VA: Teaching Company.

Sapolsky, R. M. (2000). Glucocorticoids and hippocampal atrophy in neuropsychiatric disorders. *Archives of General Psychiatry, 57*, 925–935.

Savitz, J., van der Merwe, L., Stein, D., Solms, M., & Ramesar, R. (2007). Genotype and childhood sexual trauma moderate neurocognitive performance: A possible role for brain derived neurotrophic factor and apolipoprotein E variants. *Biological Psychiatry, 62*, 391–399.

Scheeringa, M. (2014). PTSD in children younger than age of 13: Towards developmentally sensitive assessment and management. In K. Nader (Ed.), *Assessment of trauma in youths: Understanding issues of age, complexity, and associated variables* (pp. 21–37). New York: Routledge.

Schippell, P. L., Vasey, M. W., Cravens-Brown, L. M., & Bretveld, R. A. (2003). Suppressed attention to rejection, ridicule, and failure cues: A unique correlate of reactive but not proactive aggression in youth. *Journal of Clinical Child and Adolescent Psychology, 32*(1), 40–55.

Shaw, J. (2000). Children, adolescents and trauma. *Psychiatric Quarterly, 71*(3), 227–243.

Shiang, J. (2000). Considering cultural beliefs and behaviors in the study of suicide. In R. Maris, S. Canetto, J. McIntosh, & M. Silverman (Eds.), *Review of suicidology 2000* (pp. 226–241). New York: Guilford Press.

Silberg, J. L. (Ed.). (1998). *The dissociative child: Diagnosis, treatment, and management* (2nd ed.). Baltimore: Sidran Press.

Simmons, R. L., & Johnson, C. (1998). Intergeneration transmission of domestic violence. In Y. Danieli (Ed.), *International handbook of multigenerational legacies of trauma* (pp. 553–570). New York: Plenum Press.

Smyke, A., Zeanah, C. Gleason, M., Drury, S., Fox, N., Nelson, C., et al. (2012). A randomized controlled trial comparing foster care and institutional care for children with signs of reactive attachment disorder. *American Journal of Psychiatry, 169*, 508–514.

Sonderegger, R., Barrett, P. M., & Creed, P. A. (2004). Models of cultural adjustment for child and adolescent migrants to Australia: Internal process and situational factors. *Journal of Child and Family Studies, 13*(3), 357–371.

Spinazzolla, J., Blaustein, M., & van der Kolk, B. (2005). Posttraumatic stress disorder treatment outcome research: The study of unrepresentative samples? *Journal of Traumatic Stress, 18*(5) 425–436.

Stalfa, F. (2010). "Posthumous disillusionment" as a type of complicated grief. *Journal of Pastoral Care and Counseling, 64*(2), 71–78.

Taylor, J., & Harvey, S. (2010). A meta-analysis of the effects of psychotherapy with adults sexually abused in childhood. *Clinical Psychology Review, 30*, 749–767.

Terr, L. (1991). Childhood traumas: An outline and overview. *American Journal of Psychiatry, 148*, 10–20.

Thomas, P. M. (2005). Dissociation and internal models of protection: Psychotherapy with child abuse survivors. *Psychotherapy: Theory, Research, Practice, Training, 42*(1), 20–36.

Udwin, O., Boyle, S., Yule, W., Bolton, D., & O'Ryan, D. (2000). Risk factors for long-term psychological effects of a disaster experienced in adolescence: Predictors of posttraumatic stress disorder. *Journal of Child Psychology and Psychiatry, 41*(8), 969–979.

van der Kolk, B. A. (2003). Posttraumatic stress disorder and the nature of trauma. In M. Solomon & D. J. Siegel (Eds.), *Healing trauma* (pp. 168–195). New York: Norton.

van der Kolk, B. A., & Courtois, C. (2005). Editorial comments: Complex developmental trauma. *Journal of Traumatic Stress, 18*(5), 385–388.

van der Kolk, B. A., Roth, S., Pelcovitz, D., Sunday, S., & Spinazzola, J. (2005). Disorders of extreme stress: The empirical foundation for a complex adaptation to trauma. *Journal of Traumatic Stress, 18*(5), 389–399.

van Os, J., Hanssen, M., Bijl, R., & Vollebergh, W. (2001). Prevalence of psychotic disorder and community level of psychotic symptoms: An urban–rural comparison. *Archives of General Psychiatry, 58*, 663–668.

van Winkel, R., Stefanis, N., & Myin-Germeys, I. (2008). Psychosocial stress and psychosis: A review of the neurobiological mechanisms and the evidence for gene–stress interaction. *Schizophrenia Bulletin, 34*, 1095–1105.

Vila, G., Porche, L., & Mouren-Simeoni, M. (1999). An 18–month longitudinal study of posttraumatic disorders in children who were taken hostage in their school. *Psychosomatic Medicine, 61*, 746–754.

Webb, N. B. (Ed.). (2004). *Mass trauma and violence: Helping families and children cope*. New York: Guilford Press.

Weinstein, D., Staffelbach, D., & Biaggio, M. (2000). Attention-deficit hyperactivity disorder and posttraumatic stress disorder: Differential diagnosis in childhood sexual abuse. *Clinical Psychology Review, 20*(3), 359–378.

Williams, M. B., & Sommer, J. F. (Eds.). (2002). *Simple and complex post-traumatic stress disorder.* New York: Haworth Maltreatment and Trauma Press.

Wilson, J. P. (2004). PTSD and complex PTSD: Symptoms, syndromes, and diagnoses. In J. P. Wilson & T. M. Keane (Eds.), *Assessing psychological trauma and PTSD* (2nd ed., pp. 7–44). New York: Guilford Press.

Wonderlich, S., Rosenfeldt, S., Crosby, R., Mitchell, J., Engel, S. G., Smyth, J., et al. (2007). The effects of childhood trauma on daily mood lability and comorbid psychopathology in bulimia nervosa. *Journal of Traumatic Stress, 20,* 77–87.

Yates, T. M., Egeland, B., & Sroufe, A. (2003). Rethinking resilience: A developmental process perspective. In S. S. Luthar (Ed.), *Resilience and vulnerability: Adaptation in the context of childhood adversities* (pp. 243–266). New York: Cambridge University Press.

Yee, P. L., Pierce, G. R., Ptacek, J. T., & Modzelesky, K. L. (2003). Learned helplessness attributional style and examination performance: Enhancement effects are not necessarily moderated by prior failure. *Anxiety, Stress and Coping, 16*(4), 359–373.

Zelst, C. (2008). Which environments for G×E?: A user perspective on the roles of trauma and structural discrimination in the onset and course of schizophrenia. *Schizophrenia Bulletin, 34*(6), 1106–1110.

Zisook, S., Reynolds, C. F., Pies, R., Simon, N., Lebowitz, B., Madowitz, J., et al. (2010). Bereavement, complicated grief, and DSM: Part 1. Depression. *Journal of Clinical Psychiatry, 71,* 955–956.

Chapter 3

Play Therapy to Help Symptomatic Children and Adolescents after Crisis and Trauma

NANCY BOYD WEBB
JENNIFER BAGGERLY

Play therapy ingeniously undertakes the hard work of psychotherapy through nonverbal methods that appeal to children and adolescents. Since young people of all ages have difficulty talking about their problems and feelings, approaches to working with them should reflect this reality and utilize methods that are age-appropriate and appealing to their interests. Examples of play therapy approaches include art activities, doll and puppet play, and sandplay. Teenagers may enjoy musical activities, drawing, poetry or journal writing, dance, drama, and sandplay. All these have intrinsic appeal and offer nonverbal alternatives for interaction when a youngster does not want to talk.

Few young people willingly admit that they have "problems," even when they have experienced a traumatic event that causes them to have nightmares, anxiety, and major changes in their typical behavior. Their parents' or teachers' complaints about them may bring them to therapy, but once in a therapist's office, these youth cannot tolerate a discussion about their "problems" with a strange adult. The well-meaning but inexperienced therapist who asks a youngster the typical open-ended question appropriate for adults—"So can you tell me about what brings you here today?"—had better be prepared for a blank stare, a shrug of the shoulders, or (at best) "My mother said you wanted to talk to me." If it is hard for adults to seek help and discuss their emotional distress in therapy, how much more so is it for children and adolescents! Fortunately, play and expressive techniques come to the rescue, providing the necessary enticement for engaging and treating these anxious and symptomatic young persons.

In this chapter, we present a review of different play and expressive therapies that can be used with children and adolescents who are having difficulties related to stress and anxiety associated with a crisis or traumatic event. We discuss the issue of directive versus nondirective approaches, and we review empirical research that evaluates the merits of play interventions for children and adolescents after crisis and traumatic exposure.

DEFINITION, GOALS, AND NATURE OF PLAY THERAPY

Play Therapy and Expressive Therapy: Definitions

"Play therapy" is a helping interaction between a trained adult therapist and a child for the purpose of relieving the child's emotional distress by using the symbolic communication of play. "The assumption is that children will express and work through [their] emotional conflicts . . . within the metaphor of play" (Reid, 2001, p. 150). Furthermore, the play therapist not only helps bring about relief of clinical symptoms (important as this may be to the parents and youngster), but also works toward removal of impediments to the youth's continuing development, thereby enhancing prospects for future growth (Crenshaw, 2006; Webb, 2007).

The "therapy" of play therapy involves far more than merely playing. Through the interactions with the therapist, the child or adolescent experiences acceptance, catharsis, reduction of troublesome affects, redirection of impulses, and a corrective emotional experience (Chethik, 2000; James, 1994). In the safety of the "holding environment" of the playroom, the youth can express his or her feelings in fantasy and then eventually move to a state of mastery (Reid, 2001), which subsequently may carry over to everyday life. It is not play per se that produces anxiety relief for the child; rather, it is play in the context of the therapeutic *relationship* that provides the critical healing process (Chethik, 2000; Landreth, 2002). Shelby (1997, p. 149) states that "traumatized children need to be heard in the presence of another who is not afraid . . . they need someone to accept their suffering in its cruel entirety." The same statement is true of traumatized adolescents.

Although many play therapy methods can be used with adolescents, the wise clinician will avoid using the term "play therapy" with teens because "playing" may connote to them an activity for young children. In fact, Milgran (2005) makes this point in the introductory chapter of *Play Therapy with Adolescents* (Gallo-Lopez & Schaefer, 2005). Nonetheless, the avoidance of this terminology does not argue against a therapist's having play materials such as Play-Doh, and other art materials and games, available when interacting with adolescent clients.

"Expressive therapy" is a form of treatment often used with adolescents; it is similar to play therapy insofar as it employs the arts and their products to foster awareness, encourage emotional growth, and enhance relationships with others through the creative imagination (Malchiodi, 2003). This form of therapy was first recognized via a graduate program in 1974 for the purpose of integrating arts into therapy (McNiff, 2004, 2009). The basic premise is that expressive arts such as music, dance, and drama, as well as drawing, painting, sculpture, and collage, permit people of all ages to communicate their feelings nonverbally and to achieve insight and relief from anxiety as a result of this experience. Obviously, these aims and methods are very similar to the goals and methods of play therapy.

Like play therapy, expressive therapy does not require or encourage extensive verbalization, and it brings about relief from anxiety at the same time it is enjoyable. When it is used with adolescents, the challenge for the therapist is to introduce the creative activities in the form of enjoyable exercises that downplay the expectation of talking. We know that it is important not to suppress strong emotions, and that expressive therapies offer numerous ways to express one's thoughts and feelings and obtain relief and new ideas through the creative process. Expressive therapies, like play therapy, help bridge the verbal chasm that is so daunting for traumatized youth who do not have the words to verbalize their feelings.

Balance between Verbal and Play Interactions

Both play therapy and the various forms of expressive therapies combine verbal and behavioral interactions between the child and the therapist. Both therapies work toward the goal of relief from anxiety, despite the individual's stressful past and present reality. The therapist working with a child or adolescent in crisis understands that a youth whose anxiety is mounting may need to retreat from verbalized connections to his or her own life, and that playing or creating something serves as a safe refuge from his or her worries.

Play and creative activities such as art also serve as a crucial means for establishing the therapeutic relationship. Our usual procedure in the initial session with a child or teen is to say, "I am a doctor [person] who helps children [kids and families] with their troubles and their worries. Sometimes we talk, and sometimes we play, and sometimes we make something." This gives the young person permission to use verbalization or creative/play activities according to his or her particular ability, level of comfort, and preference.

Many play therapists are appropriately cautious and even reluctant about making direct verbal connections between a child's life and the symbolism they notice embedded in the child's play. When a therapist makes the child aware of the meaning behind his or her play, this deprives the youngster of the necessary distance and symbolic outlet to express his or her conflicts and anxiety. Terr (1989, p. 14) has stated that "an entire treatment through play therapy may be engineered without stepping far beyond the metaphor of the game." Our own experience has repeatedly verified that therapy conducted in a displaced fashion (e.g., through family dolls or puppets) can bring symptom relief without any [direct, or explicit] connection from the play to the child's life. This was illustrated in the case of Michael, a 4-year-old boy who developed very aggressive behavior after repeatedly witnessing his father hitting his mother. After a session in which Michael spontaneously acted out a violent, aggressive scene with family dolls, some of his troublesome interpersonal behavior diminished. During Michael's play, I (Nancy Boyd Webb) had repeatedly verbalized the *doll's* feelings (i.e., being frightened and scared), thereby helping to validate Michael's own feelings of fear and helplessness when he had witnessed a similar situation (Webb, 1999). However, I did not call attention to the similarity between the doll's experience and Michael's own life.

As a child gets older, his or her verbal communication skills usually increase, and there may be less reliance on symbolic play. Kaplan (1999) demonstrated the shifting balance among verbalization, large-muscle play activity (Nerf ball and skateboarding), and doodling in the case of an 11-year-old boy whose anxiety in discussions about his serious illness propelled him away from verbalization and toward physical activities that permitted him to temporarily deny the possible serious implications of his blood disorder. Often therapists who work with teenagers have balls and equipment available to permit the discharge of large-muscle tension during the therapy sessions.

Up to What Age Is Play Therapy Appropriate?

Play therapy can be employed across the life cycle, with different activities, according to the client's age. It is likely that the balance between verbal discussion and play content will shift gradually as a child gets older. Play usually dominates over verbalization in the preschool years, whereas the opposite situation will probably prevail as the child approaches puberty. However, there is no hard-and-fast rule about this. Art techniques, for example, may be used as a medium for therapy throughout the lifespan, as may some board and card games and visualization techniques. On the other hand, some play therapy materials such as dolls may be spurned by latency-age boys who consider them "girls' toys," although these same boys will play with animal puppets, dinosaurs, and army figures, and will engage in drawing activities such as cartooning. Doyle and Stoop (1999) present the case of 10-year-old Randy, who over several directive play therapy sessions constructed a cartoon lifeline of his very traumatic past and then brought it to life through play with animal puppets, which represented the important people and events that he had created in the lifeline.

Terr (1989, p. 15) notes that "traumatized youngsters appear to indulge in play at much older ages than do nontraumatized youngsters." This is probably because they are not able to talk about their frightening experiences. Therefore, the opportunity to play or engage in creative activities such as art must be available to facilitate the symbolic expression of experiences that are too horrible to verbalize.

More about the Functions of Play Therapy

As noted earlier, the primary purposes of play therapy are (1) to help troubled individuals express and obtain relief from their conflicts and anxieties symbolically through play in the context of a therapeutic relationship, and (2) to facilitate children's and adolescents' future growth and development. In addition, play therapy helps establish the treatment relationship and facilitates the therapist's diagnostic understanding of the child's problem. It fulfills the following functions as well:

- It provides cathartic relief from tension and anxiety (emotional function).
- It provides ways for the youth to review symbolically in play what happened, to plan ahead, and to problem-solve, thereby permitting a consideration of different outcomes (problem-solving/cognitive/educational function).
- It permits role rehearsal through play and dramatic action, which can enlarge the youth's perspective beyond the immediate situation (behavioral function).
- It provides a restorative/transformative experience of relief and hope for better times to come (spiritual function).

Each young person's situation is unique; therefore, play therapy with individual youth will have a different emphasis, depending on the specific assessment of each youngster's problem situation and his or her particular reactions. Since the focus of this book is on play therapy with children and adolescents in crisis, the discussion that follows focuses on specific therapy approaches for youth in situations of crisis and trauma.

THE PURPOSES AND FORMS OF CRISIS INTERVENTION PLAY THERAPY

Definition of the Approach

"Crisis intervention play therapy" (CIPT) is the appropriate model of treatment for children who have become symptomatic after exposure to a crisis or traumatic event. This approach, which is valid for use with adolescents as well as with younger children, employs all the usual play therapy methods, with the specific goal of helping a youth attain mastery over his or her anxiety associated with the experience. Treatment is usually short-term and directive, relying on the safety of the therapeutic relationship to permit the youngster to reenact his or her stressful experience either symbolically or directly, by using play materials. This approach is recommended as a primary intervention either for crisis situations that are distressing but not actually traumatic, or for single-event (Type I) traumas. When a child has experienced multiple

(Type II) traumas or complex traumas, CIPT will still be useful as an initial intervention, but a more extended treatment model may also be needed. (See below for further discussion.)

Promoting Mastery

Shelby (1997, p. 144) comments that "children use play to move from crisis to confidence as they learn to manage their distress." She recommends an "experiential mastery-oriented technique" based on Pynoos and Eth's (1986) posttraumatic interview, which encourages children to act out their revenge fantasies in play and then move beyond these to mastery experiences that encourage positive cognitions. The make-believe element, according to Woltmann (1955/1964, p. 24), "eliminates guilt feelings which would appear if action could result in real harm and damage and enables the child to be victorious over forces otherwise above his reach and capacity."

In a crisis or traumatic situation, the child has felt helpless and afraid. Through review of the experience in play, the child transforms his or her feelings of passivity and impotence into feelings of activity and power. For example, a child who has been subjected to painful medical procedures may earnestly play out giving injections and other treatments to a doll in doll play.

Directive versus Nondirective Play Therapy

Many of the founders of play therapy subscribed to a nondirective approach. Their philosophy emphasized that the child can and should lead the way, and that the role of the therapist is to support and follow the child's lead. This strengths-based model, labeled by Landreth (2002) as "child-centered play therapy" (CCPT), often proves to be a long-term approach that does not focus on the presenting problem, crisis, or traumatic event unless the child chooses to play this out spontaneously.

Sometimes a child's posttraumatic play takes the form of secretive, monotonous, ritualized play, which fails to bring any relief. Terr (1983) describes this type of play in 26 children in Chowchilla, California, who were overwhelmed with anxiety following the sudden and intense traumatic experience of being kidnapped and buried alive for 16 hours in a school bus. On the basis of her work with these children, as well as a review of the literature, Terr believes that a severely traumatized child needs to verbalize as well as to play. She recommends a form of directive child psychotherapy using preset or prearranged play, in which the therapist deliberately encourages the child to reenact the trauma by providing the child with play materials suggestive of the traumatic experience. This psychotherapeutic reconstruction includes a verbal review of the traumatic experience, in which the therapist helps the child obtain relief from feelings of guilt and fear associated with the trauma. Examples of such directive play reconstruction include work with a 9-year-old refugee (Bevin,

1999) and trauma-focused cognitive-behavioral therapy with a 6-year-old girl (Neubauer, Deblinger, & Sieger, 2007).

Often children and adolescents do not want to remember their frightening crisis or traumatic experiences. Avoidance is typical following a crisis or traumatic event (American Psychiatric Association, 2013), and an avoidant youth's reluctance to review his or her anxiety-evoking memories presents a challenge to the therapist, who knows that pushing worries away does not cause them to disappear. In fact, the consensus in prevailing practice is that for traumatic experiences to be resolved, some form of retrospective review is usually necessary (Amaya-Jackson & March, 1995). As we discuss in the next section, directive, crisis/trauma-focused play therapy can help a child or adolescent to gradually process anxious feelings and to learn methods to put these in the past, so that they no longer hold center stage in the youth's present emotional life.

This perspective is congruent with the views of cognitive therapists (Cohen, Mannarino, & Deblinger, 2006; Deblinger & Heflin, 1996), who emphasize not only the importance of the stressful/traumatic play reenactment, but also the need for mental reworking or "cognitive restructuring" of a trauma event. This entails a verbal review that brings about a changed outlook of the experience, through repeated guided interactions in which the therapist directs the individual to imagine and describe a different desired outcome to the stressful event. Some specific methods used in this cognitive approach include the use of calming and relaxation techniques, guided imagery, psychoeducation, positive self-talk, and instruction that the child or adolescent should rely on parents and other competent adults in dangerous situations.

Research on the Efficacy of Play Therapy

The research on the efficacy of play therapy in general has been well described by Baggerly, Ray, and Bratton (2010). Some of the most important research findings on the efficacy of play therapy were obtained via a meta-analysis, which combined the results of 93 individual studies to determine the amount of change in treatment group children versus control group children (Bratton, Ray, Rhine, & Jones, 2005). Of these individual studies, 67 examined play therapy conducted by professionals, 22 evaluated filial therapy conducted by parents, and 4 examined filial therapy conducted by teachers or mentors. The effect size (i.e., the average amount of change in standard deviation units achieved by treatment group children vs. control group children) was determined for all 93 studies, as well as for each group. For all 93 studies, the effect size was 0.80 ($p < .001$), indicating a large effect. For the 67 studies on play therapy by professionals, the effect size was 0.72 ($p < .05$), indicating a medium effect. The 26 studies on filial therapy by parents, teachers, and mentors produced a higher effect size of 1.05 ($p < .05$). However, the largest effect size was produced by the 22 studies on filial therapy by parents, at 1.15 ($p < .05$).

In addition to this meta-analysis, there are several published treatment–control research studies on play therapy with children following crisis or traumatic events. Play therapy with children following natural disasters was found to be effective by Shen (2010). After a devastating earthquake in rural Taiwan, Shen randomly assigned 30 high-risk children ages 8–12 years to an experimental treatment group or a control group. The treatment group children received 40-minute group CCPT (Landreth, 2012) two to three times a week for a total of 10 sessions. Results revealed that children in the treatment group had significant decreases in their anxiety and suicide risk, in comparison to the control group.

Play therapy with child witnesses of domestic violence also proved to be effective (Kot, Landreth, & Giordano, 1999; Tyndall-Lind, 2010). In Kot and colleagues' (1999) study, 11 child witnesses of domestic violence were assigned to the treatment group, which received 12 intensive individual CCPT (Landreth, 2012) sessions in a 3-week period; another 11 children were assigned to the control group, which received no treatment. Tyndall-Lind (2010) added to this study by comparing her results for 10 child witnesses of domestic violence at the same shelter, who received 12 intensive sibling CCPT sessions within a 2-week period. The results indicated that both the individual play therapy group and the sibling play therapy group scored significantly higher than the control group at posttest on self-concept, and significantly lower on externalizing and total behavior problems. In addition, the children in the sibling play therapy group scored significantly lower than the control group on aggressive behaviors and anxious or depressed behaviors.

Play therapy with children who were refugees (mostly from war) was shown to be effective as well (Schottelkorb, Doumas, & Garcia, 2012). Schottelkorb and colleagues (2012) randomly assigned 31 elementary school children who obtained high scores for posttraumatic stress disorder (PTSD) symptoms on the UCLA PTSD Reaction Index (see below) to either CCPT, which involved twice-weekly 30-minute sessions in the school for 12 weeks plus six 15-minute parent consultations, or a group receiving evidence-based trauma-focused cognitive-behavioral therapy (TF-CBT), which involved twice-weekly 30-minute sessions (an average of 17 sessions were completed) in the school, plus two to four parent sessions over the course of the 12 weeks. Results revealed that the war refugee children in both groups showed significant decreases in PTSD symptoms. Schottelkorb and colleagues' findings were important because they showed that CCPT was as effective in decreasing trauma symptoms as the evidence-based TF-CBT.

In another study, children experiencing chronic medical crises of insulin-dependent diabetes mellitus responded favorably to play therapy (Jones & Carnes-Holt, 2010). These researchers randomly assigned 30 children to either a treatment group (which received twelve 30-minute CCPT sessions) or a control group. Results indicated that the children receiving play therapy showed a significant increase in diabetes adaptation, compared to the control group.

Filial therapy with nonoffending parents of children who had been sexually abused was found to be effective (Costas & Landreth, 1999). In their study, Costas and Landreth (1999) randomly assigned 31 parents to either a treatment group receiving 10 sessions of filial therapy or a control group. Results indicated that the parents receiving filial therapy significantly increased their empathy and acceptance with their children and significantly decreased their parenting stress. Landreth and Lobaugh (1998) obtained similar results with 32 incarcerated fathers: The 16 fathers assigned to a group receiving filial therapy showed significant improvements in empathy and acceptance toward their children, compared to the 16 fathers in the control group. Thirteen parents of chronically ill children who received filial therapy also showed significant improvement in parental acceptance and significant decreases in parenting stress and children's behavior problems, compared to the 15 parents in the control group (Tew, 2010).

Therefore, in Bratton and colleagues' (2005) meta-analysis as well as in the above-described research studies, play therapy and filial therapy have been shown to be effective in general and for children experiencing crises and trauma. However, further play therapy studies with children in crisis and trauma need to be conducted. Baggerly and colleagues (2010, p. 468) specified that a well-designed study that would help establish play therapy as an evidence-based treatment (EBT) should include the following components:

- A comparison group receiving an EBT (preferably), or at least a placebo psychotherapy
- Randomized assignment to groups
- Adequate sample size
- Reliable and valid measures of a specific problem (e.g., trauma symptoms), administered and scored by evaluators unaware of group assignments
- Manualized treatments implemented with fidelity checks
- Therapists appropriately trained and supervised in treatment approaches
- Specific client characteristics: diagnosis or presenting problem (e.g., trauma symptoms due to natural disasters), age, and culture
- Appropriate statistical analysis (i.e., repeated-measures analysis of variance)
- Problems or limitations addressed
- Detailed description for replication by independent teams

There are numerous assessment instruments available for use in research with children who have experienced crisis or trauma. Instruments designed to screen children for trauma symptoms include the Child's Reaction to Traumatic Events Scale—Revised (Jones, Fletcher, & Ribbe, 2002), the Parent Report of Post-traumatic Stress Symptoms (Greenwald & Rubin, 1999) and the National Child Traumatic Stress Network (NCTSN) Child and Adolescent Needs and Strengths (CANS) Comprehensive—Trauma Version (Kisiel et al., 2011). PTSD symptoms can be measured with the Trauma Symptom Checklist for Young Children (Briere, 1996), the UCLA PTSD Reaction Index (Steinberg, Brymer, Decker, & Pynoos, 2004), or the Children's PTSD Inventory (Saigh, 2004). Other recommendations for assessment instruments are available from the NCTSN (*www.nctsnet.org*).

Research has not yet provided definitive conclusions about whether directive or nondirective approaches produce more favorable results in therapy with symptomatic children following crisis or traumatic events. Shelby and Felix (2005) comment that throughout the history of child trauma therapy, there has been debate about how best to intervene. Despite the lack of consensus, Amaya-Jackson and March (1995) argue for a combination of cognitive-behavioral, supportive, and psychodynamic psychotherapy to help traumatized children. However, as yet no studies have examined the efficacy of this combined approach. In view of the lack of agreement (and lack of conclusive empirical research findings), it seems understandable that few child therapists currently rely on a *purely* directive or *purely* nondirective treatment approach. An assessment of the child—tripartite assessment (see Chapter 1) and/or the use of other assessment instruments (such as those listed above)—can lead to a treatment approach that considers the child's personal attribution of meaning related to his or her crisis/traumatic experience.

This book offers examples of a variety of treatment methods that have proven to be effective with children exposed to crisis or trauma. Not all the therapeutic interventions presented here have been evaluated in controlled research studies. Ideally, more research in the future will shed light on this important topic; until then, methods that combine directive and nondirective treatment, and that are based on clinical practice experience and best judgment, will continue to be used to relieve young people's distress.

PLAY THERAPY FOR DIFFERENT TYPES OF CRISES/TRAUMAS

In Chapter 1, I (Nancy Boyd Webb) have defined the terms "stress," "crisis," and "trauma," and have presented a figure illustrating the interaction of these (see Figure 1.2). I have also discussed Terr's (1991) distinction between Type I (single-event) and Type II (multiple) traumas. As Figure 1.2 indicates, a crisis or traumatic event may be dealt with through adequate or inadequate coping. We know that many people, including children and teens, are sufficiently resilient to endure various frightening or even terrifying experiences without developing distressing symptoms (although this is more often the case with crises that are not actually traumatic and with Type I traumas than it is with Type II or complex traumas). In other cases, however, individuals' temperaments, personal histories, and/or current life situations do not permit them to cope adequately with a crisis or trauma. Figure 1.2 shows that such individuals may develop anxiety, depression, or various posttraumatic symptoms. As Nader discusses in detail in Chapter 2, the symptoms of youth exposed to traumatic events may meet formal *Diagnostic and Statistical Manual of Mental Disorders* (DSM) criteria for a diagnosis of PTSD or acute stress disorder (ASD), as well as a wide variety of comorbid disorders. CIPT is based on the hope that timely intervention may help youth who have undergone crises or traumas either to resolve their related anxieties and other symptoms before they blossom into full-blown psychiatric disorders, or to return more rapidly to normal functioning if they already meet criteria for one or more disorders.

The cases that follow illustrate the use of CIPT with children who have experienced Type I and Type II traumas (Terr, 1991). The first involves a 9-year-old girl, Susan, who was functioning well until she suffered the sudden, traumatic loss of a friend in a car accident (Type I trauma). The second case describes a series of traumatic events that occurred to a 10-year-old boy, Sergio—a refugee from Central America who almost drowned while fleeing from Mexico over the Rio Grande, and who then witnessed his mother's rape, followed by their subsequent flight to safety (Type II traumas). In both cases, the CIPT therapists acknowledged and empathized with the children's frightened feelings and attempted to clarify any cognitive distortions, while also emphasizing the children's good survival strategies, coping abilities, and current safety. Both of these cases have been previously published (Bevin, 1999; Webb, 2002) and were summarized by Webb in Carey (2006). They are presented here in greatly abridged form, to illustrate the use of directive and nondirective methods in CIPT after a single-incident trauma and after a situation of multiple traumatic events.

The Case of Susan, Age 9

Susan, age 9, was in fourth grade and active in Girl Scouts. Susan's family and Carl's had been very close for many years.

The Traumatic Event

Susan's friend, Carl, died in a car accident in which the car went off the road and a tree branch came through the car window, piercing Carl's body. The rumor in Susan's school was that the branch had decapitated the boy! Only years later did Susan learn the true cause of her friend's death—namely, that the branch had pierced his stomach and he had bled to death on the spot. The rumor was so horrible at the time that no one could discuss it.

Reason for Referral

Susan's behavior changed quite drastically after Carl's death. She became "angry, cranky, and mean"; she stopped doing her homework and after school would stay in her room, saying that she was "tired." She was also complaining of headaches and bad dreams every night. Susan refused to go to Carl's house to speak with his mother or sister, and she would become agitated and panicky whenever her mother drove anywhere near Carl's neighborhood. All of these responses qualified for a diagnosis of acute stress disorder.

Play Therapy Sessions

Although Susan had initially refused to come into my (Nancy Boyd Webb's) office, she did so after I went outside to greet her. In the first session, I told Susan that I knew about her friend's terrible death, and I explained my role as a doctor who helps kids with their troubles and worries. Susan told me about her nightmares, and I empathized with her about them, saying that sometimes daytime worries come back at night in the form of bad dreams. She denied that she had any worries.

At my suggestion, Susan willingly made some drawings, in which none of the figures looked happy. She declined my invitation to tell me anything about her pictures. She found the board game Battleship in my large collection of games and toys, and she wanted to play this repeatedly in subsequent play therapy sessions. I came to realize that the implicit theme in the game was sudden death, not unlike that of a car going unpredictably off the road. Therefore, my comments during the play reflected being scared because we never know when a bomb might hit and when our boat would sink. I also expressed concern about what would happen to the people in the boats that sank. I was, of course, referring symbolically to Carl's unexpected, accidental death.

Another time we participated in a squiggle story activity (see "Art Techniques," below), in which Susan's invented story also had themes of sudden death—with danger to a princess, and her eventual rescue by the king. I commented at the end of Susan's story that although the princess had been close to danger, she had decided to create a happy ending by having the father rescue the princess.

After about 5 weeks of therapy, Susan's headaches and nightmares stopped. We had not spoken very much about Carl, and not at all about the specific nature of his death, but Susan had spontaneously chosen play activities with death and danger themes. The therapy connected with this had apparently relieved Susan of some of her anxiety.

Discussion

The play therapy sessions with Susan were primarily nondirective and supportive, with no specific instructions to the child to draw or talk directly about her friend's tragic death. Nonetheless, this girl felt safe and understood in the therapy sessions, and she used symbolic play very effectively to convey her fears and anxieties in a disguised form. My role as the therapist was to acknowledge in a general way the frightening feelings about unexpected death, and to remark on the child's choice of a positive story outcome following danger (cognitive mastery). This process seemed to bring cathartic relief to the girl and a sense of mastery through the *symbolism* of her play.

This is an example of a single-incident trauma that was treated in a timely fashion, with nondirective, supportive CIPT that relieved the child's symptoms.

The Case of Sergio, Age 9

Sergio grew up in Central America on a farm with his parents and younger sister. Because of gunfights and unrest in their village, Sergio's father left to find work in the United States, intending to send for his family later. After 2 years, Sergio's father made arrangements for his wife to take her two children to Mexico and cross into the United States, with the help of a "coyote" (guide) who was supposed to escort the family across the Rio Grande.

The Traumatic Events

Sergio's mother was carrying a basket with clothes on her head and holding her 2-year-old daughter in her arms, while Sergio held his mother's skirts as they started to cross the river. The mother lost her footing and fell, while Sergio was dragged downstream. His mother eventually was able to rescue him, and they managed to get ashore. Then the "coyote" appeared with a gun and raped the mother, while Sergio watched helplessly in terror. The family then proceeded to a safehouse, where the father came in a few days to meet them. Sergio did not speak during the entire 2-day period until they were reunited.

Reason for Referral

Approximately 2 months after this series of traumatic experiences, Sergio was enrolled in school, in a bilingual classroom. He did not speak in school; he did not make friends; and when any of his classmates tried to interact with him, Sergio would begin to cry helplessly. In addition, Sergio was having a lot of trouble sleeping at night.

Play Therapy Sessions

The first few sessions consisted of talking, drawing, relaxation exercises, and free-play activities. The Spanish-speaking therapist told Sergio that she was someone who understood children's fears, and that she wanted to help him sleep better and have a better time in school. The therapist initially refrained from presenting Sergio with any toys that might recall memories of his traumatic experiences.

In the fifth session, the therapist decided to introduce a toy bathtub, some small plastic doll figures, and a block of wood floating in the water. She encouraged Sergio to have the figures swim in the water. The boy instead created a happy scene of a family fishing with both the father and mother present.

In the next session, the therapist provided the same toys and asked him to pretend that the water was a river that the family needed to cross. With a lot of ongoing encouragement from the therapist, Sergio eventually recreated his trauma, including the part when he felt as if he were drowning. During this reenactment, Sergio began referring to his own experience (rather than projecting onto the dolls). The therapist's response emphasized how strong he was to have endured such a terrible experience.

In the next session, the therapist decided to attempt a "role play" of the mother's rape, using rag dolls. She asked Sergio to show what happened after they crossed the river, and he did so after initially not wanting to do so. The therapist encouraged and reassured Sergio by reminding him that he and his mother were safe now. In the subsequent two sessions, the therapist encouraged Sergio to act out in play his retaliation fantasies toward the "coyote." This not only validated his anger, but permitted him a way through play to turn the passivity and helplessness he had experienced during the traumatic event into active expression of his frustration and anger. At about this time, Sergio's nightmares diminished, and he began to form new relationships with his peers.

Discussion

This boy had suffered a series of traumatic experiences, beginning in his homeland, where his family lived in a dangerous environment surrounded by gunfire. He then endured the stress involved in fleeing from his home without his father and then traveling through a strange country. His own near-drowning, followed by the witnessing of his mother's rape and her subsequent admonition not to talk about it, all resulted in a child who was suffering from multiple (Type II) traumas and met criteria for a diagnosis of PTSD.

The CIPT was directive and supportive. After the treatment relationship had developed, the therapist used sensitive persuasion to urge Sergio to reconstruct his experience. The process of CIPT illustrated here demonstrates how to build an effective relationship with a traumatized child, and then how to help him gradually face his horrible experience, at his own pace. The therapist repeatedly emphasized the boy's strengths and resilience, and the boy gradually began integrating this belief into his own self-concept. The impediments to his normal developmental course were removed through this directive CIPT.

RANGE OF PLAY THERAPY METHODS

The well-trained play therapist must be familiar with a variety of play therapy materials and techniques for working with children and adolescents in crisis or trauma. Although few offices are equipped with *all* of the play therapy materials described in the case examples in this book, it is important that a range of choices be available to each youth. The discussion that follows reviews some of the major play therapy methods, with suggestions about necessary materials. (For a video/DVD demonstration of different play therapy techniques, see Webb, 1994/2006b.)

Art Techniques

The graphic and plastic arts have broad application and appeal to children and adults of all ages. Many therapists invite children and teens to draw, both as part of the assessment and as part of the treatment process. Possible drawings might include drawings of a person, a family, a house, a tree, or whatever the person wants to draw. In the "draw-a-person" and "draw-your-family" exercises (DiLeo, 1973; Malchiodi, 1998), the play therapist learns about the individual's perceptions of his or her own body, as well as of family relationships. Training in how to assess and use drawings in therapy is typically included as part of many play therapy training programs.

Winnicott's (1971) "squiggle technique" is another drawing exercise, which can serve as excellent icebreaker with children or teens who claim they cannot draw. This exercise involves the players' taking turns making pictures out of each other's scribbles. Each youth subsequently can be asked to select two or three of his or her favorite squiggle drawings in a series and then to make up a story about it. The squiggle story method was used in the case of Susan to help reengage her in treatment when she wanted to terminate prematurely.

Modeling clay provides a safe outlet for aggressive feelings, since the clay requires pounding, poking, squeezing, and cutting to achieve whatever form is desired. This modality lends itself to family and group play as well as individual therapy, since each member may create an individual project or the group may work on a joint product.

Soft Play-Doh is easier for younger children to handle than is modeling clay, and its greater malleability lends it to being squished between the fingers, thus offering an additional sensory experience. Hurley (1991) described a young girl's anxious use of Plasticine (a material similar to Play-Doh) following her father's suicide by gunshot. The child created several heads that corresponded to the members of her family; she mutilated one head, and then anxiously turned to other play activities. She was not ready to talk about her father's death, but her play conveyed her anxious feelings and allowed the therapist to express some appropriate reactions to the mutilation.

Doll Play

Doll play holds great appeal to preschool children of both sexes and to elementary-school-age girls. Miniature bendable family dolls lend themselves to reenactment of exchanges a child has witnessed in his or her own family. The therapist can learn a great deal from watching and listening to the child's play with the family dolls. Often a preschool child unabashedly names the family dolls to correspond with his or her own family members, and/or selects their hair color and size to match those in his or her own family. Boys and teens may choose to play with toy soldiers, superhero dolls, and action figures, together with trucks and assorted army equipment.

Stuffed animals sometimes take the place of human figures in a child's or teen's representational play. Just as in doll play, the youth displaces onto the toy animals the feelings and conflicts with which he or she is struggling. The principle is to provide children and teens with an array of figures that will permit the widest possible expression of feelings, conflicts, and reenactments of traumatic events.

Puppet Play

The use of puppets in play therapy, like the use of dolls, rests on the assumption that the individual (1) identifies with a doll or puppet, (2) projects his or her own feelings onto the play figure, and (3) displaces his or her conflicts onto the doll or puppet. Both doll and puppet play allow the youth and therapist to talk about feelings and thoughts that "belong" to the doll or puppet, with no direct acknowledgment that the youth has similar feelings. Fantasy also prevails when puppets are used; a puppet that is beaten does not feel real pain, and simulated aggression and killing allow puppet play to go far beyond the limits of human endurance. Another very important feature of puppet (and doll) play is the opportunity to repeat over and over a traumatic experience and its various outcomes.

Although the use of any puppet will vary in the hands of different individuals, the provision of a wide variety of puppets gives the person choices and permits a range of emotional expressions. I have found that it is helpful to have several puppets of one type of animal or insect, so that young people can use them to enact typical family scenes. Insect hand puppets (e.g., ladybugs, spiders, bees, dragonflies, and grasshoppers) provide useful opportunities for youth to master through play their fear of insects, and to express in fantasy their "superiority" over these small creatures, which stimulate fear in many of their peers.

Storytelling

From the time of the Bible, stories have captured the human imagination through creative use of fantasy. Stories may be told, read, created or watched; all methods involve distancing, identification, and projection. Listening to stories permits the individual to exercise the power of his or her imagination as he or she envisions animal or human characters coping with situations similar in some respects to those in his or her own everyday life.

> Both storytelling and journaling were implemented with a 14-year-old female client who had been sexually assaulted by several teens when she was walking home from school. The counselor gave her a plush toy dog. Then the

> counselor told the client a story of a beautiful champion retriever dog that suffered painful wounds after being attacked by a pack of wolves. The dog limped, refused to chase balls, became skittish, and rarely ate food. Over several sessions, the counselor asked the client to discuss and write in her journal about (1) the wonderful things about the dog before the attack; (2) things the dog did to have fun and calm down before the attack; (3) the dog's thoughts, feelings, and behaviors before, during, and after the attack; (4) what the dog did to survive the attack, and who helped rescue the dog from the attack; (5) why the dog should try to recover; (6) what the dog actually did to recover; (7) what the dog's future would be once it recovered (vs. not recovering); and (8) what stayed the same and what changed in the dog after the recovery. Focusing on the storytelling of the dog provided the client with enough psychological distance to process her recovery objectively, in a way that allowed for integration.

Adaptations of storytelling involve writing down a youth's spoken stories and putting them into a "book," with a cover drawn on construction paper and the pages stapled together. Sometimes this technique is used to record a child's experiences in a natural disaster, such as a tsunami (see Baggerly, 2007); in other cases, this method has been used to record the life histories of children in foster care and adopted children. The Internet offers several "lifebook" guides and workbooks to be used by parents, caregivers, or professionals to create a record of the details of an adopted child's or foster child's past life.

Responding to the Created Story

As with other creative media (e.g., art), the therapist's use of a child's or adolescent's story productions depends on the assessment and treatment goals in each situation. An analysis of the repeated themes in stories or art provides the therapist with diagnostic or added information related to the young person's conflicts and feelings. Play therapy is both an art and a science, dependent on the skills and judgment of the therapist. Sometimes the therapist will use the fantasy material with the child in a displaced manner, keeping the disguise; at other times, the therapist may question whether the young person notices some resemblance between the fantasy the youth has created and his or her own life. The therapist's training and beliefs about working in a displaced manner versus making interpretations to the youth's life inevitably guide the treatment approach. Therapists working within a cognitive-behavioral framework believe that it is essential to make the *implicit* meaning of a story *explicit*, in order for the individual to move beyond the crisis or traumatic memory (see Neubauer, Chapter 6, this volume).

Although the techniques for uncovering a child's or adolescent's inner world through art and stories may seem deceptively simple, the therapeutic management and response to the youth's revelations depend on a thorough understanding of child and adolescent development, the nature of their typical responses to stress, and the varieties of symbolic communication. Regular supervision is essential for beginning therapists.

Sandplay

Sandplay is a method of play therapy that uses sandboxes and toy miniatures for the purpose of creating scenes in the sand, thereby combing elements of doll play and storytelling. Usually two sandboxes are available, one with dry sand and the other with damp or wet sand. The instructions to the individual are to make a "world" or a "picture" of anything he or she wants in the sand, using miniatures the person selects from a variety of choices. After the scene is completed, the therapist invites the youth to tell a story about what has been constructed. The use of sandplay as therapy requires special training and access to a rather extensive supply of materials.

Board Games

Interest in games with rules emerges between 7 and 11 years of age, when a child has achieved the level of cognitive development characterized by logical and objective thinking (Piaget, 1962). Game playing requires self-discipline (e.g., waiting for one's turn), cooperation, and obeying rules (Schaefer & Reid, 2001). These ego control functions are beyond the capabilities of most preschool children.

The use of board games with school-age children has been cited in the professional literature (Schaefer & Reid, 2001; Webb, 2007) as a means to refine diagnosis (by observing how a child plays a game), as an opportunity to enhance ego functions (by helping the child master frustration tolerance and self-control), and as a natural route to improving the child's socialization skills (Schaefer & Reid, 2001).

Board games that hold special appeal for latency-age children and teens include both standard commercial games and games that have been designed specifically for therapy purposes. Examples of the former are Candy Land, Clue, and Connect Four; examples of therapeutic games are The Talking, Feeling, and Doing Game and The Goodbye Game.

A youth's reactions to winning and losing, and his or her occasional attempts to change the rules and even to cheat, all become matters for therapeutic discussion. Although most games do not elicit extensive fantasy material from the players, they provide an interactional experience that can be simultaneously enjoyed and analyzed.

Other Assorted Play Therapy Techniques

The possibilities for using play therapeutically are limited only by the imagination and creativity of the young person and the therapist. Insofar as any object may be used symbolically and/or idiosyncratically, it would be impossible to discuss comprehensively or demonstrate, even in a book devoted in its entirety to play therapy, an exhaustive inventory of play therapy techniques. In our combined experience as play therapists, we continue to "discover" new activities to use creatively and therapeutically with children and adolescents.

A Cautionary Note

No therapy office can or should resemble a toy store! This would be overstimulating to most children and countertherapeutic. Many years ago, when renting office space on an hourly basis, I (Nancy Boyd Webb) learned that it is possible to carry "the basics" for play therapy in a large satchel. For me, this included paper, markers, scissors, tape, stapler, a few puppets, family dolls, one board game, and a small tape recorder. The selection of materials varied with the ages and interests of the particular clients who had appointments on a particular day. Children and adolescents will use their imaginations when allowed to do so, and sometimes simplicity brings benefits that diversity may confuse and obscure.

ROLE OF THE PLAY THERAPIST

In play therapy, as in every form of psychotherapy, the therapist tailors his or her interventions to the needs of each client and the specific treatment goals of each case. Following thoughtful consideration about the implications of his or her attitude and actions, the therapist chooses among the following alternative roles:

1. *Participating.* The therapist plays along with the child or adolescent, being careful to follow the youth's lead and not to jump ahead.
2. *Limiting.* The therapist serves as auxiliary ego, attempting to strengthen the child's or adolescent's own ego functioning by emphasizing rules, encouraging frustration tolerance, and setting limits.
3. *Interpreting.* The therapist gently makes connections between the child's or adolescent's symbolic play and the youth's own life. This approach should be used cautiously and only after a positive treatment relationship has been established. As previously discussed, some therapists do not interpret children's play.

The therapist's role in therapy with a traumatized child or adolescent will include the following steps:

- Establish a supportive therapeutic relationship.
- Teach the child or adolescent some relaxation methods to help keep anxiety in check.

- Provide toys that will assist the child/adolescent in recreating the traumatic event.
- Encourage a gradual reenactment of the traumatic event through drawing or with toys after the child/adolescent feels safe in the therapeutic relationship.
- Move at the child/adolescent's pace; do not attempt too much in one session.
- Emphasize the child/adolescent's strength as a survivor.
- Repeat that the traumatic experience was in the *past.*
- Point out that the child/adolescent is safe in the present.

It is clear from this discussion, and from the many case examples in this book, that the role of the play therapist varies. The therapist always tries to understand the themes and underlying meaning of the child's or adolescent's play, in order to provide communication that validates the young person's feelings while also sharing a new vision to help the youth through his or her struggles.

TRAINING IN CHILD THERAPY

Some child and adolescent therapy training programs in different areas of the United States are listed in the Appendix to this book. A supervised internship is an integral part of these programs, regardless of the number of years of experience or educational background of the trainees.

Many schools of social work, and programs in counseling and clinical psychology, offer elective courses in treatment of children and adolescents, and the internships of such programs often involve direct practice with children/adolescents and families. Fortunately, regular supervision is a hallmark of these internships, since the challenges and pitfalls of working with young clients, parents, and families demand the careful attention of seasoned practitioners.

GROUP AND FAMILY PLAY THERAPY

Many of the same techniques and materials appropriate to play therapy with an individual child or adolescent can also be used effectively with the youth and his or her family, as well as in group play therapy with children or activity groups with teens. Several chapters in this book demonstrate play therapy with children and adolescents in groups: Haen (Chapter 12) discusses the use of expressive therapies in groups for traumatized adolescents, and Schuurman and DeCristofaro (Chapter 10) describe the power of mutual-support groups with bereaved children after a parent's death.

Many chapters in this book describe parent counseling, family therapy, and/or children's group therapy, in addition to individual play therapy with a child or adolescent. When an entire family has experienced a crisis, it is logical to treat the family members together to implement mutual support and enhance their coping skills, in addition to offering individual therapy as indicated. Shelby and Felix (2005) refer to mounting research evidence indicating that parental or caregiver involvement in a child's therapy is a critical part of child trauma treatment.

The fact that this book focuses on play therapy as a method for treating *individual* children and adolescents in crisis by no means denies the validity and necessity of utilizing family therapy and group therapy approaches in conjunction with individual play therapy. Often the therapy may involve parent–child sessions in a format referred to as "filial therapy." Readers who want more information regarding family play therapy may consult Schaefer and Carey (1994) and Gil (1994). An overview of group play therapy for children and adolescents can be found in Sweeney and Homeyer 1999), and VanFleet (1994) gives a full presentation of filial therapy. Some studies of filial therapy have been described above in "Research on the Efficacy of Play Therapy."

PARENT COUNSELING

Because of their youth, therapy with children and adolescents inevitably includes work with parents, and therapists must be able to relate helpfully to them and other caregivers as well as to their young clients. All too often, treatment failure results from failure to engage parents or caregivers adequately as allies in the young person's treatment.

When a child or adolescent client lives with one or both parents, the therapist must include them in the treatment plan as a vital component of the youth's treatment. Conveying to a parent that he or she will serve as an essential ally of the therapist forms the basis for the parent–therapist alliance. Many therapists keep this alliance vital by meeting with parents once a month to discuss the young person's behavior, and by establishing a telephone policy inviting parents to notify them of any matters of concern. A therapist respects the confidentiality of a child or adolescent client by refraining from reporting verbatim comments made by the youth in treatment, and by discussing with the parent(s) only general issues related to the therapy

Sometimes it is appropriate for the therapist to meet with the parent(s) in the young person's presence. This should occur only after advance planning and involvement of the child or teen with regard to the purpose of the meeting.

Other approaches to including parents in their child's treatment are conjoint therapy (see Weinreb & Groves, Chapter 5, this volume) or filial therapy (VanFleet, 1994). Therapy with any two family members together is referred to as "conjoint therapy," whereas "filial therapy" (VanFleet, 1994) involves work with the parent(s) alone without the child to train the parent(s) to interact more effectively with the child. This training is followed by parent–child sessions with the therapist present.

In Chapter 6, Neubauer and colleagues describe a different way of including a parent when a child has suffered sexual abuse and witnessed domestic violence. This method begins with parallel individual sessions for the nonoffending parent and the child with the same therapist. After several weeks, when the parent and child have developed trust in the therapist, conjoint sessions take place to address the child's traumatic exposure. The literature addressing therapy with a traumatized child increasingly stresses the importance of including the parent as essential to accomplishing treatment goals for the child.

VERSATILE APPLICATIONS OF PLAY THERAPY

The different play therapy approaches described here can be used in a variety of health, child welfare, educational, and mental health settings by a wide range of play therapists, such as school social workers, child life specialists, early childhood educators, disaster workers, pastoral counselors, pediatric nurses, and child welfare workers, in addition to therapists from the mental health professions of psychology, clinical social work, counseling, and psychiatry. Many of these professionals do not have formal training in play therapy, although they may have knowledge about normal and pathological child and adolescent development. Our hope is that this volume will spark the interest of these professionals in delving further into the world of childhood and becoming more knowledgeable and comfortable communicating with children and adolescents through the symbolic language of play, as a means of helping the youth overcome the effects of crises and achieve optimal growth.

CONCLUSIONS

Play therapy has a long history of effectiveness in helping children and adolescents with their conflicts and anxieties. In recent years, there has been growing interest in developing methods to help youth who have undergone traumatic or crisis experiences. CIPT uses a combination of directive and nondirective methods to assist a child or adolescent to regain his or her previous level of functioning. In the context of a supportive therapeutic relationship, the play therapist uses a variety of cognitive, psychotherapeutic, and supportive methods to help the youth achieve mastery of his or her distressing or traumatic memories through symbolic and reconstructive play. The goal is to help the young person recognize that the crisis or trauma occurred in the past, so that his or her normal development can proceed on course.

STUDY QUESTIONS

1. How can the play therapist explain the value of play therapy to parents who state that "All my child does with you is play"?
2. Discuss the pros and cons of using directive play therapy approaches with children and adolescents who have been traumatized.
3. What safeguards can and should a play therapist use to avoid retraumatizing a young person?
4. Discuss the issue of verbalization in crisis intervention play therapy. How can the play therapist decide whether to make a connection between the youth's play and his or her traumatic experiences? Do you believe that it is necessary to make this connection, or do you agree with Lenore Terr that the child is capable of understanding through the symbolism of the play?

REFERENCES

Amaya-Jackson, L., & March, J. S. (1995). Posttraumatic stress disorder. In J. S. March (Ed.), *Anxiety disorders in children and adolescents* (pp. 276–299). New York: Guilford Press.

American Psychiatric Association. (2013). *Diagnostic and statistical manual of mental disorders* (5th ed.). Arlington, VA: Author.

Baggerly, J. (2007). International interventions and challenges following the crisis of natural disasters. In N. B. Webb (Ed.), *Play therapy with children in crisis: Individual, group, and family treatment* (3rd ed., pp. 345–367). New York: Guilford Press.

Baggerly, J. N., Ray, D. C., & Bratton, S. C. (Eds.). (2010). *Child-centered play therapy research: The evidence base for effective practice.* Hoboken, NJ: Wiley.

Bevin, T. (1999). Multiple traumas of refugees—near drowning and witnessing of maternal rape: Case of Sergio, age 9, and follow-up at age 16. In N. B. Webb (Ed.), *Play therapy with children in crisis: Individual, group, and family treatment* (2nd ed., pp. 164–182). New York: Guilford Press.

Bratton, S., Ray, D., Rhine, T., & Jones, L. (2005). The efficacy of play therapy with children: A meta-analytic review of the outcome research. *Professional Psychology: Research and Practice, 36*(4), 376–390.

Briere, J. (1996). *Trauma Symptom Checklist for Children.* Odessa, FL: Psychological Assessment Resources.

Carey, L. (Ed.). (2006). *Expressive and creative arts methods for trauma survivors.* London: Kingsley.

Chethik, M. (2000). *Techniques of child therapy: Psychodynamic strategies* (2nd ed.). New York: Guilford Press.

Cohen, J. A., Mannarino, A. P., & Deblinger, E. (2006). *Treating trauma and traumatic grief in children and adolescents.* New York: Guilford Press.

Costas, M., & Landreth, G. (1999). Filial therapy with nonoffending parents of children who have been sexually abused. *International Journal of Play Therapy, 8*(1), 43–66.

Crenshaw, D. (2006). Neuroscience and trauma treatment. Implications for creative arts therapists. In L. Carey (Ed.), *Expressive and creative arts methods for trauma survivors* (pp. 21–38). London: Kingsley.

Deblinger, E., & Heflin, A. H. (1996). *Treating sexually abused children and their non-offending parents: A cognitive behavioral approach.* Thousand Oaks, CA: Sage.

DiLeo, J. H. (1973). *Children's drawings as diagnostic aids.* New York: Brunner/Mazel.

Doyle, J. S., & Stoop, D. (1999). Witness and victim of multiple abuses: Case of Randy, age 10, in a residential treatment center, and follow-up at age 19 in prison. In N. B. Webb (Ed.), *Play therapy with children in crisis: Individual, group, and family treatment* (2nd ed., pp. 131–163). New York: Guilford Press.

Gallo-Lopez, L., & Schaefer, C. E. (Eds.). (2005). *Play therapy with adolescents.* Lanham, MD: Aronson.

Gil, E. (1994). *Play in family therapy.* New York: Guilford Press.

Greenwald, R., & Rubin, A. (1999). Brief assessment of children's post-traumatic symptoms: Development and preliminary validation of parent and child scales. *Research on Social Work Practice, 9*, 61–75.

Hurley, D. (1991). The crisis of paternal suicide: Case of Cathy, age 4½. In N. B. Webb (Ed.), *Play therapy with children in crisis: A casebook for practitioners* (pp. 237–253). New York: Guilford Press.

James, B. (Ed.). (1994). *Handbook for treatment of attachment-trauma problems in children.* New York: Free Press.

Jones, E. M., & Carnes-Holt, K. (2010). The efficacy of intensive individual child-centered play therapy for chronically ill children. In J. N. Baggerly, D. C. Ray, & S. C. Bratton (Eds.), *Child-centered play therapy research: The evidence base for effective practice* (pp. 51–67). Hoboken, NJ: Wiley.

Jones, R. T., Fletcher, K., & Ribbe, D. R. (2002). *Child's Reaction to Traumatic Events Scale-Revised (CRTES-R): A self-report traumatic stress measure.* (Available from Russell T. Jones, Department of Psychology, Stress and Coping Lab, 4102 Derring Hall, Virginia Tech University, Blacksburg, VA 24060)

Kaplan, C. (1999). Life-threatening blood disorder: Case of Daniel, age 11, and his mother. In N. B. Webb (Ed.), *Play therapy with children in crisis: Individual, group, and family treatment* (2nd ed., pp. 356–379). New York: Guilford Press.

Kisiel, C., Lyons, J. S., Blaustein, M., Fehrenbach, T., Griffin, G., Germain, J., et al. (2011). *Child and adolescent needs and strengths (CANS) manual: The NCTSN CANS Comprehensive—Trauma Version: A comprehensive information integration tool for children and adolescents exposed to traumatic events.* Chicago: Praed Foundation/Los Angeles, CA & Durham, NC: National Center for Child Traumatic Stress.

Kot, S., Landreth, G., & Giordano, M. (1998). Intensive child-centered play therapy with child witnesses of domestic violence. *International Journal of Play Therapy, 7*(2), 17–36.

Landreth, G. (2002). *Play therapy: The art of the relationship* (2nd ed.). New York: Brunner-Routledge.

Landreth, G. (2012). *Play therapy: The art of the relationship* (3rd ed.). Muncie, IN: Accelerated Development.

Landreth, G., & Lobaugh, A. (1998). Filial therapy with incarcerated fathers: Effects on parental acceptance of child, parental stress, and child adjustment. *Journal of Counseling and Development, 76*(2), 157–165.

Malchiodi, C. A. (1998). *Understanding children's drawings.* New York: Guilford Press.

Malchiodi, C. A. (Ed.). (2003). *Handbook of art therapy.* New York: Guilford Press.

McNiff, S. (2004). *Art heals. How creativity cures the soul.* Boston: Shambhala.

McNiff, S. (2009). *Integrating the arts in therapy.* Springfield, IL: Charles C Thomas.

Milgran, C. (2005). Introduction. In L. Gallo-Lopez & C. E. Schaefer (Eds.), *Play therapy with adolescents* (pp. 3–17). Lanham, MD: Aronson.

Neubauer, F., Deblinger, E., & Sieger, K. (2007). Trauma-focused cognitive-behavioral therapy for child sexual abuse and exposure to domestic violence: Case of Mary, age 6. In N. B. Webb (Ed.), *Play therapy with children in crisis* (3rd ed., pp. 107–132). New York: Guilford Press.

Piaget, J. (1962). *Play, dreams, and imitation in childhood.* New York: Norton.

Pynoos, R., & Eth, S. (1986). Witness to violence: The child interview. *Journal of the Academy of Child Psychiatry, 25,* 306–319.

Reid, S. E. (2001). Therapeutic use of card games with learning-disabled children. In C. E. Schaefer & S. E. Reid (Eds.), *Game play* (2nd ed., pp. 146–164). New York: Wiley.

Saigh, P. A. (2004). *A structured interview for diagnosing posttraumatic stress disorder: Children's PTSD Inventory.* San Antonio, TX: Psych Corp.

Schaefer, C. E., & Carey, L. (Eds.). (1994). *Family play therapy.* Northvale, NJ: Aronson.

Schaefer, C. E., & Reid, S. E. (Eds.). (2001). *Game play* (2nd ed.). New York: Wiley.

Schottelkorb, A. A., Doumas, D. M., & Garcia, R. (2012). Treatment for childhood refugee trauma: A randomized, controlled trial. *International Journal of Play Therapy, 21*(2), 57–73.

Shelby, J. S. (1997). Rubble, disruption, and tears: Helping young survivors of natural disaster. In H. G. Kaduson, D. Congelosi, & C. E. Schaefer (Eds.), *The playing cure: Individualized play therapy for specific childhood problems* (pp. 143–169). Northvale, NJ: Aronson.

Shelby, J. S., & Felix, E. D. (2005). Posttraumatic play therapy: The need for an integrated model of directive and nondirective approaches. In L. A. Reddy, T. M. Files-Hall, & C. E. Schaefer (Eds.), *Empirically based play interventions for children* (pp. 79–103). Washington, DC: American Psychological Association.

Shen, Y. (2010). Effects of postearthquake group play therapy with Chinese children. In J. N. Baggerly, D. C. Ray, & S. C. Bratton (Eds.), *Child-centered play therapy research: The evidence base for effective practice* (pp. 85–103). Hoboken, NJ: Wiley.

Steinberg, A. M., Brymer, M., Decker, K., & Pynoos, R. S. (2004). The UCLA PTSD Reaction Index. *Current Psychiatry Reports, 6,* 96–100. Available from *http://springer.com/medicine/psychiatry/journal/11920.*

Sweeney, D. S., & Homeyer, L. E. (Eds.). (1999). *Group play therapy: How to do it, how it works, and whom it's best for.* San Francisco: Jossey-Bass.

Terr, L. C. (1983). Play therapy and psychic trauma: A preliminary report. In C. E. Schaefer & K. J. O'Connor (Eds.), *Handbook of play therapy* (pp. 308–319). New York: Wiley.

Terr, L. C. (1989). Treating psychic trauma in children: A preliminary discussion. *Journal of Traumatic Stress, 2,* 3–20.

Terr, L. C. (1991). Childhood traumas: An outline and overview. *American Journal of Psychiatry, 148*(1), 10–20.

Tew, K. (2010). Filial therapy with parents of chronically ill children. In J. N. Baggerly, D. C. Ray, & S. C. Bratton (Eds.), *Child-centered play therapy research: The evidence base for effective practice* (pp. 295–309). Hoboken, NJ: Wiley.

Tyndall-Lind, A. (2010). Intensive sibling group play therapy with child witnesses of domestic violence. In J. N. Baggerly, D. C. Ray, & S. C. Bratton (Eds.), *Child-centered play therapy research: The evidence base for effective practice* (pp. 69–83). Hoboken, NJ: Wiley.

VanFleet, R. (1994). *Filial therapy: Strengthening parent–child relationships through play*. Sarasota, FL: Professional Resource Press.

Webb, N. B. (1999). The child witness of parental violence: Case of Michael, age 4, and follow-up at age 16. In N. B. Webb (Ed.), *Play therapy with children in crisis: Individual, group, and family treatment* (pp. 49–73). New York: Guilford Press.

Webb, N. B. (Ed.). (2002). *Helping bereaved children: A handbook for practitioners* (2nd ed.). New York: Guilford Press.

Webb, N. B. (2006a). Crisis intervention play therapy to help traumatized children. In L. Carey (Ed.), *Expressive and creative arts methods for trauma survivors* (pp. 39–56). London: Kingsley.

Webb, N. B. (2006b). *Play therapy techniques: A clinical demonstration* [DVD]. New York: Guilford Press. (Original work released on videotape 1994)

Webb, N. B. (2007). (Ed.). *Play therapy with children in crisis* (3rd ed.). New York: Guilford Press.

Winnicott, D. W. (1971). *Playing and reality*. New York: Basic Books.

Woltmann, A. G. (1964). Varieties of play techniques. In M. R. Haworth (Ed.), *Child psychotherapy* (pp. 20–32). New York: Basic Books. (Original work published 1955)

Part II

CRISES AND TRAUMA IN THE FAMILY

Chapter 4

Children and Teens with Substance-Abusing Parents

SHULAMITH LALA ASHENBERG STRAUSSNER
ROBIN DONATH

According to recent U.S. government data, an estimated 22.2 million Americans age 12 or older (8.5% of the population) met the clinical criteria for substance use disorder. Of these, 14.9 million were dependent on or abused alcohol; 4.5 million were dependent on or abused illicit drugs; and 2.8 million were dependent on or abused both alcohol and illicit drugs (Substance Abuse and Mental Health Services Administration [SAMHSA], 2012). Illicit drugs included marijuana/hashish, cocaine (including crack), heroin, hallucinogens, and inhalants—as well as the nonmedical use of prescription psychotherapeutics, such as pain relievers (e.g., OxyContin), tranquilizers (e.g., Valium), sedatives (e.g., Ambien), and stimulants (e.g., Adderall). In addition, 42.1 million people, or 18.1% of all adults, smoked cigarettes, accounting for one of every five deaths in the United States (Centers for Disease Control and Prevention, 2014).

Many of these individuals are parents of young children and adolescents. According to the National Association for Children of Alcoholics (NACoA, n.d.), one in four children under the age of 18 is affected by parental alcohol and/or drug use—a conservative figure because it does not include children who are not residing in households or who are homeless. An estimated 54% of children ages 3–11 years are exposed to secondhand smoke (Richter & Richter, 2001).

Numerous research studies have found that children of substance-abusing parents (COSAPs) are at great risk for a variety of problems. These children are found in every socioeconomic, ethnic, and racial group in the United

States (Straussner, 2001), and in every educational, health care, mental health care, and community setting. Because COSAPS exhibit not only problematic behaviors but also strengths and resilience, careful individual assessment is warranted.

This chapter focuses on the impact of parents' abuse of selective substances, such as alcohol, heroin/other opiates, cocaine/methamphetamines, tobacco, and marijuana, on their children. It provides an overview of the dynamics of families with substance-abusing parents, the impact on their children at different ages, and evidence-based treatment approaches for children and their parents. Case examples of interventions with children of different ages are included.

DEFINITIONS OF TERMS

Before we discuss the dynamics of substance-abusing families, it is important to clarify the various terminologies used in regard to problematic use of different substances. Every day millions of Americans use alcohol and other psychoactive substances; however, not everyone experiences problems due to such use. It is therefore helpful to conceptualize alcohol and other drug (AOD) use as ranging on a continuum from nonproblematic experimental and social use (e.g., having a glass of wine with dinner) to substance misuse (e.g., using pain medication to get high) to abuse (excessive use of a substance that results in a negative impact on the life of the individual and those around him or her), and finally to AOD dependence or addiction (which may require physical detoxification and/or formal treatment) (Straussner, 2014a). The potential for addiction of different substances varies greatly; for example, narcotics or crack cocaine have a much higher potential for addiction than alcohol or marijuana does.

The terms "alcoholism" and "drug addiction," though no longer used for diagnostic purposes (Straussner, 2014b), imply a progressive deterioration of an individual's social, physical, and mental status. These terms refer to continued use of a substance despite experiencing a variety of medical and psychosocial problems with various degrees of severity. The extensive use of some substances, such as opiates or alcohol, leads to "physical dependence," which means that the user cannot wait too long between doses without experiencing craving and symptoms of physical withdrawal; in most such cases, the person will require detoxification under medical supervision. The use of other psychoactive substances, particularly cocaine (including crack), methamphetamine, or tobacco, can lead to severe psychological dependence but may not require formal medical detoxification.

In this chapter, we use "substance abuse" as a catchall term for problems related to AOD use. Research studies have not identified a single etiological factor that accounts for why some individuals abuse or become addicted to a substance and others do not. Among the most frequently cited factors are genetic and neurobiological differences, psychodynamic factors, severe psychological stress and trauma, and social and environmental dynamics (see Straussner, 2014a, for a fuller discussion of these factors).

IMPACT OF PARENTAL SUBSTANCE ABUSE ON THE FAMILY

A parent's abuse of a psychoactive substance has a profound impact on all family members. Such abuse is a multifaceted issue, resulting in ongoing controversy as to whether it is a disease, a mental health or psychological disorder, or a behavior or bad habit that can be controlled by the individual. This controversy underlies many of the conflicting policies and treatments. It also leads to the confusion and shame that both substance-abusing parents and their children feel in attempting to understand and deal with the constant crises in their lives. What is clear is that because AOD use can impair judgment, cognition, and motor skills, substance abuse can directly reduce a caregiver's ability to provide a safe and nurturing home for his or her children. Substance abuse may thus be seen as a "highjacking of parental capacity to invest in parenting" (Suchman, Rounsaville, DeCoste, & Luthar, 2007, p. 8).

In addition to differential biological, physiological, and psychological impacts of different substances, the legal status of a substance affects both parents and children. For example, many substances, such as alcohol; sleeping pills and tranquilizers; prescribed opioid pain medications; tobacco; and, in an increasing number of U.S. states, marijuana, can be obtained legally. Consequently, the lifestyles and ethnic backgrounds of individuals using these substances vary widely, reflecting the population at large. Moreover, as indicated above, addiction to alcohol develops slowly, and thus the insidious impact of alcohol abuse is most commonly seen after adult independence has been achieved and the individual has married and become a parent. Although the effects of alcohol abuse by a parent vary considerably from family to family, common dynamics include communication problems, conflict, and chaos/unpredictability; inconsistent messages to children; breakdown in rituals and traditional family rules and boundaries; and emotional, physical, and (at times) sexual abuse (Straussner, 2011).

Unlike the use of alcohol, the use of nonprescription opiates is illegal. Although the number of middle-class individuals who abuse opioid-based prescription pain relievers has grown, those who abuse opiates have typically tended to be members of disenfranchised low-income groups, with many of them characterized as having antisocial personality disorder. Many opiate-abusing individuals grew up in dysfunctional and often physically abusive families, with alcohol- and/or opiate-abusing parents and even grandparents. Since opiates are highly addictive, individuals tend to be affected at a younger age, often before completing their education and functioning as self-supporting adults. Consequently, they may have difficulties in forming and/or maintaining stable families of procreation of their own and remain connected to their dysfunctional families of origin (Straussner, 2011).

Given that the time and effort necessary to obtain illegal drugs and to pay for them are considerable, the lifestyle associated with opiate addiction is highly unstructured and characterized by criminal activities. A series of live-in partners, prostitution, and incarcerations are fairly common and have a severely negative impact on family life. The children in these families are often reported to child welfare services and some may be removed from their parents and familiar surroundings. Moreover, many persons who use intravenous opiates and their partners are infected with HIV/AIDS and other sexually transmitted diseases, as well as exposed to various systemic infections, including hepatitis C. Life expectancies tend to be lower than in other families, resulting in children who need to deal with the trauma of dying or dead parents.

Parental use of stimulants such as methamphetamines and cocaine (including crack) can also lead to various medical complications, including sudden death; severe financial problems; and negative psychological effects, such as increased paranoia and suicidal ideation—all of which, again, have a major negative impact on family life. The legal repercussions of using these illicit drugs can be severe.

The growing legalization of marijuana is likely to lead to increased use among some parents and adolescent children (Palamar, Ompad & Petkova, 2014). Although little research has been done on the impact of parental marijuana use on family life, marijuana-abusing individuals tend to be more inner-focused and less socially interactive, making them less physically and emotionally available to their families (Straussner, 2011).

Whereas it was more common in the past for fathers to abuse drugs and alcohol, currently it is not unusual to find families in which both parents have substance use problems. In such situations, a child is essentially parentless and likely learns to take care of him- or herself. Unfortunately, depending on the child's age, he or she may become a "parentified child" (Fitzgerald et al., 2008)—functioning as a caregiver for the parents and younger siblings, even at the cost of his or her own development.

Finally, it is not uncommon for family members to engage in behaviors that maintain and perpetuate substance abuse by protecting the abusing individual from any negative consequences. For example, the wife of a husband suffering from a hangover may call his employer to say that he is sick with the flu and will not be able to come to work that day. This dynamic has been termed "enabling" (Zelvin, 2014) and adds to the confusion experienced by many COSAPs. Moreover, it is important to keep in mind that many mothers, whether they have substance abuse problems themselves or not, tend to remain in relationships with substance-abusing men. Men, on the other hand, are more likely to leave women who have substance abuse problems, leaving the women with limited financial and emotional resources that make it difficult to care for themselves, much less their children. In addition, many substance-abusing women come from homes where they were physically and/or sexually abused, and where parenting was poor or nonexistent. As a result, their own parenting behavior may be deficient, and they may have difficulty in developing a healthy attachment to their children. Many such women get reported to child welfare services and often lose custody of their children.

Although the descriptions above focus on traditional families with heterosexual parents, similar dynamics may occur in families where the parents are gay or lesbian. Unfortunately, although there is a growing body of literature on gay and lesbian individuals who abuse substances (Senreich & Vairo, 2014), the literature on gay/lesbian families with a substance-abusing parent is sparse.

Given the dynamics described above, familiarity with the pharmacological actions of different substances of abuse, their impact on individuals and families, and the kinds of medical and psychosocial interventions that are needed for those who are addicted, should be required for anyone trying to help children and teens of substance-abusing parents.

IMPACT OF PARENTAL SUBSTANCE ABUSE ON CHILDREN

Although the ramifications of parental substance abuse may vary, and some COSAPs are relatively well adjusted, growing up with a substance-abusing parent is generally a painful experience with increased risk for a variety of emotional, behavioral, physical, cognitive, academic, and social problems (Anda et al., 2006). Parental substance abuse is one of the top reasons why children enter the child welfare system (Barnard & McKeganey, 2004).

Recent neurological and psychological studies reveal that children who grow up in violent and otherwise traumatizing households, as is often seen in families with substance-abusing parents, suffer not just from the psychological impact, such as emotional dysregulation and difficulties in social relationships (Fewell, 2011); they may also have permanent neurological changes (D'Andrea, Ford, Stolback, Spinnazzola, & van der Kolk, 2012). Moreover, many COSAPs run a high risk of developing their own substance abuse and/or establishing their own substance-abusing family systems in adulthood.

The degree of familial dysfunction depends on many factors, including whether the substance-abusing parent is the mother, father, or both; the coping abilities of the nonaddicted parent; the physical and psychological status of parents and other family members; the child's age when the parental substance use is or was most problematic; the economic resources of the family; the availability of extended family and other support systems; the existence of sexual and physical abuse; and the inborn ego strength or resilience of the child.

In order to better understand the impact of parents' substance abuse on their children, it is useful to look at the children through a developmental lens. The following sections explore the impact on children of different ages, and identify the best interventions for children and their families.

Impact of Prenatal Substance Abuse on Newborns and Infants

Studies show that biological, environmental, and systemic risk factors commence in pregnancy and are compounded by the postnatal caregiving environment (Tsantefski, Humphreys, & Jackson, 2014). Substances used by the mother are transmitted to the fetus during pregnancy and may result in the birth of an addicted baby, or, depending on the substance used and the timing, in permanent physiological and neurological damage (Azmitia, 2001). It is important to note that although substance use during pregnancy can be very destructive, for many women pregnancy and motherhood can function as motivating factors in seeking treatment. Conversely, fear of losing child custody and lack of child care resources are frequent treatment obstacles.

One of the most destructive substances affecting the embryo is alcohol. Fetal alcohol syndrome (FAS) was first identified in the early 1970s (Jones & Smith, 1973). Subsequent research revealed a continuum of developmental outcomes, currently known as fetal alcohol spectrum disorder (FASD), ranging from subtle neurobehavioral effects, facial deformities, hyperactivity, central nervous system deficits, and information-processing problems to profound intellectual disability. FASD is believed to affect approximately 2–5% of school-age children in the United States (May et al., 2009; Smith, 2011).

The use of illicit drugs, particularly opiates such as heroin, is also associated with prenatal and childbirth complications and with adverse outcomes for infants and children. Although some babies appear to suffer no ill effects, others may be premature or small for gestational age and may have resulting complications such as respiratory problems. Some newborns suffer from drug withdrawal, known as neonatal abstinence syndrome, and have symptoms such as excessive crying and irritability; hypertonia (stiff muscles); tremors; sleep disturbances; and increased sensitivity to light, sound, and touch. As the child develops, other physiological effects may become evident, including developmental delays such as failure to thrive; cognitive deficits; and speech, language, and motor delays. Physical problems such as asthma may develop in connection with respiratory deficiencies. During the school years, learning disabilities and behavioral problems such as attention-deficit/hyperactivity disorder (ADHD) and conduct disorder may become evident (Azmitia, 2001; Nadel & Straussner, 2006). It is not hard to understand the difficulties that a substance-abusing parent may have in trying to deal with such a child.

Although there has been some research on the effects of cocaine, marijuana, and tobacco on newborns, it has been difficult to disentangle the unique effects of each from nutritional deficiencies as well as polysubstance use. Prenatal smoking has been found to increase the chances of sudden infant death syndrome and orofacial clefts.

Impact of Parental Substance Abuse on School-Age Children

School-age COSAPs can range from those known as "resilient children," who do very well in school and are rarely recognized as having any problems at home, to those exhibiting severe emotional and behavioral problems.

More recent studies have focused on children, particularly boys, with externalizing behavior problems (Eiden, Edwards, & Leonard, 2007). Such children exhibit ADHD (or attention deficits and hyperactive behaviors not quite meeting diagnostic criteria), conduct disorder, and academic problems; they also cause difficulties for teachers and other students, and thus may become scapegoated by their peers. Consequently, not only do these children lack basic supports at home, but they also may not obtain the support from peers and teachers that could ameliorate some of the emotional pain they experience in growing up with a substance-abusing parent. Other children, most commonly girls, are more likely to exhibit internalizing behaviors and feelings, such as social withdrawal, low self-esteem, and feelings of loneliness. These feelings can predispose these children toward depression, suicidality, and addictions, which become more noticeable during adolescence.

In an early study of children of alcoholic parents, the author Claudia Black (1981) identified the dynamics of "don't talk, don't trust, and don't feel" as being at the core of their personalities. Although Black's ideas lack a strong research base to support them, these dynamics do have some clinical value and are seen as having a lifelong impact on COSAPs.

Impact of Parental Substance Use on Adolescents

An estimated 10% of adolescent children live with a substance-abusing parent (SAMHSA, 2008). It is important to keep in mind the great variability among early, middle, and late adolescence, as well as the differences among individual adolescents. For example, a 14-year-old girl can be as physically developed as an 18-year-old, but may have the cognitive and emotional development of a 12-year-old. Generally, younger adolescents are more dependent on peers for a sense of identity, are more loyal to their families, and are much more concrete in their thinking (Freshman, 2014). In contrast, older adolescents' newly developing capacity for abstract reasoning makes them better able to understand the impact of their parents' substance abuse and recovery on their own behavior. At times the physical and psychological changes faced by adolescents may play a more critical role in their lives than the parental substance abuse does; therefore, understanding the developmental issues of adolescents is crucial to effective interventions (Fenster, 2011). Specifically, it is important to remember that the prefrontal cortex of the adolescent brain is not fully developed, so these youth do not yet have a well-developed capacity to control emotions and make good judgments. Also, the hormonal changes during adolescence affect the amygdala (the part of the brain that controls emotions), causing emotions to be intensified. It is common for adolescents to experience everything as a crisis; to have mood swings; to be impulsive, self-absorbed, and overly sensitive; and not to be able to plan ahead or understand cause and effect (Corzolino, 2006).

In addition to their emotional instability, adolescents are likely to confront a constellation of stress factors both within and outside their families. Preexisting internalizing and externalizing problems become more evident, placing these youth at increased risk for emotional, familial, social, academic, and legal problems. Of particular concern is the increased risk of intergenerational transmission of substance use problems during the adolescent years. Studies have shown that more than half of all children who were exposed to parental substance use disorders during adolescence developed their own substance use disorders, compared with 15% of those who were not so exposed (Rothman, Edwards, Heeren, & Hingson, 2008). Moreover, like younger children, adolescents often experience feelings of guilt and shame about their parents' substance use and may be reluctant to discuss it with peers, authority figures, or even helping professionals.

TREATMENT APPROACHES

Given the challenges to disclosure of familial substance abuse, it is important for a clinician to assess in a respectful and nonjudgmental fashion for parental substance use, regardless of a child's age or the nature of the referral. Once a parental substance abuse problem is identified, interdisciplinary collaboration is often required, as the clinician will often need to connect with multiple other systems, such as the child welfare system, substance abuse agencies, the criminal justice system, schools, and other mental health care settings and clinicians.

The following sections focus on the best interventions for children and youth of different ages, and provide examples for each (the cases are composites of different clients we have seen).

Interventions for Infants and with Young Children

There is no cure for FASD, but certain interventions have proven to be helpful for children with FASD and other prenatal substance-related disorders. Such interventions, which will vary depending on the severity of their problems, may include referral for medication to help with behavioral symptoms, educational and behavioral therapy (for both children and their caregivers), and play therapy. The use of pediatric occupational therapy may help with body organization and modulation.

The Case of Billy, Age 5½

Billy, a 5½-year-old boy of mixed Native American and European American background, was adopted shortly after his first birthday, following the death of his mother in a drunk-driving accident. His father, who was imprisoned for drug dealing at that time, relinquished his parental rights. Billy was recently referred for psychological assessment by his first-grade teacher, who found it difficult to control him in the classroom; he consistently disrupted the class by throwing things, biting, and hitting other kids. He was initially diagnosed with ADHD, but as the psychologist and social worker obtained more information about his background, his diagnosis was changed to FASD.

According to medical records and information from the adoption agency, Billy's mother had a history of heavy drinking and, initially unaware of her pregnancy, continued drinking until her fourth month of pregnancy with Billy. There were no problems noted during the pregnancy or childbirth. A few months after his birth, Billy's father was arrested and sentenced to 10 years in prison for selling methamphetamines, and his mother resumed drinking. Following the death of his mother, he was put into kinship foster care with a distant relative until arrangements were made for a legal adoption with a couple in another state. According to his adoptive parents, Billy was a "difficult" child with developmental delays, including difficulty with toilet training and poor fine motor coordination. His kindergarten teachers noted that he had "poor socialization skills, poor memory and inability to concentrate, poor language comprehension, poor problem-solving skills, and behavioral problems, especially regarding any change in routine." Because he was seen as capable of doing better if he only tried, he was seen as a child with "bad behavior," which he internalized as being a "bad boy." Despite these identified problems, Billy was not referred for any professional help because his parents saw his problems as related to his being adopted and as "something he will outgrow."

By the time Billy entered first grade, his problems had intensified. It was noted that his judgment was impaired and that he often did not understand the consequences of his destructive actions in relation to other children. Moreover, he had low frustration tolerance and difficulties with language and sensory processing, especially in sensory modulation and regulation; he would run into objects and trip when negotiating uneven surfaces, requiring constant verbal prompts to watch where he was going.

After a comprehensive psychological, social, and medical evaluation, Billy was referred to a community mental health agency and seen by a pediatric psychiatrist and a social worker. He was provided with play and behavioral therapy aimed at teaching him appropriate social skills as well as improving his self-image. His parents refused to have him put on medication for hyperactivity as recommended by the psychiatrist, but they agreed to consider this for the future. Billy was also provided with weekly pediatric occupational therapy to help him regulate his body. His parents were seen on a regular basis, to provide them with psychoeducation regarding his condition and to help them utilize appropriate supportive and disciplinary measures. In addition, family therapy was provided every 6 weeks to address communication and emotional issues between Billy and his adoptive parents.

Interventions with Preteen Children

For a preteen child, it is important to assess the child's relationship with peers and look for such dynamics as bullying and other antisocial behaviors, as well as changes and/or difficulties in school performance (Johnson, Gryczynski, & Moe, 2011). Group intervention can provide a critical source of support and an arena for the development of appropriate social skills (Peleg-Oren & Teichman, 2006).

Psychoeducation for both a non-substance-abusing parent and a parent who is in the process of recovery needs to focus on stages of child development (to help both parents understand what to expect from their child at different ages) and on parenting skills (to help parents understand how to set limits appropriately and how to reward and discipline their child) (Johnson et al., 2011). Moreover, as we discuss later, adolescent COSAPs are particularly susceptible to developing their own substance abuse problems; therefore, preadolescence is a prime period in which to provide family systems interventions, as preadolescents are more open to parenting influences than older adolescents are (Lam et al., 2007). In addition, opportunities to engage extended family members who are not struggling with addiction, as well as community supports (e.g., teachers, ministers, sports coaches), should be sought at this time. Some evidence-based treatment programs, such as the Strengthening Families Program and Celebrating Families!, are discussed in more detail in the next section.

The Case of Sean, Age 9

Sean, age 9, was the older of two children in a middle-class family of Irish background. He was referred by the school psychologist to a social worker in private practice because he was refusing to go to school. His parents were convinced that their child was being bullied in school, and their ambivalence about sending Sean to school contributed to this battle. Sean also suffered from a myriad of somatic complaints that required frequent visits to the nurse's office on the days he did attend school.

Sean's mother revealed that Sean's father had been in a rehab facility for treatment of his alcoholism the previous year, but that since then he had continued to drink. The father had previously worked in finance, but had been unemployed for almost 2 years, which was putting a severe financial strain on the family. The mother had recently started a part-time job in the nursery school attended by Sean's younger sister. The mother described the family life as "chaotic," with frequent verbal fights between her and her husband—fights that Sean attempted to mediate. Nonetheless, she was adamant that the presenting problem was that her son was being bullied in school and needed to learn to stand up for himself.

During his first visit, Sean bounced into the treatment room with a smile, excited about all the toys and games in the office. When asked whether he knew why he was there, he frowned and said that his classmates were bullying him; the latest incidents included his finding several anonymous notes on his desk and in his locker, telling him that his classmates wanted him out of their school. The social worker stated how terribly upsetting this must have been. Sean's response was that he would like to play a game—a sign that he was no longer able to tolerate speaking about his feelings. The game he chose was Sorry!.

Sean's need to win every game was an indication that he rarely "won" in the world outside. It was important to let him lead the play without challenging his methods. The next few weeks were spent playing either Sorry! or another game called Bananagrams. Reminding the clinician of how few games she won seemed to make him feel better. Sean's mother gave the social worker permission to speak with his teachers and the assistant principal about the bullying. The school personnel presented a very different picture: A recent investigation had revealed that Sean was writing the threatening notes to himself, and the teachers and principal were very concerned, as they saw Sean becoming increasingly isolated. They described his "injuries" as appearing only when he was in classes he didn't like or classes in which he was falling academically behind. The school staff was also very concerned about his academic achievement; although he was very bright, he seemed unable to focus, and his grades were suffering.

Over time, Sean's refusal to go to school increased, and he indicated that the fighting between his parents was getting worse. He was worried about his little sister, who was afraid to sleep alone and would often come to his bed in the middle of the night. His parents would fluctuate from being angry/punitive and forcing him to go to school, to letting him stay home. This inconsistency was exacerbating Sean's acting-out behavior, as he felt if he was "sick" or "upset" enough, he would be able to stay home and play video games. The clinician's assessment was that Sean felt he needed to stay home because he was worried about what would happen to his mother and sister when his parents fought. He often spoke in treatment about his father's "anger management issues" (a term he had heard his mother use). His development was being stalled emotionally, socially, and academically; an intervention needed to be made.

The clinician began to work closely with Sean's parents about the need to set clear, consistent limits for him. Sean's mother was asked to tell him, in a calm moment, that no matter what Sean said or did, he would be going to school. Sean's father was asked to leave the limit setting to the mother, as he admitted that he was unable to control his temper when he was angry (and drinking). At that point, however, the father decided that he did not want to come to family sessions any more, and that it was up to his wife to "manage" the children. The resulting relationship with the mother allowed the worker to discuss her husband's drinking and to recommend that the mother attend Al-Anon meetings, a support group for family members of alcoholics. Another important component in the work with Sean's mother was to elicit empathy for Sean; she needed to see his acting-out behavior as a symptom of his sadness, lack of control, and anger—a view that would bring her to a more attuned place with her son. The school was also asked to set limits by not allowing Sean to leave class several times a day to go to the nurse's office. Sean resisted the limit setting, but the tears and pleas stopped once he realized the limits were firm. Sean's schoolwork and his ability to self-regulate improved now that there was a clear structure both at home and at school.

Sean became more engaged in treatment and asked that the clinician talk to his father about his temper. The clinician and Sean decided that both of his parents would be invited to a session, and they made a plan about the topics that would be discussed. During the meeting with the parents, with the help of his social worker, Sean was able to articulate to his father how he felt when his father was angry and threatened his mother, and to state that he wished his father would not drink so much. His father denied at first that his drinking was a problem, and insisted that the problem was Sean's classmates. However, when Sean's mother said that she agreed with Sean, and that the father needed to get help if they were going to remain a family, he became thoughtful and agreed to go to Alcoholics Anonymous (AA).

Over time, Sean's increasing ability to self-regulate; his improved situation at school; and a more open, attuned relationship with his mother (and, to a lesser extent, with his father) all enhanced his resilience, and he was able to return to an age-appropriate path of development.

Interventions with Adolescents

Comprehensive assessment of an adolescent with a substance-abusing parent needs to focus on the previously identified psychological, behavioral, cognitive, social, and physical aspects, as well as family dynamics. The clinician also needs to attend carefully to the teen's strengths, attitudes, aspirations, and resources.

Two screening tools that have been shown to be appropriate for use with adolescent children of alcoholic parents are the Children of Alcoholics Screening Test (CAST) and the Family Drinking Survey. The CAST (Pilat & Jones, 1985) is a 30-item self-report measure that gauges the experiences and feelings of adolescents regarding their parents' drinking behaviors. The Family Drinking Survey (Whitfield, 1991), which assesses the effect of a parent's drinking on an adolescent's physical, emotional, and social health, can help clarify the impact on a teen of a parent's substance use. In addition, standardized instruments designed specifically for adolescents can also help determine the existence, extent, and impact of the adolescent's own substance misuse. One such instrument, the CRAFFT (a mnemonic acronym of the first letters of the six questions), which consists of six age-appropriate screening questions related to substance use, has been found to have good reliability and validity (Knight et al., 1999).

School- and community-based individual, group, and family counseling approaches, as well as self-help groups, are all helpful for this population. One of the most widely available and free community-based programs for teenage children of alcoholic parents are the Alateen self-help groups offered under the auspices of Al-Anon Family Groups. Utilizing the principles of AA and of Al-Anon, Alateen teaches youth about the progressive nature of alcoholism, as well as the importance of detaching from the alcoholic parent's pathological behavior and focusing on their own functioning. Another free resource is a Web-based discussion board run by the National Association of Children of Alcoholics (NACoA; *www.nacoa.org*), where teens can go online to discuss their experiences of living with AOD-abusing parents. In addition, books, booklets, and movies about COSAPs are readily available and should be used in conjunction with other interventions.

Individual insight-oriented treatment and cognitive-behavioral therapies are frequently used with this age group (David-Ferdon & Kaslow, 2008; Eyberg, Nelson, & Boggs, 2008). Regardless of the approach utilized, the overarching goal of treatment is to enhance adolescents' abilities to care for themselves—emotionally, physically, and socially. They need to be helped to develop coping strategies to deal with their emotions; develop awareness of their own thinking processes; and build skills in problem solving, interpersonal communication, conflict resolution, and negotiation. Relaxation techniques, exercises, and other strategies for self-soothing can diminish anxiety or other negative mood states. Helping teens set and follow through with educational and vocational goals is also important (Fletcher, Harden, Brunton, Oakley, & Bonell, 2008).

Group treatment is a commonly utilized format for intervention with adolescent COSAPs (Fenster, 2011). Groups are helpful in teaching adolescents that they are not alone in dealing with the consequences of having a substance-abusing parent, and thereby reducing feelings of guilt and shame. Moreover, group members also share helpful strategies for living with an addicted parent.

The parents of an adolescent may need to be helped to establish appropriate and effective discipline and expectations. Of particular value is help in reinstituting or creating such family routines and rituals as family meals, holiday/religious celebrations, and school events (National Center on Addiction and Substance Abuse at Columbia University, 2005). If needed, a referral for substance abuse treatment for the parent(s) should be made.

As mentioned in the preceding section, several evidence-based family programs are increasingly being used in different settings. One such program is the Strengthening Families Program (Kumpfer, Williams, & Baxley, 1997; *www.strengtheningfamiliesprogram.org*). This widely used family skills training program is designed to increase resilience and reduce risk factors for high-risk families with both younger children (ages 3–5) and teens (ages 12–16). It is designed specifically for parents who have a history of substance abuse but are now in the early stages of recovery. It teaches parents and teenagers skills in problem solving, interpersonal communication, and conflict resolution. Each of the 14 weekly sessions begins with a family group dinner, followed by separate group meetings for parents and youth, and ends with a family session. Both parents and children receive age-appropriate education and experiential learning, focusing on multiple themes such as goal setting, health, and communication. This program has shown a great deal of success with multiple ethnic groups and in both rural and urban settings (Kumpfer, Pinyuchon, Teixeira de Melo, & Whiteside, 2008).

Another evidence-based, family-oriented treatment model (particularly when an adolescent is also using substances) is multidimensional family therapy (MDFT; Liddle, 2002). MDFT views adolescent substance abuse as a result of multiple interacting factors, including failure to meet developmental challenges, abuse, or trauma. The primary goals of treatment are to improve adolescent, parental, and overall family functioning, which in turn will affect intergenerational alcohol abuse and other problematic behavior. MDFT is a very flexible approach; treatment length is determined by the provider, the setting, and the family, and may include a combination of individual and family sessions. MDFT begins with a thorough multisystem assessment of both developmental and environmental risk and protective factors. This information identifies the strengths and weaknesses in the adolescent's multiple systems and becomes the basis of treatment. The assessment and intervention modules include five distinct components: interventions with the adolescent; interventions with the parent(s); interventions to change the parent–adolescent interaction; interventions with other family members; and interventions with systems external to the family, such as educational and legal systems.

A final treatment program is Celebrating Families!, which was originally developed for parents involved in drug court proceedings and was later adapted for use with alcohol-involved families in which there is a high risk for domestic violence, child abuse, or neglect. The Celebrating Families! curriculum, currently distributed by the NACoA, is an evidence-based, cognitive-behavioral, support group model that works with every member of the family, from ages 3 through adulthood (see *www.celebratingfamilies.net/getting-started.htm* for more details).

Regardless of the treatment methods used, a clinician working with adolescents should possess good engagement skills and have the ability to tune in to the indirect and nonverbal signals often used by adolescents. Moreover, the issue of confidentiality needs to be clearly addressed by informing adolescent clients early of their right to confidentiality, as well as any limits to it (such as when there is potential for harm to either self or others, or when there is court involvement). It is also essential to address any concerns adolescents may have about discussing their own and their parents' problems, and to make them aware of their increased risk of inheriting a substance use problem. Finally, it is important to help young people to develop relationships with caring adults who can model healthy behaviors.

The Case of Tiffany, Age 14

Tiffany, age 14, lived in an inner-city housing project and attended the 10th grade at a local school. She was an only child and lived with her Caribbean-born mother; she had never met her father, and there were no other family members living in the city. Tiffany's mother, who used to work as a home attendant, had contracted HIV through risky sexual behavior related to her use of crack cocaine. After receiving her diagnosis, she was referred by a hospital social worker to an agency that served families affected by HIV/AIDS. She stopped using crack on her own after being diagnosed with HIV, although she still used marijuana and alcohol on an irregular basis.

At the intake, Tiffany requested to speak privately with a social worker. During her first session, despite seeking treatment, Tiffany did not initiate any conversation and gave short but polite responses to any queries. As she did not seem ready to talk, the social worker asked whether she would like to play Uno, a card game often used in therapy. Many early adolescents like to play games, and while playing they begin to express themselves.

Over the course of a few weeks, Tiffany began to relax and to open up about her life. First she spoke about school (she was doing well academically and had started thinking about going to a local college to study nursing), and then spoke about her peer relationships. It was in the context of speaking about a boy she liked that she began to speak about her mother.

Tiffany told the worker that she was sneaking out to meet her boyfriend after school and was terrified that her mother would discover this. As Tiffany seemed unusually fearful, the clinician asked Tiffany, "What would happen if your mother did find out? What are you afraid of?" Tiffany burst into tears, and after a while she began to talk about her physical abuse, which had begun at the age of 5 at the height of her mother's addiction. She spoke of being left alone in their apartment for days at a time, often running out of food. Her mother had told Tiffany she was not to leave the apartment for any reason while she was gone. Moreover, whenever she cried that she was hungry or did not listen to her mother, her mother would make Tiffany kneel on rice (a punishment used in some Caribbean cultures). There were times when she had been made to kneel overnight, without being allowed to use the bathroom, and was further punished with extra time if she cried. Even though she missed school for days at a time, no one had ever questioned her mother about her daughter's absences or noticed that she was being abused. Tiffany said that things had been better for a while, but since her mother's HIV diagnosis, she was drinking more often and the abuse had increased; her mother had recently started to hit her with the cord of an electric iron.

Tiffany wore a skirt to the next session and showed the social worker the permanent rice imprints on her knees. The marks from the cord could be seen as well. The clinician asked whether Tiffany had ever told anyone else about this. Tiffany said that she had recently met with her school counselor, and had told her that her mother was drinking heavily and had hit her several times with the cord. The counselor told her that because Tiffany's mother had been diagnosed with HIV, this was her way of dealing with the stress, and that Tiffany was now old enough to "just deal" with this situation.

The social worker did not think that Tiffany could or should learn to "just deal" with the physical abuse and her mother's drinking. Because the social worker was a mandated reporter, and because she felt that she had a responsibility to protect Tiffany, she checked with her supervisor and then called child welfare services to report the mother. An investigation was begun immediately. Two days later, Tiffany's mother came to the agency, enraged and smelling of alcohol. She told the social worker that she would no longer allow Tiffany to have any contact with the worker or anyone else in the agency.

Although child welfare workers did find evidence of the physical abuse, they did not remove Tiffany from the home. Instead, they required weekly therapy for both Tiffany and her mother with a social worker from the child welfare system, which had recently begun to implement the Celebrating Families! program. Tiffany's mother was also required to attend AA meetings to deal with her drinking. Monthly home visits were put into place as well.

CONCLUSION

According to numerous studies, healthy child development requires a safe and stable environment and a caring family that provides acceptance, trust, a sense of autonomy, and security. COSAPs are often unable to experience such an environment and are at an increased risk for lifelong problems, including a relatively high level of acting-out behaviors, depressive and anxiety symptoms, low self-esteem, feelings of guilt and loneliness, and their own abuse of substances.

In assessing and intervening with COSAPs, it is important to bear in mind that each child is unique, and that each has some strengths to be acknowledged and reinforced, as well as difficulties and deficits. Conversely, even seemingly well-functioning COSAPs need help at different times in their lives, so that the same family patterns do not continue into future generations. A child's age is another critical factor in determining the kind of intervention that is offered. What is appropriate for a preschool child is different from what is needed by an adolescent.

Moreover, it is important that clinicians be aware of research showing that those COSAPs who entered adulthood with self-esteem and a sense of self-efficacy had at least one person who provided them with unconditional love and support (Werner & Johnson, 2004). Furthermore, studies identified the three key factors contributing to COSAPs' resilience as being able to express their feelings and having someone to talk to about their feelings; knowing the truth about their parents' substance problems; and having a positive attitude about the future (Johnson et al., 2011). Given these findings, it is critical for clinicians to help COSAPs (regardless of their age) by listening to them regarding what is going on at home, by educating them about parental substance abuse, and by helping them plan for a healthy future.

STUDY QUESTIONS

1. How would intervention with an adolescent differ when the worker knows the parent has an active substance use problem, compared to working with a child of the same age without a substance-using parent?
2. In the case of Billy, despite the adoptive parents' knowledge of their child's difficulties, they did not seek services until the child was in first grade. How different do you think the child's development would have been if he had received a diagnosis of FASD and started to receive services earlier in his life?
3. If a clinician knows that a child's parent has a drug problem, but the child does not bring up this issue during treatment sessions, should the clinician bring it up for discussion or not? What would be the rationale for your decision?
4. Treatment is often abruptly terminated in cases where parental substance abuse is present. How can clinicians who work with this population deal with their countertransference and prevent burnout?

REFERENCES

Anda, R., Felitti, V., Bremner, J., Walker, J., Whitfield, C., Perry, B., et al. (2006). The enduring effects of abuse and related adverse experiences in childhood. *European Archives of Psychiatry and Clinical Neuroscience, 256*(3), 174–186.

Azmitia, E. C. (2001). Impact of drugs and alcohol on the brain through the life cycle: Knowledge for social workers. *Journal of Social Work Practice in the Addictions, 1*(3), 41–64.

Barnard, M., & McKeganey, N. (2004). The impact of parental problem drug use on children: What is the problem and what can be done to help? *Addiction, 99*(5), 552–559.

Black, C. (1981). *It will never happen to me.* Bainbridge Island, WA: M.A.C. Printing.

Centers for Disease Control and Prevention. (2014). Current cigarette smoking among adults—United States, 2005–2012. *Morbidity and Mortality Weekly Report, 63*(2), 29–34.

Corzolino, L. (2006). *The neuroscience of human relationships.* New York: Norton.

D'Andrea, W., Ford, J., Stolbach, B., Spinazzola, J., & van der Kolk, B. A. (2012). Understanding interpersonal trauma in children: Why we need a developmentally appropriate trauma diagnosis. *American Journal of Orthopsychiatry, 82*(2), 187–200.

David-Ferdon, C., & Kaslow, N. (2008). Evidence-based psychosocial treatments for child and adolescent depression. *Journal of Clinical Child and Adolescent Psychology, 37*(1), 62–104.

Eiden, R. D., Edwards, E. P., & Leonard, K. E. (2007). A conceptual model for the development of externalizing behavior problems among kindergarten children of alcoholic families: Role of parenting and children's self regulation. *Developmental Psychology, 43*(5), 1187–1201.

Eyberg, S. M., Nelson, M. M., & Boggs, S. R. (2008). Evidence-based psychosocial treatments for children and adolescents with disruptive behavior. *Journal of Clinical Child and Adolescent Psychology, 37*(1), 215–237.

Fenster, J. (2011). Treatment issues and intervention with adolescents from substance-abusing families. In S. L. A. Straussner & C. H. Fewell (Eds.), *Children of substance-abusing parents: Dynamics and treatment* (pp. 117–141). New York: Springer.

Fewell, C. H. (2011). An attachment and mentalizing perspective on children of substance-abusing parents. In S. L. A. Straussner & C. H. Fewell (Eds.), *Children of substance-abusing parents: Dynamics and treatment* (pp. 29–47). New York: Springer.

Fitzgerald, M. M., Schneider, R. A., Salstrom, S., Zinzow, H. M., Jackson, J., & Fossel, R. V. (2008). Child sexual abuse, early family risk, and childhood parentification: Pathways to current psychosocial adjustment. *Journal of Family Psychology, 22*(2), 320–324.

Fletcher, A., Harden, A., Brunton, G., Oakley, A., & Bonnell, C. (2008). Interventions addressing the social determinants of teenage pregnancy. *Health Education, 108*(1), 29–39.

Freshman, A. (2014). Assessment and treatment of adolescents with substance use disorders. In S. L. A. Straussner (Ed.), *Clinical work with substance-abusing clients* (3rd ed., pp. 395–420). New York: Guilford Press.

Johnson, J. L., Gryczynski, M. S., & Moe, J. (2011). Treatment issues and intervention with young children and their substance-abusing parents. In S. L. A. Straussner & C. H. Fewell (Eds.), *Children of substance-abusing parents: Dynamics and treatment* (pp. 101–120). New York: Springer.

Jones, K. L., & Smith, D. W. (1973). Recognition of the fetal alcohol syndrome in early infancy. *Lancet, ii*, 999–1001.

Knight, J. R., Shrier, L. A., Bravender, T. D., Farrell, M., Vander Bilt, J., & Shaffer, H. J. (1999). A new brief screen for adolescent substance abuse. *Archives of Pediatrics and Adolescent Medicine, 153*, 591–596.

Kumpfer, K. L, Pinyuchon, M., Teixeira de Melo, A., & Whiteside, H. O. (2008). Cultural adaptation process for international dissemination of the Strengthening Families Program. Retrieved from *http://ehp.sagepub.com/cgi/content/abstract/31/2/226*

Kumpfer, K. L., Williams, M. K., & Baxley, G. (1997). *Drug abuse prevention for selective groups: The Strengthening Families Program. Resource manual* (National Institute on Drug Abuse, Technology Transfer Program, NCADI No. BKD201.NTIS, BP No. 98-113103). Bethesda, MD: National Institute on Drug Abuse.

Lam, W. K., Cance, J. D., Eke, A. N., Fishbein, D. H., Hawkins, S. R., & Williams, J. C. (2007). Children of African-American mothers who use crack cocaine:

Parenting influences on youth substance use. *Journal of Pediatric Psychology, 32*, 877–887.

Liddle, H. A. (2002). Multidimensional family therapy. Retrieved from *www.strengtheningfamilies.org/html/programs_1999/10_MDFT.html*

May, P. A., Gossage, J. P., Kalberg, W. O., Robinson, L. K., Buckley, D., Manning, M., et al. (2009). Prevalence and epidemiologic characteristics of FASD from various research methods with an emphasis on recent in-school studies. *Developmental Disabilities Research Reviews, 15*(3), 176–192.

Nadel, M., & Straussner, S. L. A. (2006). Children in substance abusing families. In N. Phillips & S. L. A. Straussner (Eds.), *Children in the urban environment: Linking social policy and clinical practice* (2nd ed., pp. 169–190). Springfield, IL: Charles C Thomas.

National Association for Children of Alcoholics (NACoA). (n.d). What is NACoA? Retrieved from *www.nacoa.org/aboutnacoa.htm*

National Center on Addiction and Substance Abuse at Columbia University. (2005). Family matters: Substance abuse and the American family. Retrieved from *www.casacolumbia.org/absolutenm/articlefiles/380-family matters_report.pdf.*

Palamar, J. J., Ompad, D. C., & Petkova, E., (2014). Correlates of intentions to use cannabis among U.S. high school seniors in the case of cannabis legalization. *International Journal of Drug Policy, 25*(3), 424–435.

Peleg-Oren, N., & Teichman, M. (2006). Young children of parents with substance use disorders (SUD): A review of the literature and implication for social work practice. *Journal of Social Work Practice in the Addictions, 6*(1–2), 49–61.

Pilat, J. M., & Jones, J. W. (1985). A comprehensive treatment program for children of alcoholics. In E. M. Freeman (Ed.), *Social work practice with clients who have alcohol problems* (pp. 141–159). Springfield, IL: Charles C Thomas.

Richter, L., & Richter, D. (2001). Exposure to parental tobacco and alcohol use: Effects on children's health and development. *American Journal of Orthopsychiatry, 71*(2), 182–202.

Rothman, E. F., Edwards, E. M., Heeren, T., & Hingson, R. W. (2008). Adverse childhood experiences predict earlier age drinking onset: Results from a representative U.S. sample of current or former drinkers. *Pediatrics, 122*(2), 298–304.

Senreich, E., & Vairo, E. (2014). Assessment and treatment of lesbian, gay and bisexual clients with substance use disorders. In S. L. A. Straussner (Ed.), *Clinical work with substance-abusing clients* (3rd ed., pp. 466–494). New York: Guilford Press.

Smith, I. E. (2011). Prevention and intervention programs for pregnant women who abuse substances. In S. L. A. Straussner & C. H. Fewell (Eds.), *Children of substance abusing parents: Dynamics and treatment* (pp. 161–184). New York: Springer.

Straussner, S. L. A. (Ed.). (2001). *Ethnocultural factors in substance abuse treatment.* New York: Guilford Press.

Straussner, S. L. A. (2011). Children of substance-abusing parents: An overview. In S. L. A. Straussner & C. H. Fewell (Eds.), *Children of substance-abusing parents: Dynamics and treatment* (pp. 1–27). New York: Springer.

Straussner, S. L. A. (2014a). Assessment and treatment of clients with substance use disorders: An overview. In S. L. A. Straussner (Ed.), *Clinical work with substance-abusing clients* (3rd ed., pp. 3–38). New York: Guilford Press.

Straussner, S. L. A. (2014b). The DSM-5 diagnostic criteria: What's new? *Journal of Social Work Practice in the Addictions, 13*(4), 448–453.

Substance Abuse and Mental Health Services Administration (SAMHSA). (2008). *NSDUH Report: Children living with substance-dependent or substance-abusing parents: 2002 to 2007.* Rockville, MD: Author.

Substance Abuse and Mental Health Services Administration (SAMHSA). (2012). National Survey on Drug Use and Health (NSDUH). Retrieved from *www.samhsa.gov/data/NSDUH/2012SummNatFindDetTables/National Findings/NSDUHresults2012.htm*

Suchman, E., Rounsaville, B., DeCoste, C., & Luthar, S. (2007). Parental control, parental warmth, and psychological adjustment in a sample of substance-abusing mothers and their school-age children. *Journal of Substance Abuse Treatment, 32*, 1–10.

Tsantefski, M., Humphreys, C., & Jackson, A. C. (2014). Infant risk and safety in the context of maternal substance use. *Children and Youth Services Review, 47*(1), 10–17.

Werner, E. E., & Johnson, J. L. (2004). The role of caring adults in the lives of children of alcoholics. *Substance Use and Misuse, 39*(5), 699–720.

Whitfield, C. (1991). *Co-dependence: Healing the human condition.* Deerfield Beach, FL: Health Communications.

Zelvin, E. (2014). Treating the partners of individuals with substance use disorders. In S. L. A. Straussner (Ed.), *Clinical work with substance-abusing clients* (3rd ed., pp. 326–347). New York: Guilford Press.

Chapter 5

Child–Parent Psychotherapy after Child Exposure to Parental Violence

MAXINE L. WEINREB
BETSY McALISTER GROVES

This chapter describes the course of treatment for a young child who witnessed her father's physical abuse of her mother. The episodes of actual physical abuse were interspersed with loud arguments and threats of abuse, which had occurred with regularity since the child's birth. This family was seen at the Child Witness to Violence Project at Boston Medical Center, a program that provides developmentally informed trauma-focused counseling for young children and their parents who are exposed to violence. The chapter presents an overview of research and clinical findings about the impact of domestic violence on children, and then focuses on assessment and intervention strategies as demonstrated in the detailed case example.

PREVALENCE OF DOMESTIC VIOLENCE

"Domestic violence," also referred to as "intimate-partner violence," is defined as a pattern of behaviors incorporating a range of abusive tactics—emotional, physical, and/or sexual—that result in the coercive control of one partner over the other. The large majority of victims are women. Approximately 25% of women have been affected by intimate-partner violence at some point in their lifetimes (Walters, Chen, & Breiding, 2013). Children are often the hidden victims of domestic violence (Groves, Zuckerman, & Marans, 1993). It is estimated that as many as 15 million children live in dual-parent families in which some form of intimate-partner violence occurred at least once in the past year, and that 7 million of these children live in homes where there is severe (i.e., repeated) violence (McDonald, Jouriles, Ramisetty-Mikler, Caetano, & Green, 2006). This is more than twice the number of children who suffer from asthma (Bair-Merritt & Groves, 2014). Young children (ages 6 and younger) are disproportionately represented in this population (Fantuzzo & Mohr, 1999).

THE IMPACT OF DOMESTIC VIOLENCE ON CHILDREN

Hundreds of studies have focused on the consequences of domestic violence for children. These studies indicate that domestic violence may affect children's emotional and cognitive development, their physical health, their social functioning, their ability to learn and function in school, and their ability to negotiate intimate relationships in adolescence and adulthood (Enlow, Egeland, Blood, Wright, & Wright, 2012; Kitzmann, Gaylord, Holt, & Kenny, 2003; Wolfe, Crooks, Lee, McIntyre-Smith, & Jaffe, 2003).

Research on early brain development and the impact of toxic stress underscores the vulnerability of young children to chronic exposure to domestic violence. "Toxic stress" is defined as events that are chronic, long-lasting, severe, and intense, and that occur without access to the buffering relationship of a parent or caregiver (National Scientific Council on the Developing Child, 2014). Such stress affects the structure of the developing brain and the stress response system, establishing a series of negative outcomes that persist into adulthood (Bair-Merritt, Zuckerman, Augusytn, & Cronhelm, 2014). Children who are exposed to domestic violence are also at greater risk for poor health outcomes in adulthood, including heart disease, cancer, sexually transmitted diseases, substance abuse, and depression (Anda, Block, & Felitti, 2003).

Perhaps the greatest distinguishing feature of domestic violence for young children is that it psychologically robs them of both parents. One parent is the terrifying aggressor; the other is the terrified victim. For young children, who depend exclusively on their parents to protect them, there is no refuge. In a study of children under the age of 4, Scheeringa and Zeanah (1995) found that witnessing domestic violence was a stronger predictor of posttraumatic stress disorder (PTSD) than direct abuse was. Young children's perception of their own safety is closely linked to the perceived safety of their caregivers. They cannot trust that their caregiving environment will reliably protect them, and this increases their psychological vulnerability (Groves, 2002; Osofsky, 1999). Cassie, the young child discussed later in this chapter, provides a vivid example of the confusion, fear, and anxiety that mark many children who live with domestic violence.

Children who grow up with domestic violence learn powerful lessons about the use of intimidation and force in relationships. In violent homes, children learn that aggression is a part of intimate relationships, or that it is acceptable to relieve stress by yelling at or threatening another family member.

These lessons do not work well for children in other social contexts; they may misinterpret other children's behavior or behave in distrustful and aggressive ways. Studies document the strong association between exposure to interparental violence in early childhood and dating-violence perpetration and victimization in early adulthood, with early exposure directly predicting dating-violence perpetration in adolescence (Narayan, Englund, Carlson, & Egeland, 2014). Although research enumerates many adverse effects of domestic violence on children, several variables may mediate the intensity and severity of a child's response. These variables include the chronicity and severity of the domestic violence; the proximity of the child to the violence; and the existence of other risk factors in the child's and family's lives, such as substance abuse, poverty, and mental illness (Pynoos & Eth, 1985). Children are affected in different ways, and not all children are equally affected. Protective factors may include the child's temperament, his or her achievement in school, parental attunement, and the child's relationship with other caring adults. Studies on resilience in children exposed to domestic violence point to several key variables that enhance resilience: easy temperament in the child, the amount of violence witnessed, parenting effectiveness and responsiveness, family cohesion, and the absence of depression or traumatic stress in the mother (Graham-Bermann, Gruber, Howell & Ginz, 2009; Howell, 2011).

These findings highlight the importance of effective parenting and maternal mental health, and suggest avenues for a comprehensive approach to working with vulnerable children. Services for children affected by domestic violence should offer a range of supports that include parenting education/support and assessment/intervention for parental mental health issues.

CLINICAL FINDINGS ON CHILDREN EXPOSED TO DOMESTIC VIOLENCE

The Child Witness to Violence Project at Boston Medical Center, a clinical mental health intervention program for children ages 8 and younger who have been exposed to violence, was founded in direct response to the high prevalence of young children exposed to violence in Boston (Taylor, Harik, Zuckerman, & Groves, 1994). The majority of children referred to the program have been exposed to domestic violence.

An in-house retrospective analysis of clinical data from 149 children under the age of 7 seen in the Child Witness to Violence Project gives an interesting profile of young children whose parents decide to seek help for exposure to domestic violence. The majority (73%) of referred children were boys. Nearly two-thirds of the children had been exposed to violence chronically since birth, according to parental reports. The most common symptoms mentioned by parents were increased aggression, impulsivity, temper tantrums, sleep dysregulation, and separation anxiety. In addition, parents mentioned preoccupation with the violent events, as seen in play, verbalizations, and avoidance/withdrawal.

In our clinical work with young children, we have learned about the importance of understanding the violence from a child's perspective. Children make unique meanings out of events in their lives; these meanings are in part based on age, developmental stage, and prior life experiences. Furthermore, children's understandings of events may differ significantly from the adults' appraisals of the same events. Understanding the child's subjective experiences of trauma, assisting them with distortions they may have, and helping the caregiving adults better understand the children's perspective are essential components of successful therapeutic interventions.

The Child Witness to Violence Project uses an evidence-based intervention model: child–parent psychotherapy (CPP), developed by Alicia Lieberman and Patricia Van Horn (Lieberman & Van Horn, 2005; Lieberman, Van Horn, & Ippen, 2005) at the Child Trauma Research Project at San Francisco General Hospital. This intervention has demonstrated its effectiveness in reducing symptoms and improving functioning of both children and their mothers who are involved with the treatment. This intervention has been recognized as an effective and evidence-based intervention by the National Child Traumatic Stress Network and is being disseminated to sites across the country.

CPP recognizes the centrality of the child's relationship with a parent in the early years; it targets the parent–child relationship, rather than the individual child. CPP builds on the premise that the attachment system is the main organizer of a child's response to safety and danger in early childhood, and that emotional or behavioral problems can best be addressed within the context of the attachment relationship. The intervention seeks to strengthen the parent–child relationship, recognizing that this relationship is the most important protection a child can have.

CPP focuses on the development of both the parent and the child. Infants, toddlers, preschoolers, and school-age children are in a rapidly developing process of growth and learning. The impact of trauma on their lives will be dependent on their ages and developmental stages. CPP allows developmental issues to guide the treatment. This model enables parents and children to increase their understanding of the other's perspective and to build stronger mutual relationships.

PRINCIPLES OF INTERVENTION WITH CHILDREN AFFECTED BY DOMESTIC VIOLENCE

The Child Witness to Violence Project treats children and mothers affected by domestic violence in flexible combinations of parent–child meetings and meetings with a parent alone. The specific arrangement of sessions may depend on the age of the child, the presentation of the mother, and the topics to be discussed.

The initial phase of the assessment includes an evaluation of each family's safety and immediate needs. In this phase, families may need referrals for legal assistance, housing, or other concrete services. This case management and advocacy constitute an essential component of the intervention. If family members are not safe, or if the violence is ongoing, trauma-focused work cannot begin. Once these issues have been dealt with, the assessment focuses on the child's symptoms that are interfering with daily functioning, the parent's concerns about the child, the child's experience with the violent event, the child's understanding of these events, the parent's emotional strengths and vulnerabilities, and the child's strengths.

The goals of treatment include relieving symptoms that interfere with functioning; increasing the parent's and child's skills at recognizing and regulating affective states; creating a trauma narrative and shared understanding of the meaning of the trauma; increasing the child's and parent's ability to understand each other's perspectives; and strengthening the child–parent relationship.

The following case example, which was formulated from a composite of several families with whom we worked, illustrates efforts to translate those principles and issues into therapeutic practice.

THE CASE OF CASSIE, AGE 4 YEARS, 2 MONTHS

Cassie, age 4 years and 2 months, was referred by an advocate for battered women from a nearby health center, where her mother, Carolina, had sought help for the increasing tension, violence, and fear in the household. Six months earlier, Cassie's father, Michael, had been arrested for assaulting Carolina. Carolina sought a restraining order, barring Michael from coming to the home or having contact with Cassie.

Presenting Problem

Carolina reported that Cassie had not been the same since the assault and arrest. For 2 months after these incidents, Cassie was afraid to move about the apartment independently. She also became very bossy and aggressive, and had trouble leaving her mother. Carolina described that Cassie was most aggressive when limits were set on her behavior or when she was told "no." In addition, Cassie continued to have separation problems, difficulty with transitions, and hypervigilance. She had a recurrent nightmare from which she woke up yelling, "Stop it!", and then begged her mother to let her sleep in Carolina's bed.

Family Information

Carolina, age 30, had emigrated with her family from a Central American country when she was an infant. Her father, whom she described as a domineering man, could be violent and aggressive and would not allow her to engage in social activities without a chaperone or to date until she was 25.

At 23, Carolina met Michael and secretly began to date him, but her father learned of it and prohibited her from seeing him again. He threatened to ban her from his home if she continued to see him, proclaiming that such conduct would dishonor him and be a disgrace to their religion. Nevertheless, Carolina continued to date Michael, and she was indeed subsequently banned from the home. The couple eloped and had no further contact with Carolina's family.

Two years later, just as Carolina became pregnant with Cassandra, Michael was laid off from his job as a mortgage broker. His income from unemployment hardly met the family's needs, even with Carolina's salary from her work as a bank teller. Humiliated by not being able to provide for his family, Michael became increasingly controlling, irritable, and angry. Carolina's pregnancy was stressful, and she constantly worried about her safety and that of her unborn daughter. At birth, Cassie was reported to be healthy, alert, and robust.

Carolina stayed at home until Cassie was 3 months old and then enrolled her in a day care center, which she was continuing to attend and enjoy. She was very attached to her caregivers there, and by Carolina's report, they "love her to pieces." However, by the time Cassie was 3½ years old, Michael's abuse of Carolina had escalated to slapping, pushing, and choking. On one occasion, Michael tripped over Cassie's favorite stuffed bear, Teddy, and threw it against the wall, causing it to burst so that the stuffing spilled all over the floor. When Cassie began to cry, Michael demanded that she stop crying, declaring that it was all her mother's fault because she was a bad mother who didn't know how to keep their house neat. Cassie ran to her room. Michael then hit Carolina across the mouth, causing substantial bleeding. One of their neighbors became concerned when she heard Michael assaulting Carolina and called the police. Cassie heard the commotion, came running out of her room, and hid behind her mother, yelling, "Daddy, stop it!" The police arrested Michael. As they escorted him out of the house, Cassie cried, "Don't go, Daddy! Daddy won't do it again." Cassie then brought her mother a tissue and put it on her wound. Later, Cassie begged her mother to fix Teddy. Carolina sewed the stuffed bear back together, but the mend left a large ridge, which Carolina described as resembling a large scar. She said that Cassie continued to talk about this incident and regularly declared, "Daddy hurt Teddy."

Currently, Carolina worked in a bank, and Cassie continued to attend her day care program; as described above, Cassie was reported to be doing well there.

Parent Interview: First Session

Given that young children's development occurs in relationship to their caregivers, it is critical to work with a child in the context of the family. In fact, caregivers are often the central therapeutic agents for change in children. However, when caregivers are themselves traumatized as a result of domestic violence (as Carolina was), it is not uncommon for them to have difficulty being fully emotionally available, sensitive, and responsive to their children. Therefore, when a clinician is interviewing a battered mother, it is important to consider the mother's symptoms, her ability to maintain an empathic relationship with her child (which may have been ruptured as a result of the trauma), her skill in recognizing danger or stress, and her capacity to support the child. This sort of assessment requires that the clinician be familiar with the effects of violence on children and their parents, and for the clinician to be highly responsive to the mother from the very first contact.

Carolina presented as a somewhat anxious and depressed woman, with symptoms of hyperarousal and feelings of helplessness and hopelessness about her life and Cassie's. Her helplessness was intensified by profound feelings of guilt about her perceived failure to protect her child; she kept saying, "I failed Cassie, just as my own parents failed me." Carolina stated that her estrangement from her parents was a source of emotional pain, and that she had expected more from Michael. She said that it was common in her religion and culture for women to be subservient. Although she rejected that idea, nonetheless she worried that she was as passive and submissive a parent as her own mother. She feared that as a result, Cassie might be damaged forever. She felt ashamed and guilty that she had stayed with Michael for as long as she had, and she doubted her skills as a parent to help Cassie grow up to be a good and kind person. I (Maxine L. Weinreb, the clinician in this case and the "I" in what follows) acknowledged and validated Carolina's feelings, and added that such feelings are commonly held when there have been traumatic experiences like those that Carolina and Cassie had endured.

As Carolina told more of the story, she began to sob and said softly that she did not want to think about the violence she had endured and to which Cassie had been exposed. I remarked that it was understandable and natural that she would want to forget such an ordeal. I then asked whether it was OK to ask her about what happened when she did think about it. Carolina replied, "I feel very sad and fall apart, just like now. I can never handle any relationship well, including with my parents, my husband, and my daughter." When I asked more about her relationship with Cassie, Carolina expressed pride in her child, saying that when she wasn't "bossing me around," she was adorable, smart, outgoing, and affectionate. Her facial expression changed as she talked about her daughter's strengths, and it was clear that she felt a strong bond with her daughter. She added that Cassie was doing well in day care, had a great relationship with her teachers, and had friends at school. Carolina reported that she never hit Cassie, but that when Cassie was aggressive and bossy (which she felt that Cassie had learned from her father), she yelled back and said "mean" things to Cassie, about which she was often sorry.

I offered information about the effects of trauma on children, and explained that young children's behavior often tells us about the feelings and challenges in their lives. I stressed that it is not uncommon for children's behavior to change when they have witnessed scary events such as those to which Cassie was exposed, and I reassured her that her thoughtful decision to seek therapy for Cassie was a significant way to help her. As I provided emotional support and validation, Carolina abruptly stopped crying and whispered that this was one of the few times that someone had understood her. I commented that she deserved to be heard and understood, and asked whether she had considered getting help just for herself.

Parent Interview: Second Session

During the second session, I shared information about CPP and its emphasis on working with the parent and the child together. I also talked about our use of play as part of the therapy, explaining that it is through their play that children learn and express their feelings. Carolina was somewhat skeptical that playing would help Cassie "get better," but agreed to give it a try. I asked Carolina about the kinds of activities that she and Cassie enjoyed doing together. She said that as a child she had always loved playing with dolls, and that she used to enjoy doing that with Cassie. She noted that they didn't engage in such play very often anymore because Cassie usually became domineering and rude, which angered and frightened Carolina. She added that in her family of origin she was never allowed to be disrespectful to her parents, and she had tried to maintain that rule with her daughter. However, no matter what she did, Cassie continued to be rude. I said I understood that she was trying to raise Cassie to be a good person, as any caring and loving parent would. I asked her why she thought Cassie talked to her rudely, and she said she believed Cassie had learned it from her father.

At the end of the session, I asked Carolina whether she had talked to Cassie about the violence to which she had been exposed. She said she had not mentioned it because she hoped that if she didn't bring it up, Cassie would forget about it. She added that Cassie was probably "too young to understand, anyhow." Carolina then commented that she was probably kidding herself and quietly asked if I thought she should talk to her about it. I said that not only can it be very difficult for a parent to talk about such horrifying events with a child, but when caregivers have experienced trauma, it can bring out strong reactions and reminders for them. I asked Carolina how her family had dealt with difficult family issues when she was growing up. She replied that no one ever talked about them. I wondered whether one reason it might be hard for Carolina to talk about what had happened was that this was not the style in which she was raised. I said that it is helpful to children to talk about the violence because the absence of an explanation can give rise to confusion about the cause of the violence, including the children's feeling that they themselves are responsible for it. I explained that part of our work together would be to help Cassie talk and play about her experiences. We ended by talking about how to explain to Cassie why they were coming to see me. I reassured Carolina that therapy was an important way to help Cassie, and that I expected—as was the case with other children exposed to domestic violence—that with help she would develop well.

Dyadic Therapy: First Session

Cassie came into the playroom with her mother and stayed close by her side. She looked longingly at the toys. Carolina suggested that Cassie play with them, but she remained close to her mother. I wondered aloud whether Cassie understood that her mommy would be staying with her. Once Carolina reassured her that she would remain in the room, Cassie immediately went to the toys. Initially she explored them in a disorganized fashion, moving quickly from toy to toy. Although the room was relatively quiet, she became preoccupied with noises from outside the office. When I opened the door and showed her that what she was hearing was a man emptying the trash, she seemed to be relieved. Cassie spent some time focusing on the infant toys, but eventually began to use toys such as baby dolls, human figures, the doctor kit, and play food. At one point, Cassie engaged in pretend play with her mother and me, stating that she was the "mother" and her mother and I were the "kids." She went on to "cook" the toy food for us as her children, often reprimanding us for being "bad."

When I asked Cassie whether she knew why she and her mother came to talk to me, she vehemently replied "no." Carolina looked at me and blurted out that even though we had talked about it, she couldn't get out the words to tell Cassie why they were coming. I inquired if she would like to try it or if she needed my help. She asked that I do it, and I agreed, asking that she correct me or add anything that should be said. I said to Cassie, "Your mommy and I talked, and she told me that some scary things happened with your daddy. She thinks you are pretty mad and scared, and she wants to help you feel better." At that point, Cassie picked up the baby doll and began to lightly hit her mother's leg with it. Carolina looked at her lap and began to cry. I asked Carolina if we could take a look at what had just happened, and asked her how she understood it. Carolina shook her head in bewilderment, and Cassie brought her a tissue. I commented, "Mommy seems to really need it [the tissue] because she seems very sad." I commented that Cassie seemed to have some big feelings too. Cassie jumped on Carolina's lap. Carolina reciprocated and stroked her hair.

Cassie returned to playing with the dolls, explaining that the babies were at day care and that she was their teacher. Shortly before she left, she noticed a book on the shelf and asked her mother what it said. She replied that the book was called *There's a Nightmare in My Closet* (Mayer, 1968). Cassie seemed to freeze, and her mother did not seem to know how to respond. I said, "You know what, Cassie and Carolina? This is a book about a child who learned how to keep a nightmare from scaring her. "Cassie asked her mother to read it, and they both giggled when the child scolded the nightmare. When it was time to go, Carrie asked her mother to read it again, but her mother said it was time to go. Cassie began to have a tantrum; she hit her mother and screamed. Carolina reprimanded her. I commented that both of them were upset, and asked Carolina if she needed my help. She responded angrily that it was Cassie who needed my help. I asked Carolina whether she minded if I talked with Cassie, and I then said to Cassie, "Cassie, please listen. You cannot hit your mommy, and you have to listen to her. You were having so much fun with Mommy, and you wanted to stay and read the book again, but it is time to go. Even though it makes you sad and mad about going, it is never OK to hit Mommy. And sometimes when that happens, Mommy gets sad and mad too, and says thing that make you both feel bad. Is that right, Carolina?" Carolina nodded. Cassie stopped hitting and became silent. The fact that she recovered so quickly suggested that helping Cassie and Carolina pay attention to what they were feeling and giving names to their feelings would help them avoid their mutual emotional dysregulation. The following interaction than occurred:

CAROLINA: Yes. I am sorry I yelled, but you have to listen.

CASSIE: I want to read the book. I want to. I want to.

CAROLINA: I know, but we have to go. Maybe we can read it next time.

CASSIE: Promise?

CAROLINA: Yes, baby. I'm sorry.

Carolina kissed Carrie, and they left.

Dyadic Therapy: Second Session

Cassie ran excitedly into the playroom and headed for the baby dolls. She asked excitedly, "Are all these babies for me?" When I commented that it was kind of hard for her to believe that it was all for her to play with, she smiled broadly and yelped, "Hooray!" She then "invited" her mother and me to play, and gave us very explicit directions involving dressing the dolls and combing their hair. When Carolina attempted to help Cassie tie a bow on a doll's clothing, she protested loudly, stating that she wanted to do it herself.

As the session progressed, Cassie eagerly played with the toy food and included her mother in the play. As in the previous session, she became the mother feeding the children, and Carolina played the part of the daughter. At one point, Cassie asked Carolina to play the part of the mommy. Carolina became quite animated and "made" an elaborate and delicious meal for Cassie. Cassie proved to be engaging and friendly, and they both seemed to derive gratification from the interaction. I commented that her mommy sure knew how to feed the babies.

Cassie then explained to the babies that they were at day care and that she was their teacher. She elaborated further that she was taking care of them because she did not know when their mothers were returning. She also said, "They don't know what happened to their daddy because he went away." When I said that I wondered if the babies were a little scared and worried, she agreed that they were and said that they were also mad. She then abruptly said, "Let's play food now. I'm going to cook supper now." Carolina sat quietly as she observed this play.

After the "supper" was cooked, Cassie said, "Mommy, you have to read me the nightmare book. You promised." Carolina agreed, reminding her that then they would have to leave. As they read the book together, once again they both giggled with delight at the point in the story when the child scolds the nightmare. Watching their shared enjoyment, I could see that the joy of their joint experience was as therapeutic in itself as was Carolina's attunement to Carrie's need to manage her nightmares.

Preliminary Assessment and Treatment Goals

Cassie presented as a bright and feisty child who was able to play spontaneously and to use that play to make meaning of her experience. She was doing well in many spheres of her life, but could become quite dysregulated when she felt emotionally or physically unsafe in the environment. She was able to re-regulate her emotions fairly quickly with empathy and support, and could sustain task involvement, but remained hypervigilant to potential sources of danger.

There were recurrent themes in Cassie's play about small children who needed protection. Possibly Cassie identified with these vulnerable figures and wished that adults would take care of her. However, when she reversed the roles in her play and chose to be the adult and represented her mother as the child, this suggested that she felt a need to be in control and to fend for herself where nurturance issues were concerned. She also wanted to protect her mother.

Initially, Cassie demonstrated mild separation anxiety. When reassured, she settled in, and her play became more orderly and precise. She expressed confusion about the separation in her family, particularly in regard to her father. Separation distress is often an expression of a child's fear of losing the parents. Cassie's aggression might be her way to protect herself from feeling vulnerable, anxious, and fearful. The strong feelings she experienced, which her mother could not currently help her modulate, were another source of anxiety. It would be important to restore Cassie's trust that her mother could protect her, and to reestablish her mother as a safe authority figure. Until Carolina's authority could be restored, it was likely that Cassie's emotional stability would continue to be at risk.

Feedback Session with Carolina

The purpose of the feedback session was to share observations and ideas about what might be helpful to Cassie, and to discuss the treatment plan with Carolina. I asked Carolina what she had learned about herself and Cassie. She said that she was experiencing a mixture of intense sadness, dismay, and humiliation that Cassie had been so aware of so much. I replied that Cassie might need her to help make sense of her own experience so she could feel calmer. I hoped that giving a different explanation for Cassie's play would alleviate some of Carolina's fear that Cassie would grow up to be "mean" and violent like her father. I also wondered out loud with Carolina whether she had been sad for a long time, and whether that made it harder to parent Cassie.

I commented that Cassie was pretty feisty, and noted that if that trait could be rechanneled, she would never have to worry that Cassie would become a subservient woman. We shared a laugh together, and it was the first time I had seen her so animated, other than when she read to Cassie. I wondered whether Cassie acted like the" boss" because she was scared and worried that the violence might happen again. I said that what Cassie really wanted was for Carolina to take back the role of boss—albeit a nice boss. We agreed (laughingly, again) that this would be a challenge. I was struck that the sad and anxious woman I had seen in previous sessions was quite a warm person who could demonstrate humor I had not seen before.

At the end of the session, Carolina said that since they had been reading *There's a Nightmare in My Closet*, Cassie had been having fewer nightmares. She had purchased a copy of the book and planned to surprise Cassie with it that evening at bedtime. I commented about how supportive Carolina was to Cassie in the face of her own difficulties, and she revealed that she had recently found a therapist who was helping her feel stronger.

Treatment Goals

I formulated the following list of treatment goals:

- Continue to form an alliance with Carolina and Cassie.
- Relieve Cassie's symptoms.
- Help Carolina understand the meaning of Cassie's behavior.
- Increase Carolina's self-esteem and confidence as a parent.
- Strengthen the parent/child relationship.
- Restore Carolina's role as protector.
- Help Carolina and Cassie increase their ability to talk about the trauma.

Dyadic Therapy: Third Session

Cassie bounced in with a stuffed bear in her arms and put it in my face.

Content of Session	*Rationale/Analysis*
THERAPIST: Oh, this must be Teddy. Mommy told me about him. Hi, Teddy!	I want her to know that I know what happened with Teddy, but I don't know how much or exactly what to say.
CARRIE: (*Sadly*) Look at his boo-boo!	Part of me wants to eliminate her pain (and mine) and point out that

	he is fixed now. That will come later. Right now, I need to bear witness.
THERAPIST: You want me to see that he got hurt right there.	Carolina's description that the ridge looks like a scar is highly accurate. What a traumatic reminder this must be for both of them.
CARRIE: Right there. (*Runs her finger across it.*)	It *is* a traumatic reminder.
THERAPIST: Yes. Right here. May I touch it?	I want to let Cassie and Carolina know that I can tolerate this, but Carolina seems to shudder a bit as I do so. Did I go too far, too fast?
THERAPIST: I wonder if this reminds you of the time when Mommy and Daddy were fighting.	I must acknowledge this. Is Teddy a metaphor for their shared trauma?
CARRIE: (*Puts Teddy on the floor.*) Time to read the nightmare story.	Carrie is getting anxious and uses avoidance to manage it.
THERAPIST: You are telling Mommy and me that you are done with Teddy right now. I wonder if we should put him on the shelf, so he is safe and nothing will happen to him.	I want to gently acknowledge her avoidance, and to give the message that it is safe to talk about Teddy and what he represents.
CASSIE: Yes!	
CAROLINA: That's a good idea. I'll get a blanket to keep him warm. (*Gets a doll blanket.*)	Carolina has also had enough, but is still able to soothe Carrie.
THERAPIST: Looks like Mommy is doing everything she can to make sure that Teddy is safe and warm.	I want to support and highlight Carolina's nurturing and protective actions.

Shortly after, Cassie asked for Teddy. She pointed to the ridge and said, "Daddy hurt Teddy, and then he hurt Mommy. He scared me." When I asked whether she might want to draw a picture about what she was telling me, she drew a picture of her mother, her father, and her standing in a line. She said about it sadly, "I miss Daddy." This sort of ambivalent feeling about a perpetrating parent is common among children exposed to intimate-partner violence. However, since children at Cassie's developmental level find it cognitively difficult to integrate two conflicting feelings at one time, I felt it especially important to clarify and reflect those feelings. It also gave me an opportunity to explain my role in a context that was concrete:

THERAPIST: Sometimes you feel afraid of Daddy. Sometimes you miss seeing him. Sometimes you feel both things all together.

CASSIE: Yes. Teddy, too.

THERAPIST: I bet that can be confusing. It can make kids worry, too. Lots of children who come here have worries like that, and it is my job and Mommy's to help with those worries. We can all talk or play about worries if you decide you want to.

CASSIE: Oh. [She falls silent and does not elaborate further. I understand this as her way of managing very strong feelings and do not pursue it.]

Shortly after that dialogue, Cassie shifted her play to day care and the babies. She said to them, "Don't worry. Mommy will be back soon." It appeared that she was starting to see her mother as a protective parent.

Dyadic Therapy: Middle Sessions

Cassie continued to bring Teddy to every session and to talk about her father's hurting Teddy. With support, Carolina was able to explain to Cassie that because Michael had hurt his family, he wasn't allowed to come home any more. During every session, Cassie also asked her mother to read *There's a Nightmare in My Closet* to her. This pattern continued for several weeks, and I recognized this repetitive play and reading as common reactions in a child exposed to violence and other trauma: The experience is relived in order to make sense of it. As the weeks went by, Cassie began using the play to express both her external and internal feelings and to clarify her role in relationship to her mother. I was able to use their joint play as a way to address the themes of attachment, nurturance (the food metaphor), and protection in the dyad. Carolina and Cassie continued to play together and to get enjoyment from one another.

Carolina reported that the individual therapist she was seeing had recommended antianxiety medication. She found both the sessions with this therapist and the medication to be helpful, saying that she now had more patience with Cassie. She also reported that Cassie also seemed calmer and was sleeping better.

Dyadic Therapy: Final Sessions

Near the end of the fifth month of treatment, Cassie came to the session obviously distressed and preoccupied. She snuggled up next to her mother, holding Teddy tightly. I remembered that the 1-year anniversary of her father's arrest for assaulting her mother fell during this month.

Content of Session	*Rationale/Analysis*
THERAPIST: You seem worried today.	I am attempting to identify feelings and affect.
CASSIE: (*Finds a police figure.*) No. Well—a little. I am a policeman, and I am going to arrest the bad little girl. Her father was hitting. She was sad for a whole day. She didn't go to school. She had a giant time out. She cried.	
THERAPIST: The little girl is going to be punished because she did something bad? Can you tell Mommy and me more about it?	
CASSIE: She *is* bad. (*Begins to touch Teddy's "boo-boo."*) Her daddy hit her mommy.	Now I have it! I had previously understood that play with Teddy was Cassie's way of processing her parents' violent separation. With Cassie in the role of aggressor, I suddenly understand that there are multiple meanings, thoughts, and feelings associated with Teddy.
THERAPIST: Carolina, I wonder if Cassie is worried that she made her daddy hit her mommy.	When young children are exposed to intimate-partner violence, it is common for them to feel responsible.
CAROLINA: (*Horrified and stunned*) Cassie, you think it is your fault that Daddy hit me?	
CASSIE: (*Suddenly sobbing*) Yes. It is. I cried because he hurt Teddy. He hit you. I am bad. I made him hit you because I cried about Teddy.	The trauma that Cassie experienced and her developmental understanding of events has likely disrupted her view about safety.
THERAPIST: Maybe we need to hear from Mommy about this. What do you think?	Cassie needs direct reassurance from her primary attachment figure—her mother. Can Carolina do it? I am acutely aware that I am taking the chance that Carolina may not be emotionally available at this time. I am somewhat anxious

about whether this suggestion may backfire and be more upsetting to Cassie. I need to address both Carolina's state of mind and Cassie's developmental needs.

CASSIE: (*Whimpering*) Mommy, are you going to tell me and Teddy not to live in our house anymore?

CAROLINA: (*Visibly upset, starts to shake.*) What, Cassie? Did your father tell you that? What did he tell you (*angrily*)?

I think Carolina's strong reaction to Cassie's question is related to her own fears and anxieties about Michael.

THERAPIST: Cassie, I think your mommy is feeling very worried and mad about your daddy. She might be remembering when he did scary things to her and you. Carolina, I know you are worried, but that isn't quite what Cassie wants to tell you. Cassie thinks it is her fault that Michael hurt you because she was crying after he hurt Teddy, and Michael had told her not to cry.

I feel it is important to help mother and daughter understand each other's behavior and perspective, and to support and label the affective experiences of both members of the dyad.

CAROLINA: (*To Cassie, crying*) Oh, baby, it wasn't your fault. It is never all right to hit anyone. Your father is a grown man and should know that rule. It is his fault. I don't like it when you are rude, but I love you. You are a wonderful, smart little girl, and you are not bad.

I know this isn't easy for Carolina, and I am touched by her resolve to talk about what is likely to be very difficult material.

CASSIE: (*Runs to her mother and snuggles in her arms.*)

After witnessing this warm encounter, I feel that some trust has been restored.

THERAPIST: When bad things happen, everyone gets confused and scared. It is good to talk about it and figure it out together.

I attempt to provide information about the effects of exposure to violence. I also hope they both get the message that talking about their shared experience can help them make meaning of it.

Final Sessions

Cassie was seen in treatment for a total of 8 months. Throughout the process, I was alert to further disruptions in the parent–child attachment, the cognitive distortions in Cassie's understanding of the events, and the need to tell all or part of the trauma story several times. The bond between Cassie and Carolina continued to strengthen, and Cassie found it easier to separate from her at school and to sleep through the night. Cassie did remain somewhat hypervigilant to loud noises, but with her mother's help, she was able to label them as "surprise noises" that couldn't hurt her. Although Cassie still needed to take the role of the protector in her play, she became much less controlling and less punitive toward her mother, showed physical affection, and usually allowed her mother to take care of her and even be "the boss"—sometimes.

CONCLUDING COMMENTS

Cassie's presentation was similar to that of many children exposed to violence: She experienced symptoms of sleep dysregulation, had difficulty with transitions, demonstrated some mildly aggressive and controlling behavior, and was troubled by separation anxiety. She had ambivalent feelings about her father and was unsure that the world was safe or that adults could be reliable protectors. Cassie eventually became able to express her feelings and worries; her symptoms decreased; and she was able to recover a sense of mastery (i.e., her separation issues decreased to ones that were age-appropriate) and make meaning of her experiences through play.

Carolina's participation was a critical factor in Cassie's recovery from the trauma of exposure to violence. As she began her own recovery, she was able to provide more adaptive, calm, and nurturing interchanges with Cassie. She was also able to help Cassie talk about what had happened—an essential step in facilitating Cassie's mastery of the traumatic events. As Cassie played out her fears and fantasies related to the violence she had witnessed, made meaning of the events in her life, and came to see her mother as a strong protector, her emotional regulation began to stabilize. She was also able to integrate her feelings about her father and subsequently focus on the appropriate developmental tasks of childhood, including feeling less anxiety about separation, developing more confidence in navigating the world, and controlling her aggression. On the other hand, as Cassie grew older and her developmental understanding of the traumatic events in her life changed, it was possible that she would need to come back to revisit her feelings about the events.

A therapist's abilities to be intentional about each step of the therapeutic process and to be self-reflective about the therapeutic encounters are essential aspects of the treatment process in cases like Cassie's. Even the most experienced clinicians find it difficult to acknowledge that very young children are subjected to such frightening and even life-threatening experiences. There are times when children's and/or family members' stories are difficult to hear and evoke feelings of sadness, anger, or helplessness in therapists. At the Child Witness to Violence Project, there is an "open-door" policy among the staff, so that there is usually another staff member available to talk with after a difficult session. This helps the clinicians reflect on intense feelings, explore countertransference, and/or prevent vicarious traumatization. Certainly it was this support that helped me deal with the strong feelings elicited by this darling little girl, Cassie, and her heroic mother, Carolina. As discussed more fully by Maschi in Chapter 20 of this book, we recommend strongly that this kind of peer support be available to all clinicians who work with traumatized children and their families.

STUDY QUESTIONS

1. Discuss the effects of exposure to violence in the preschool years on a child's future functioning.
2. How would you expect Cassie to understand her experiences with violence and loss, given her developmental level?
3. The therapist notes that parental involvement is critical in work with young children. What are the advantages and challenges of bringing a parent into the session?
4. There are varied opinions about whether it is essential in treatment to have the child retell or reenact the trauma. Discuss whether or not this is a necessary treatment goal.
5. Discuss the role of culture in this case and the issues surrounding it that the therapist might have explored. How would learning more about the cultural outlook and traditions of this family have helped the therapist learn more about the family's child-rearing values and practice? How does the culture of the therapist affect the relationship?

REFERENCES

Anda, R., Block, R., & Felitti, V. (2003). *Adverse Childhood Experiences Study*. Centers for Disease Control and Prevention, Kaiser Permanente's Health Appraisal Clinic in San Diego. Retrieved from *www.cdc.gov/NCCDPHP/ACE/index.htm*

Bair-Merritt, M., & Groves, B. M. (2014, January 28). *Screening and intervention for IPV in pediatric settings*. Paper presented at the 2014 International Conference on Child and Family Maltreatment, San Diego, CA.

Bair-Merritt, M., Zuckerman, B., Augustyn, M., & Cronhelm, P. (2014). Silent victims: An epidemic of childhood exposure to domestic violence. *New England Journal of Medicine, 369*(18), 1673–1675.

Enlow, M. B., Egeland, B., Blood, E. A., Wright, R. O., & Wright, R. J. (2012). Interpersonal trauma exposure and cognitive development in children 0–8 years: A longitudinal study. *Journal of Epidemiology and Community Health. 66*(11), 1005–1010.

Fantuzzo, J. W., & Mohr, W. K. (1999). Prevalence and effects of child exposure to domestic violence. *The Future of Children, 9*(3), 21–32.

Graham-Bermann, S. A., Gruber G., Howell, K. H., & Girz, L. (2009). Factors discriminating among profiles of resilience and psychopathology in children exposed to intimate partner violence. *Child Abuse and Neglect, 33*, 648–660.

Groves, B. M. (2002). *Children who see too much.* Boston: Beacon Press.

Groves, B. M., Zuckerman, B., & Marans, S. (1993). Silent victims: Children who witness violence. *Journal of the American Medical Association, 269*(2), 262–265.

Howell, K. (2011). Resilience and psychopathology in children exposed to family violence. *Aggression and Violent Behavior, 16*, 562–569.

Kitzmann, K. M., Gaylord, N. K., Holt, A. R., & Kenny, E. D. (2003). Child witnesses to domestic violence: A meta-analytic review. *Journal of Consulting and Clinical Psychology*, 71, 339–352.

Lieberman, A. F., & Van Horn, P. (2005). *Don't hit my mommy.* Washington, DC: Zero to Three Press.

Lieberman, A. F., Van Horn, P., & Ippen, C. G. (2005). Toward evidence based treatment: Child–parent psychotherapy with preschoolers exposed to marital violence. *Journal of the American Academy of Child and Adolescent Psychiatry, 44*(12), 1241–1247.

Mayer, M. (1968). *There's a nightmare in my closet.* New York: Dial Press.

McDonald, R., Jouriles, E. N., Ramisetty-Mikler, S., Caetano, R., & Green, C. E. (2006). Estimating the number of American children living with partner-violent families. *Journal of Family Psychology, 20*(1), 137–142.

Narayan, A. J., Englund, M. M., Carlson, E. A., & Egeland, B. (2014). Adolescent conflict as a developmental process in the prospective pathway from exposure to interparental violence to dating violence. *Journal of Abnormal Child Psychology*, 42(2), 239–250.

National Scientific Council on the Developing Child. (2014). Excessive stress disrupts the architecture of the developing brain: Working Paper 3 (rev. ed.). Retrieved from *www.developingchild.harvard.edu*

Osofsky, J. D. (1999). The impact of violence on children. *The Future of Children,* 9(3), 33–49.

Pynoos, R. S., & Eth, S. (Eds.). (1985). *Post-traumatic stress disorder in children.* Washington, DC: American Psychiatric Press.

Scheeringa, M. S., & Zeanah, C. H. (1995). Symptom expression and trauma variables in children under 48 months of age. *Infant Mental Health Journal, 16*(4), 259–269.

Taylor, L., Harik, V., Zuckerman, B., & Groves, B. (1994). Exposure to violence among inner city children. *Journal of Developmental and Behavioral Pediatrics, 15*, 120–123.

Walters, M. L., Chen, J., & Breiding, M. J. (2013). *The National Intimate Partner and Sexual Violence Survey (NISVS): 2010 findings on victimization by sexual orientation.* Atlanta, GA: National Center for Injury Prevention and Control, Centers for Disease Control and Prevention.

Wolfe, D. A., Crooks, C. V., Lee, V., McIntyre-Smith, A., & Jaffe, P. (2003). The effects of children's exposure to domestic violence: A meta-analysis and critique. *Clinical Child and Family Psychology Review, 6*(3), 171–187.

Chapter 6

Trauma-Focused Cognitive-Behavioral Therapy for Child Sexual Abuse and Exposure to Domestic Violence

FELICIA NEUBAUER
ESTHER DEBLINGER
KARIN SIEGER

Interpersonal violence experienced in childhood is highly prevalent and has repeatedly been found to be associated with negative psychosocial consequences; multiple exposures increase the risk of adverse effects (Felitti et al., 1998; Teicher, Samson, Polcari, & McGreenery, 2006). Moreover, children who have experienced sexual victimization often endure other types of victimization as well (Finkelhor, Ormrod, Turner, & Hamby, 2005). Although there are indications of recent significant declines in some forms of childhood victimization, including child sexual abuse (CSA) and exposure to domestic violence (DV), it is important to note that overall rates of these childhood traumas remain quite high (Finkelhor& Jones, 2006, 2012).

After briefly reviewing the potential effects of exposure to CSA and DV in childhood, this chapter offers an overview of a treatment approach, trauma-focused cognitive-behavioral therapy (TF-CBT), that has been found to be highly efficacious in helping children overcome the aftereffects of such exposure (Cohen, Mannarino, & Deblinger, 2006). The implementation of TF-CBT is presented in the form of a case study of a 15-year-old girl who experienced both CSA and DV.

Research has repeatedly demonstrated that children exposed to CSA (Bal, Crombez, De Bourdeaudhuij, & Van Oost, 2009; Beitchman, Zucker, Hood, daCosta, & Akman, 1992; Deblinger, McLeer, Atkins, Ralphe, & Foa, 1989; Perez-Fuentes et al., 2013; Trickett, Noll, & Putnam, 2011) and/or DV (Fantuzzo & Mohr, 1999; Graham-Bermann, 2001; Groves, 1999; Rossman,

2001) may experience significant psychosocial difficulties. Moreover, research findings have indicated that different forms of abuse in the home are interrelated, and children of battered women are at risk for other abusive experiences (McCloskey, Figueredo, & Koss, 1995). A child exposed to DV, for example, is 12–14 times more likely to experience sexual abuse at the hands of his or her mother's partner, and 7 times more likely to be sexually abused by a perpetrator outside the home (McCloskey et al., 1995). Fifty-two percent of children and adolescents being evaluated in a sexual abuse clinic reported DV in their homes (Kellogg & Menard, 2003). Indeed, studies have demonstrated that being exposed to both DV and child abuse may have a greater adverse impact on children than exposure to either DV or child abuse alone (Levendosky & Graham-Bermann, 2001; Sternberg et al., 1993).

TRAUMA-FOCUSED COGNITIVE-BEHAVIORAL THERAPY

Given the documented negative effects of trauma in childhood, steps should be taken to provide early, effective interventions to forestall and/or alleviate the possible negative emotional effects of such experiences. TF-CBT has been proven efficacious in over a dozen randomized trials and has been cited in numerous reviews of the literature as having the strongest record of empirical support (Deblinger, Cohen, & Mannarino, 2012; Silverman et al., 2008). TF-CBT incorporates ideas from varied psychological theories, including cognitive-behavioral, humanistic, psychodynamic, family systems, and attachment theories. Though TF-CBT is not a traditional play therapy approach, it is a treatment model that often incorporates play, art, music, and other creative activities for engaging clients in the treatment process. The outcome findings of randomized trials as well as other quasi-experimental studies have documented the benefits of TF-CBT in helping children overcome posttraumatic stress disorder (PTSD), depression, feelings of shame, and other emotional/behavioral difficulties in the aftermath of CSA, exposure to DV, natural disasters, and human-made disasters, as well as traumatic losses (Cohen et al., 2006; Deblinger et al., 2012).

TF-CBT begins with the child and parent participating in separate individual sessions; a portion of therapy time is also devoted to conjoint parent–child work when appropriate over the course of therapy. The TF-CBT model incorporates treatment components that are summarized by the acronym PRACTICE: Psychoeducation and parenting, Relaxation, Affect expression and modulation, Cognitive coping, Trauma narration and processing, *In vivo* exposure, Conjoint sessions, and Enhancing safety and future development. Treatment includes three phases; it begins with stabilization and skill building, then focuses on trauma narration and processing, and ends with skill consolidation and closure. During the first phase, in a gradual fashion, a child and parent are engaged in trauma education and skill-building exercises that incorporate playful and fun activities. The parent is simultaneously supported in learning and practicing effective parenting and communication skills throughout the course of treatment. During the middle phase of treatment, trauma narration helps children directly confront traumatic memories through a variety of reading, writing, and creative methods that ultimately help them to process feelings, thoughts, and sensations. The goal of these sessions is to help children become more comfortable acknowledging and coping with traumatic memories and reminders, so they no longer need to avoid trauma cues. As children's avoidance diminishes, they can often more effectively process the disturbing thoughts and worries that may underlie their difficulties. Parents continue to practice the parenting and coping skills learned while working through and processing their own feelings and thoughts associated with the trauma(s) endured by their children. In the final phase of treatment, after assessment and preparation, conjoint parent–child sessions involve the sharing of the narrative when that has been determined to be of clinical benefit. In addition, the final phase focuses on an overall review and consolidation of skills learned and trauma experiences processed in the context of therapy.

THE CASE OF ASHLEY, AGE 15

This case is a composite of several cases involving adolescents referred to us for treatment in the aftermath of similar traumatic experiences.

Ashley was a 15-year-old girl who resided with her younger sister, Keisha, and their grandmother, Ms. Langley. Ashley and Keisha had been placed with Ms. Langley 2 years ago when their mother began neglecting the children as a result of her substance abuse. Ashley had had inconsistent contact with her mother after that, as well as with her father due to his incarceration. Ashley attended a charter school in the city and generally received passing grades. She was particularly interested in music, singing, art, and dancing. She also enjoyed spending time on social media. Ashley's grandmother, Ms. Langley, was widowed and worked long hours as a home health aide. While in her mother's care, Ashley had witnessed her mother's experiences of DV by several boyfriends, including Keisha's father. Prior to being referred for therapy, Ashley disclosed to her grandmother that she had been sexually abused by Keisha's father when she was 10 years old. Although Ms. Langley hadn't suspected that Ashley had experienced CSA, she knew Ashley had been exposed to this man's abusive behavior toward Ashley's mother. In fact, the disclosure helped Ms. Langley make sense of some of her granddaughter's behaviors when she was younger, such as being relieved when her sister's father wasn't around and engaging in sexualized behaviors that seemed beyond her years. Texts indicated that Ashley was smoking marijuana and that her current boyfriend had been pressuring her for sex. Ms. Langley reported being fearful that if her granddaughter continued to smoke marijuana and did not make better choices, she would end up "on the street and drug-addicted" like her mother. Ms. Langley's attempts to talk to Ashley about these concerns had not gone well. Ashley defended her boyfriend, who, according to the texts, had slapped and pushed her. Ashley told her grandmother that this behavior was "nothing."

After seeing a man who looked like Keisha's father, Ashley began thinking more about the CSA. She subsequently disclosed to her grandmother that when she was 10 years old, Keisha's father had begun to find ways to spend time alone with her. After Ashley's disclosure, Ms. Langley contacted the police, who contacted child protective services (CPS). Following the investigation and substantiation of the CSA allegations, the CPS worker recommended that Ashley receive treatment to address the impact of the CSA, as well as the exposure to DV and drug abuse in her mother's home.

Assessment and Treatment Overview

Before treatment began, an assessment was conducted, including the use of standardized measures to assess Ashley's and Ms. Langley's psychosocial functioning. Ashley reported experiencing posttraumatic stress symptoms, including intrusive thoughts (about the DV and CSA) and avoidant behaviors, as well as nightmares about the CSA. She, however, minimized her own drug use and her boyfriend's abusive behavior. Ashley reported that she would frequently sneak out to be with her boyfriend when she was feeling distressed and/or angry at her grandmother. This often led to instances in which the boyfriend mistreated her or pressured her for sex and encouraged drug use. Ashley stated that if she broke up with her boyfriend, all of the other boys who seemed interested in her would "only pick up where he left off."

Ms. Langley reported depressive symptoms and tended to avoid focusing on the traumas endured by her daughter and granddaughter. She said that Ashley avoided discussions about her life prior to moving in with her grandmother, and barely talked about her mom or about her current boyfriend. Ms. Langley's completion of a child behavior report indicated that Ashley was exhibiting clinically significant internalizing and externalizing behavior problems. Specifically, she would become emotionally dysregulated and lose her temper easily, would blame others for her mistakes, would talk back to authority figures, and at times would isolate herself in her room and cry. Ms. Langley also noted that Ashley was increasingly disrespectful, was not complying with chores and requests, and often seemed agitated and on edge at home.

Ms. Langley agreed to participate in treatment to support her granddaughter's healing, and to learn how to communicate and respond more effectively to Ashley's behavior problems and poor choices. Ms. Langley expressed mixed feelings about how she could talk with Ashley about these issues without becoming very upset. The therapist indicated that these topics would initially be addressed during separate individual sessions, which would be designed to help her cope; later they would consider the potential benefits of conjoint sessions with Ashley. Ashley was unsure about her grandmother's participation in therapy, but acknowledged that she needed help and accepted that this treatment approach was most successful when a caregiver participated.

Treatment Plan

The goals for the initial phase of treatment included continued education and skill building with both Ashley and her grandmother. Ashley received age-appropriate education about DV, CSA, date rape, and substance abuse. In addition, she learned and practiced relaxation, affective expression and modulation skills, and cognitive coping skills. The middle phase of treatment increasingly focused on the traumas Ashley experienced. Though initially uninterested in writing about her traumatic experiences, Ashley became engaged in the trauma narration process when she realized how many musicians describe traumatic life experiences in their lyrics. In addition, the therapist made a point of leaving time at the end of each trauma narrative session to discuss music and/or listen to a song. Ashley received age-appropriate sex education earlier in treatment than usual because of her ongoing sexual relationship with her boyfriend. Assertiveness and personal safety skills were also discussed and practiced with respect to everyday circumstances and dating relationships, as well as potentially threatening or abusive encounters.

Treatment with Ms. Langley focused on similar skill-building and educational goals, including learning about the prevalence of and common reactions to CSA and witnessing DV in childhood. Ms. Langley was encouraged to practice the same coping skills Ashley was learning to help her cope more effectively herself, while also serving as an effective coping role model for her granddaughter. Sessions with Ms. Langley also focused on learning and practicing behavior management skills and enhancing caregiver–child communication, so Ms. Langley could assist and support Ashley, potentially increasing the chance Ashley would seek her grandmother out to avoid making poor choices as well as to process trauma-related memories and reminders.

Initial Phase of Treatment: Stabilization and Skill Building

First Contact with Child and Caregiver

Ms. Langley and Ashley met briefly with the therapist for introductions, an age-appropriate review of the assessment and general treatment plan, and an explanation about confidentiality. The therapist shared that most children and their families successfully complete treatment in approximately 12–16 sessions, and that due to the complex nature of Ashley's traumatic experiences, treatment might be extended beyond 16 sessions, but the therapy could be completed by summer break if they worked hard to attend sessions and follow through on practice assignments at home. Many families appreciate the length-of-treatment discussion, as it gives them a sense of control and optimism about the future.

The therapist then met with Ms. Langley and Ashley individually. The therapist engaged the grandmother by emphasizing her important role in treatment and reviewing any potential concrete or attitudinal barriers to weekly participation. In addition, the results of the standardized assessment measures were reviewed. It was explained that Ashley had elevated levels of behavior problems in some areas, which were not surprising, given what Ashley had witnessed and experienced. The therapist also shared that Ashley had symptoms of depression and posttraumatic stress—very common responses to traumatic events experienced in childhood and adolescence. The therapist also reviewed Ashley's report of PTSD symptoms about which Ms. Langley was unaware, while emphasizing that caregivers are often not aware of some of their children's internal fears and difficulties. The strengths of both Ms. Langley and her granddaughter (e.g., their close relationship, Ashley's ability to maintain passing grades in school) were emphasized as well. The therapist also explained that the measures would be administered again at the end of treatment, to determine whether the problems initially reported had diminished. Ms. Langley's self-report measures were reviewed as well, and her moderate levels of depressive symptoms were acknowledged. Finally, the therapist explained that when an adolescent experiences the sort of trauma Ashley did, it is natural for a loving caregiver to focus on the disturbing symptoms and problem behaviors. Ms. Langley was asked to refocus her attention on her granddaughter's strengths. Together, Ms. Langley and the therapist listed ways in which Ashley was showing strengths and healthy behaviors (maintaining friends, getting passing grades, sometimes cooperating with her grandmother, etc.). Ms. Langley was given a practice assignment to pay attention to all of the behaviors Ashley did fairly well over the next week; to come up with a list of two or three things that Ashley sometimes did well, but that Ms. Langley would like to see more often; and to bring the list to the next session.

Therapeutic engagement was the focus of the initial individual treatment session with Ashley as well. The therapist elicited a spontaneous positive narrative by asking Ashley to describe a recent activity she had enjoyed. This not only seemed to build rapport, but revealed that Ashley had fairly strong expressive skills and particularly enjoyed artwork and music—activities that could be incorporated into treatment. Conversely, Ashley minimally acknowledged why she was referred for treatment, sharing only what she had mentioned during the PTSD assessment. This provided a natural segue for the therapist to provide an age-appropriate explanation of the assessment findings, which helped Ashley understand how the distressing PTSD symptoms she was reporting would be addressed through treatment. During this initial session, Ashley was also taught relaxation skills. She thought it was silly to learn skills such as deep breathing, but she conceded that focused breathing helped her physically relax.

Psychoeducation and Skill-Building Sessions

During this initial phase of treatment, the therapist helped Ms. Langley better understand the impact of trauma on children and determine how Ashley's problem behaviors might have developed. Ms. Langley noted that when Keisha was born and for some years later, Ashley was cooperative and helpful and was a good older sister. However, at some point, Ashley began to act differently, vacillating between ignoring Keisha and exhibiting anger and aggression that was more intense than situations would dictate. The therapist helped Ms. Langley understand that interactions with Keisha likely reminded Ashley of the sexual abuse, and thus created feelings of anger and irritability. Ms. Langley seemed to understand this and reported that Ashley would sometimes belittle her sister the way Keisha's father and other men would talk to their mother. As Ms. Langley began to understand the etiology of some of Ashley's behaviors, she was able to have more patience and compassion for her granddaughter.

Throughout this phase of treatment, the therapist reviewed Ms. Langley's interactions with Ashley and her efforts to apply the coping and parenting skills she was learning. Ms. Langley often seemed eager to complain about Ashley's behavior during the week. The therapist then emphasized that while Ashley's behavior problems would be discussed, the focus would be on *Ms. Langley's* behavior and her responses to both the positive and negative behaviors Ashley exhibited. This was important because parenting behavior changes would be the most direct route to producing change in Ashley's acting-out behaviors. Ms. Langley was therefore encouraged to share instances in which Ashley exhibited positive behaviors, and to describe how she herself responded to those behaviors. Upon discussion, Ms. Langley noted that she didn't attend to the positive behaviors as much as the negative ones, and she agreed to focus more attention on Ashley's helpful behaviors. Ms. Langley was given guidance on using praise effectively, being specific, avoiding "negative tags," and staying purely positive when offering praise. Ms. Langley was asked to praise Ashley every time she demonstrated cooperative or helpful behavior at home over the next week. To help Ms. Langley understand her granddaughter's traumas, she was given two information sheets about CSA and DV, which emphasized their impact on children. Although the basic facts were reviewed in session with Ms. Langley, she was asked to read both handouts in full and to bring any questions she had to the next session. The relaxation skills Ashley was learning were reviewed and practiced with Ms. Langley also.

Psychoeducation and skill building constituted the focus of the initial sessions with Ashley as well. Throughout this phase, the therapist engaged Ashley in discussions about CSA and DV in the abstract, using game formats. Coping skills activities were also introduced, via playful exercises that required Ashley to participate actively in role plays and dramatic scenes during which she would employ the newly learned coping skills.

Content of Session	*Rationale/Analysis*
THERAPIST: Now I'd like to have you tell me some of the current ways you relax and calm yourself down.	Let's see what her baseline is. I want to find out what strengths and skills she already possesses to help herself.
ASHLEY: I listen to music and I dance. Sometimes I journal in my book. But the negative thoughts are still there sometimes and really bother me.	
THERAPIST: OK, so listening to music sometimes helps you. That's great. I want to give you a couple of metaphors to think about your feelings when the negative thoughts come in your mind. If your radio or iPod is turned up too high for your comfort, what do you do?	Let's see how she does with the metaphors—to see if she can relate to the idea that emotions can feel very intense but they don't stay very intense, and she can learn to feel more in control of her strong emotions.
ASHLEY: Turn it down.	
THERAPIST: Yes. And have you ever been to the beach and been knocked down by a wave? If so, what do you do?	
ASHLEY: Yes, and I get back up.	
THERAPIST: OK, so managing emotions is like that. I can teach you skills so that you learn to turn the volume down to make your emotions less intense. You can think about the wave, too. If an intense emotion feels like it's going to knock you down, it will subside, just like the ocean. If lots of stressful things occur quickly together, that can make the intensity build higher too. Does that ever happen to you?	She seems genuinely interested and is answering spontaneously, so I think it will be useful to monitor what skills work and when. Then we can target the situations that are most difficult. I have to remember to focus on strengths and praise those, not just focusing on any difficulty in doing this because it may take practice for her. And I have to remember to tell her later that she may have negative thoughts later on in life when she is highly stressed, and she can use these skills successfully then too.
ASHLEY: A lot. I get upset easily.	
THERAPIST: What are some things you can do when you are	

experiencing a great deal of distress to help manage those emotions?

ASHLEY: Music. Draw. (*Therapist writes these down.*)

THERAPIST: I think those things could be very helpful in many situations. But what would you do if you were so distressed that drawing or listening to music wasn't helping?

ASHLEY: That's harder. Maybe go to sleep? I don't know.

THERAPIST: Who could you reach out to for help in coping if it got really hard?

ASHLEY: I guess I could call a good friend. I am not sure I would go to my grandmother.

THERAPIST: Would you try if it was bad enough?

Great! She is able to understand the concept of this. I will continue to encourage Ms. Langley to use these skills as well.

ASHLEY: I guess so. (*Therapist writes those down.*)

THERAPIST: OK, so we are starting a list of coping tools. Over the next week, I want you to keep this list somewhere safe and use it if you are feeling distressed or have negative thoughts. We'll talk about when these strategies worked and when they didn't. And we'll keep adding to it. I will explain it to your grandmother, too.

Sharing Ashley's list with Ms. Langley will help her to support Ashley, and perhaps down the road they can talk together about the strategies that work best to reduce the intensity of distressing feelings. The list of coping strategies will also help Ashley when she finds herself struggling with distressing feelings.

ASHLEY: Do I have to talk with her about my problems?

THERAPIST: Actually, there may be many times when you can choose one of the other coping strategies you mentioned. But this way she can support your efforts, and if you need to go to her, she will understand and better know how to help you.

The therapist also helped Ashley expand her emotional vocabulary. For example, Ashley was asked to create a list of as many feeling words as she could. Ashley was then given scenarios that elicited additional feeling words, including "embarrassed" and "brave." Ashley was also asked to give examples for several of the feeling words (situations that made her happy, sad, etc.). Gradual exposure to trauma memories was pursued through asking Ashley to indicate the different feelings she had during the CSA and DV episodes by circling those feelings with two different-colored pens.

The therapist consistently praised Ashley's efforts to practice the coping skills. She also provided age-appropriate psychoeducation about CSA and DV through use of a card game with trauma-related as well as neutral questions on the cards (Deblinger, Neubauer, Runyon, & Baker, 2006). Ashley picked cards from a pile, read each question aloud, and then answered the questions herself, allowing the therapist to assess what accurate information as well as inaccurate information or dysfunctional thoughts she had. The therapist praised her for each answer and provided accurate information when necessary. The exercise allowed Ashley to talk about the traumas she experienced in an abstract manner, which was much less anxiety-provoking at this stage than discussing it directly, and was good preparation for the trauma narration and processing work to come.

Content of Session	*Rationale/Analysis*
THERAPIST: You're really doing a great job with this, Ashley. Now tell me, what are some of the feelings kids and teens in general have when they have been sexually abused?	She's really doing great with this, and she appears much more at ease than she did last week. That makes sense, since she just met me and she has trust issues, given how much trauma she has been through.
ASHLEY: Sad (*pauses*). Scared. Betrayed. Damaged.	
THERAPIST: That's true. Some kids do feel sad or scared or betrayed, or as if they have been damaged in some way from the abuse. Others feel worried or embarrassed, or like it was their fault. Great job. Now tell me how children feel if they have seen or heard their father or another man hurt their mother.	

Dialogue	Commentary
ASHLEY: Scared. Really angry. Upset.	Her answers are age-appropriate, so let's fill in some other information, and then see if she'll relate it to her own experience. She does with some of the other questions, but not with others.
THERAPIST: Yes, some kids do feel really angry and upset, or scared their mom might get really hurt. Other children might feel sad or worried or embarrassed. The important thing is that no matter how a child feels about sexual abuse or domestic violence, all of the child's feelings are OK. How did you feel when you were sexually abused?	I suspect it will be easier to talk about the DV than the CSA because she barely answered the assessment questions about that.
ASHLEY: Betrayed. Angry, sad, and scared. Damaged.	
THERAPIST: How about when you saw Keisha's dad hurt your mom?	
ASHLEY: Really, really angry. I wanted to get back at him.	
THERAPIST: I know that a lot of other kids feel that way, too. Thank you for sharing your feelings with me. You're doing a really great job.	Great job, Ashley! This is why we don't just back off when a child or teen is reluctant or avoidant initially.

Ms. Langley was very pleased with how praise was working. More specifically, she noticed Ashley being more helpful over the week and was pleasantly surprised that Ashley shared her feelings on one occasion. The therapist encouraged Ms. Langley to continue offering specific and purely positive praise for these behaviors (e.g., "I like when you do your chores when I ask" and "It makes me happy when you tell me how you feel" vs. "Why don't you act like this all the time?").

From functional analyses the therapist conducted to assess the circumstances surrounding caregiver–child interactions, it appeared that Ms. Langley vacillated between being overly indulgent with Ashley because of everything she had been through and being overly strict and punitive. Thus the therapist continued to work with Ms. Langley to identify the thoughts that were underlying her own distress and inconsistent caregiving responses.

Ms. Langley was then asked to tell whether there was a time during the past week when she had been feeling particularly distressed about what Ashley had been through in terms of the CSA and DV. Ms. Langley was able to pinpoint a time when her own daughter (Ashley's mother) contacted her, and she subsequently experienced a lot of worry about Ashley. After describing and getting in touch with the feelings she was experiencing, the therapist asked Ms. Langley to try to capture the thoughts that were racing through her mind at that time. After reviewing Ms. Langley's feelings and thoughts, the therapist helped Ms. Langley identify thoughts in the list that were accurate and helpful, as well as those that were unhelpful. The therapist then engaged in Socratic questioning to help Ms. Langley challenge the accuracy of some of her unhelpful thoughts. Ms. Langley was asked to record distressing feelings during the week, as well as the thoughts experienced at those times. The therapist gave Ms. Langley this practice assignment to help her identify and begin challenging trauma-related thoughts that might be inaccurate or unhelpful (e.g., "My child's life is ruined," "My granddaughter will turn out just like her mother"), while replacing them with more helpful, accurate thoughts on her own.

Over the sessions that followed, the therapist helped Ms. Langley more consistently apply behavior management in response to Ashley's noncompliant behavior and poor choices. The therapist also continued to help Ms. Langley develop her own cognitive coping skills by discussing a few examples of helpful and unhelpful ways of thinking about problem situations. The therapist then looked at Ms. Langley's list of thoughts from the prior week, to identify and praise healthy, productive thoughts, while also identifying and examining the accuracy of distressing and/or dysfunctional thoughts. The following dialogue illustrates this process.

Content of Session	*Rationale/Analysis*
THERAPIST: OK, Ms. Langley. Here you said that you think Ashley will grow up to be just like her mother because you were never in a violent situation but your daughter always chose bad boys and made bad relationship decisions no matter what you did to try to help her. Based on what you learned last week, do you think those thoughts are helpful and accurate? Whose fault was the violence and the abuse?	This is a common thought. It's tricky because I want to reframe this to validate her concerns; after all, her daughter did make poor decisions with relationships. But for Ashley, that behavior, learned by observation, can be unlearned. And I can help Ms. Langley focus on the courage she had to try to have different results and protect her granddaughters when she agreed to take them to live with her, so they'd have a better life.
MS. LANGLEY: All the men's fault. And Keisha's dad in particular,	

for also sexually abusing Ashley. But my daughter has some responsibility, too.

THERAPIST: Yes, it is the men's fault, Keisha's dad's in particular. And, Ms. Langley, you are right; your daughter has some responsibility for the choices she kept making. But we have to separate out a grown woman from a young teen who can still learn differently. Ashley is living with you now, without violence, and learning about healthy relationships. So how might you change that thought to make it more accurate and helpful?

MS. LANGLEY: I guess I could say I know Ashley learned to accept sexual pressure and violence by the experiences she had in her mother's care. But since she left that environment, I showed her that it isn't OK to be violent or accept violence, and now that we are all safe, she can learn other, better ways to handle relationship choices and to keep herself safe.

Nice job! That's exactly it. I hope that if she can get the others this easily, analyzing and changing her thoughts can come somewhat naturally to her and will start helping her right away.

THERAPIST: That's great, Ms. Langley. If you think that way, how do you feel?

MS. LANGLEY: Better. At least like it's not definite that she will follow in her mother's footsteps. But I have to say, I am still very unsure.

THERAPIST: That makes sense. But do you think that from now on when you have that worry, you can replace that thought with a more helpful one, so you can feel better and be more optimistic?

The therapist informed Ms. Langley that she was teaching similar skills to Ashley, and how she would go about this. However, the therapist noted that initially she would practice these cognitive coping skills with Ashley only with regard to nontraumatic events. Ms. Langley was asked to encourage the use of these important skills by modeling them and praising Ashley's efforts to use the skills with everyday stressors. The therapist then spent some time explaining to Ms. Langley the rationale for beginning to encourage Ashley to write or draw about her traumatic experiences. It was explained that the therapist would help Ashley share traumatic memories, including her thoughts, feelings, and sensations. After Ashley completed a trauma narrative, the therapist could then help Ashley challenge any unhealthy thoughts or beliefs she had developed as a result of the traumatic experiences and write a final chapter about what she was learning in therapy, thereby reinforcing healthier beliefs about herself, relationships, and expectations for the future. Ms. Langley was pleased that Ashley would be processing her experiences, but she remained skeptical about her granddaughter's willingness to cooperate.

Middle Phase of Treatment: Trauma Narration and Processing

The gradual exposure and skill-building process continues in the middle phase of treatment, with an increasing focus on the client's traumatic experiences. In this case, sessions with Ms. Langley continued to emphasize the importance of practicing the coping skills and behavior management skills (e.g., praise, differential attention, reflective listening and mild negative consequences) with Ashley at home. At the start of each session, the therapist and Ms. Langley reviewed caregiver–child interactions during the prior week, in order to support the grandmother's efforts to model effective coping skills while implementing effective parenting skills. During this phase, the therapist also assessed Ms. Langley's therapy progress and stability to determine whether she was emotionally prepared to review her granddaughter's narrative, first in individual sessions and later in conjoint sessions with Ashley.

During this phase, the therapist introduced the idea of writing a narrative to Ashley by suggesting that she could write a better book than the one about CSA they had read together. Though Ashley responded well to this idea, the therapist needed to periodically review the rationale for Ashley to talk, write, and/or create a narrative book about her experiences throughout these sessions. Trauma narration and processing extended a little beyond the usual four to five sessions because Ashley had experienced chronic exposure to DV as well as CSA. There were a few sessions in which Ashley shut down and refused to work on her trauma narrative. The therapist did not abandon the trauma focus in response to this avoidance, however. Instead, she took one step back in the gradual exposure process by talking with Ashley about popular entertainers who had trauma histories and reading about them.

Ashley chose to create a "book" (i.e., narrative) about her experiences, drawing pictures for each chapter as well as writing some poetry. Using art, like play, often makes it easier for youth of any age to talk about traumatic issues. Some teens write poetry or song lyrics to share and/or process their traumatic experiences. Ashley's book included an introduction; chapters on when she told her grandmother about the CSA, as well as when she talked with the police about it; chapters about the first time she was sexually abused; chapters on the first, last, and most scary incidents of DV; and a chapter about positive and negative interactions with her boyfriend. Finally, Ashley wrote a closing chapter about what she had learned from therapy about herself and her relationships with her grandmother and her boyfriend, as well as what she had learned about the world. She ended this final chapter with her expectations for her future. The following is an excerpt from a trauma narrative session.

Content of Session	*Rationale/Analysis*
THERAPIST: Ashley, we are going to continue with your book today. Last time, you did a nice job talking about when the domestic violence happened to your mom. Today I would like you to either draw or tell me about the scariest time when there was domestic violence or when Keisha's dad sexually abused you.	Ashley has been doing great with the trauma narrative, after some initial avoidance. It makes sense that she would not choose to discuss the sexual abuse first, as that is the most anxiety-provoking for her. She really illustrates the idea that for many teens, as long as they are fairly stable, it is best to share trauma-related thoughts and feelings rather than avoid them, so the teens can get some support in making sense of the experiences. Ultimately, it is my hope that when Ashley is reminded of these traumatic experiences in the future, she will remember with pride the strength she had in disclosing to her grandmother, coping with the aftermath, and using her artistic talents to draw and write about her experiences.
ASHLEY: The scariest violence to my mom.	
THERAPIST: Let's change chairs so you can type about the domestic violence. Here is paper and the colored pencils, so you can draw a picture of the scariest time you saw Keisha's dad hurt your mom.	

ASHLEY: (*After a few minutes*) I'm done.

THERAPIST: (*Reading*) This is really a good chapter, Ashley. You did a great job adding thoughts, feelings, and body sensations, too. Now just like before, I want you to draw a picture to go with it.

ASHLEY: OK.

THERAPIST: You do really beautiful artwork, Ashley. When I showed your last picture to your grandmother, she said the drawings looked just like your mom. How does it feel to write and draw about this?

ASHLEY: Good.

THERAPIST: I'm very proud of you.

As Ashley continued to develop her book, the therapist reviewed the narratives between sessions, looking for dysfunctional thoughts (inaccurate and/or unhelpful thoughts) to process and potentially correct. As Ashley was able to change the dysfunctional thoughts, more helpful thoughts were incorporated into several chapters (e.g., "Because of what happened to me before and to my mom, I thought if more bad stuff happened, oh well. Now I realize that was wrong, and I can choose to be with a man who is not violent.").

Preparing Ms. Langley and Ashley for Conjoint Sessions

Earlier in treatment, the therapist had explained to Ashley why having open communication with her grandmother was important, and how therapy would help with that. The therapist explained that she would share (in a developmentally appropriate manner) what her grandmother was working on in therapy, and would also share some of Ashley's work with her grandmother in their separate individual sessions. Like many teenagers, Ashley was originally self-conscious about having her private information shared with her grandmother. She said that the idea felt embarrassing and uncomfortable, particularly the sharing of details about the CSA. She also expressed that she didn't like upsetting her grandmother in any way. The therapist reassured Ashley that she would prepare Ms. Langley so that it wasn't too upsetting for her. She also emphasized that her grandmother was committed to attending therapy because she wanted the best for Ashley, and that Ms. Langley was eager to read her work (especially since she had been so impressed with Ashley's artwork), though she knew it would be distressing.

The therapist shared Ashley's narrative during an individual session with the grandmother, after determining that Ms. Langley was emotionally prepared to review it. Ms. Langley was surprised to learn how much DV her grandchildren had been exposed to while in their mother's care. During this emotionally challenging session, the therapist supported Ms. Langley in using her coping skills, as the material she was reading was upsetting for her in terms of the DV's impact on her daughter as well as her grandchildren. Despite the distress she experienced upon hearing the narrative, Ms. Langley was determined to review it together with Ashley during a conjoint session. The therapist prepared Ms. Langley for such a conjoint session by encouraging Ms. Langley to share and process her own thoughts and feelings in reaction to hearing Ashley's narrative, and by role-playing the planned conjoint activities. Ms. Langley was initially quite distressed in response to her granddaughter's narrative, but was reassured when she read the final chapter, which highlighted all that Ashley had learned as well as her positive expectations for the future.

Final Phase: Consolidation and Closure

The final phase of TF-CBT included a review of psychoeducational materials and coping skills, as well as the sharing of the trauma narrative with Ashley and her grandmother together. By this stage of treatment, Ashley was beginning to show greater willingness to open up to her grandmother about her interactions with her boyfriend. Thus Ashley was open to having a conjoint session focused on reviewing the sex education that had been provided earlier in individual sessions with Ms. Langley, who now sensitively provided input in terms of family and cultural values. This was particularly important, given that Ashley had been introduced to sexuality in an abusive, inappropriate context. Ms. Langley seemed surprised that Ashley's preferences for how and when a sexual relationship might ideally progress reflected her family values more closely than she anticipated.

By this stage of treatment, both Ashley and Ms. Langley appeared to be emotionally ready to engage in conjoint caregiver–child sessions in which the trauma narrative would be shared. These sessions were designed to achieve four objectives. First, they would allow Ms. Langley to demonstrate her ability to hear and talk about the traumas. Second, the sessions would give Ashley an opportunity to experience a sense of pride in sharing her narrative, further alleviating her feelings of shame and distress associated with the traumas. Third, the sessions would enhance caregiver–child communication regarding the traumas, and would clear up misunderstandings and areas of confusion. Finally, these sessions would lay the groundwork for therapeutic caregiver–child interactions and the practicing of effective skills to continue after formal therapy ended.

Before the conjoint sessions began, the therapist helped Ms. Langley process and overcome her anxiety about these sessions. Ms. Langley was worried that she might start crying when Ashley read the narrative, and she thought that Ashley would be angry at her for not knowing about the CSA. The therapist helped Ms. Langley work through these emotions while practicing how she wanted to respond to Ashley prior to the conjoint sessions. Ms. Langley identified helpful and supportive statements that she could make to Ashley during their conjoint sessions. In her sessions with the therapist, Ms. Langley role-played responding to Ashley in a supportive and validating way.

Ashley's readiness to engage in conjoint sessions with her grandmother was assessed as well. Ashley stated that she felt nervous about sharing her narrative with her grandmother because she didn't want her to cry. Ashley was reassured that it was OK to cry when thinking about something sad that happened, and that her grandmother was prepared and really wanted to hear Ashley read her narrative.

During the first conjoint session, Ashley and Ms. Langley talked about CSA and DV in general, as some children find it easier to speak generally about traumas before they are able to talk with caregivers about their specific experiences. Ashley and Ms. Langley played a question-and-answer game in which the therapist asked the two of them questions about CSA and DV and each earned points for correct answers. Ms. Langley expressed pride in Ashley's ability to answer so many questions. This created a fun atmosphere that allowed both Ashley and Ms. Langley to relax, despite the seriousness of the subject matter.

In the next conjoint session, Ashley read her trauma narrative. Ms. Langley praised her work and her confidence in writing and reading her book. After Ashley read her narrative, Ms. Langley asked Ashley open-ended, nonthreatening questions, such as "What did it feel like to write about the sexual abuse and the domestic violence?" and "What would you tell your friends if they went through this too?" When the final chapter was shared, both Ashley and her grandmother were moved to tears. With a little prompting from the therapist, Ms. Langley emphasized that her tears were a reflection of her happiness that Ashley had learned so much and seemed so much stronger that she had when they started therapy together.

Prior to completing therapy, Ashley and her grandmother also learned body safety skills to reduce the likelihood of future victimization. The therapist emphasized to Ashley that most children don't know what to do when they are sexually abused, and that they cannot be expected to stop adults from engaging in violence or abuse. The therapist also reminded Ashley that she did tell her grandmother about the abuse after she felt safe, and that telling is the most important personal safety skill. Other safety skills covered included discussing peer pressure related to drugs, sex, and other risky behaviors.

During the final conjoint sessions, Ashley and Ms. Langley reviewed their safety plan and practiced personal safety skills together. As part of the safety plan, Ashley created a "contract" that she and her grandmother agreed to and signed; this listed safe places both inside and outside their home, as well as safe people (with their phone numbers) that Ashley could talk to in case she needed help. Ms. Langley emphasized that Ashley could call her anytime to pick her up, with no questions asked, if she was ever feeling pressure from her boyfriend or others to engage in unhealthy or risky behaviors. In addition, Ms. Langley agreed to support Ashley by listening to her and not trying to solve all of her problems. Ashley expressed relief to have her grandmother's support, and she added that she was finding herself less interested in spending as much time with her boyfriend as she had in the past. Finally, Ashley and her grandmother were given scenarios that helped them to practice implementing the proposed safety skills and plans, while simultaneously receiving support and constructive feedback from the therapist. The therapist planned the conjoint sessions to end on a positive note by helping Ashley and Ms. Langley prepare praise for one another. Ashley praised her grandmother for helping her talk about the CSA and for always believing in her. Ms. Langley praised Ashley for working hard in therapy and for being a wonderful granddaughter and older sister to Keisha.

Ending Therapy

Upon completion of the planned course of therapy, the battery of standardized measures that Ashley and Ms. Langley had completed before therapy was readministered. The results showed that Ashley's symptoms had diminished significantly, and that Ms. Langley was no longer reporting significant depressive symptomatology or blaming herself for her daughter's and granddaughter's situations. During the last phase of therapy, the final session was planned for Ashley and her grandmother to celebrate their accomplishments in therapy. During the final session, Ashley received her therapy completion certificate from the therapist, and she contributed to the celebration by bringing her favorite music to play. Both Ms. Langley and the therapist praised Ashley for her hard work in therapy. Although Ms. Langley anticipated that she and Ashley would face significant challenges in the future she was very happy with her granddaughter's progress and was open to the therapist's request that they call or schedule booster sessions if necessary in the future.

CONCLUDING COMMENTS

Ashley and her grandmother seemed to benefit from TF-CBT's structure and focus on trauma, as well as its incorporation of critical skill-building components. Their success over a relatively short time frame (20 sessions) was reflective of many complex trauma cases. The parenting sessions were particularly important to the family's recovery in supporting more effective caregiver–child communication. Trauma-focused work was done individually with the child and caregiver until the caregiver could effectively support the child's healing process in conjoint sessions. Both Ashley and her grandmother learned how the traumas Ashley had experienced had influenced her choices and behaviors. Moreover, they both felt reassured that the skills they learned in therapy would help them cope during times of stress and in response to possible symptom relapse in the future. In addition, they were encouraged to contact the therapist as a resource if they felt the need for guidance or booster sessions in the future.

It is worth noting that in the case composite scenario described here, the case went fairly smoothly, as both Ashley and her grandmother were generally accepting of the overall treatment plan. This may not always occur. Early in treatment, some teens state firmly that they aren't going to talk about their personal traumatic experiences at all. It is preferable not to debate this issue in the early stages of treatment, but rather to engage these teenagers in some gradual exposure activities from the start of treatment. Most teens do not object to brief trauma-related discussions, as long as these discussions are not personal. In fact, many teens find trauma-related educational information helpful and will respond to some more personal but limited trauma-related questions during the skill-building sessions. When teens continue to be avoidant during the middle phase of treatment, they may respond to the use of metaphors in explaining the value of writing about or discussing their personal abuse experiences. For instance, a therapist can discuss getting into a swimming pool gradually and working up to total immersion, not just diving in, and can then observe that trauma work is like that. Another helpful metaphor is noting that cleaning out a cut in order to prevent infection may sting a little, but that if the cut is left alone and it becomes infected, it hurts much more later. Offering teens some control over the trauma narrative development process can also be helpful; for example, they can be given a choice between dictating to the therapist and typing their own narratives on the therapist's computer so they don't say the words out loud (at least initially). Many therapists have also found that teens' creative interests can provide the vehicle for overcoming avoidance. For instance, a musically inclined teen can be engaged in writing a rap song about the traumatic experiences (rather than a narrative in prose), similar to what many famous musicians have done.

In summary, it is important to note that TF-CBT has been found to be effective as a short-term treatment model with diverse children and adolescents who have experienced multiple and complex traumas (Cohen, Mannarino, & Deblinger, 2012). As an evidence-based treatment model, TF-CBT continues to be evaluated and applied to many other populations, including children who have experienced traumatic grief, war exposure, and other traumas (Cohen et al., 2012). Moreover, TF-CBT will continue to evolve in response to ongoing research, which may further elucidate critical therapy ingredients and optimal doses of treatment needed to help children, teens, and their parents effectively heal in the aftermath of trauma.

STUDY QUESTIONS

1. It was noted that after the abuse, Ashley's behavior changed. She began to act differently, either ignoring her sister or demonstrating increasing anger and aggression. What other behaviors might one see an adolescent exhibit after experiencing abuse?
2. How might a therapist tailor TF-CBT to a much younger child who has gone through the same type of abuse? What developmental factors come into play?
3. How might a clinician respond if a teen refuses to engage with the parent/caregiver and says, "She will never understand, and she will just blame me for what happened"?
4. What psychoeducational information could the therapist in this case have provided to Ashley and her grandmother about CSA and DV?
5. How might the therapist have conducted therapy differently if Ashley's mother wanted to be involved too?

REFERENCES

Bal, S., Crombez, G., De Bourdeaudhuij, I., & Van Oost, I. (2009). Symptomatology in adolescents following initial disclosure of sexual abuse: The roles of crisis support appraisals and coping. *Child Abuse and Neglect, 33*, 717–727.

Beitchman, J. H., Zucker, K. J., Hood, J. E., daCosta, G. A., & Akman, D. (1992). A review of the short-term effects of child sexual abuse. *Child Abuse and Neglect, 15*, 537–556.

Cohen, J. A., Mannarino, A. P., & Deblinger, E. (2006). *Treating trauma and traumatic grief in children and adolescents*. New York: Guilford Press.

Cohen, J. A., Mannarino, A. P., & Deblinger, E. (Eds.). (2012). *Trauma-focused CBT for children and adolescents: Treatment applications*. New York: Guilford Press.

Deblinger, E., Cohen, J. A., & Mannarino, A. P. (2012). Introduction. In J. A. Cohen, A. P. Mannarino, & E. Deblinger (Eds.), *Trauma-focused CBT for children and adolescents:Treatment applications* (pp. 1–26). New York: Guilford Press.

Deblinger, E., McLeer, S., Atkins, M., Ralphe, D., & Foa, E. (1989). Post-traumatic stress insexually abused, physically abused, and nonabused children. *Child Abuse and Neglect, 13*(3), 403–408.

Deblinger, E., Neubauer, F., Runyon, M., & Baker, D. (2006). *What do you know?: Atherapeutic card game about child sexual and physical abuse and domestic violence*. Stratford, NJ: CARES Institute.

Fantuzzo, J. W., & Mohr, W. K. (1999). Prevalence and effects of child exposure to domestic violence. *The Future of Children, 9*, 21–32.

Felitti, V. J., Anda, R. F., Nordenberg, D., Williamson, D. F., Spitz, A. M., Edwards, V., et al. (1998). Relationship of childhood abuse and household dysfunction to many of the leading causes of death in adults: The Adverse Childhood Experiences (ACE) Study. *American Journal of Preventive Medicine, 14*, 245–258.

Finkelhor, D., & Jones, L. (2006). Why have child maltreatment and child victimization declined? *Journal of Social Issues, 62*(4), 685–716.

Finkelhor, D., & Jones, L. (2012). *Have sexual abuse and physical abuse declined since the 1990s?* (Report No. NCJ 199298). Durham, NH: Crimes against Children Research Center.

Finkelhor, D., Ormrod, R., Turner, H., & Hamby, S. L. (2005). The victimization of children and youth: A comprehensive, national survey. *Child Maltreatment, 10*(1), 5–25.

Graham-Bermann, S. A. (2001). Designing intervention evaluations for children exposed to domestic violence: Applications of research and theory. In S. A. Graham-Bermann& J. L. Edleson (Eds.), *Domestic violence in the lives of children: The future of research, intervention, and social policy* (pp. 237–267). Washington, DC: American Psychological Association.

Groves, B. M. (1999). Mental health services for children who witness domestic violence. *The Future of Children, 9*, 122–132.

Kellogg, N. D., & Menard, S. W. (2003). Violence among family members of children and adolescents evaluated for sexual abuse. *Child Abuse and Neglect, 27*, 1367–1376.

Levendosky, A. A., & Graham-Bermann, S. A. (2001). Parenting in battered women: The effects of domestic violence on women and their children. *Journal of Family Violence, 16*, 171–192.

McCloskey, L. A., Figueredo, A. J., & Koss, M. P. (1995). The effects of systemic family violence on children's mental health. *Child Development, 66*, 1239–1261.

Perez-Fuentes, G., Olfson, M., Villegas, L., Morcillo, C., Wang, S., & Blanco, C. (2013). Prevalence and correlates of child sexual abuse: A national study. *Comprehensive Psychiatry, 54*(1), 16–27.

Rossman, B. B. (2001). Longer term effects of children's exposure to domestic violence. In S. A. Graham-Bermann & J. L. Edleson (Eds.), *Domestic violence in the lives of children: The future of research, intervention, and social policy* (pp. 35–65). Washington, DC: American Psychological Association.

Silverman, W. K., Ortiz, C. D., Viswesvaran, C., Burns, B. J., Kolko, D. J., Putnam, F. W., et al. (2008). Evidence-based psychosocial treatments for children and adolescents exposed to traumatic events. *Journal of Clinical Child and Adolescent Psychology, 37*(1), 156–183.

Sternberg, K. J., Lamb, M. E., Greenbaum, C., Cicchetti, D., Dawud, S., Cortes, R. M., et al. (1993). Effects of domestic violence on children's behavior problems and depression. *Developmental Psychology, 29*, 44–52.

Teicher, M. H., Samson, J. A., Polcari, A., & McGreenery, C. E. (2006). Sticks, stones, and hurtful words: Relative effects of various forms of childhood maltreatment. *American Journal of Psychiatry, 163*(6), 993–1000.

Trickett, P., Noll, J., & Putnam, F. (2011). The impact of sexual abuse on female development: Lessons from a multigenerational, longitudinal research study. *Development and Psychopathology, 23*, 453–476.

Chapter 7

Multiple Losses, Crises, and Trauma for Children in Foster Care or Residential Treatment

ATHENA A. DREWES

This chapter discusses the impact of complex trauma from multiple life events—such as attachment difficulties and separations, sexual abuse, exposure to domestic violence, and *in utero* drug exposure—experienced by children in the foster care and residential treatment systems. It also addresses how a therapist can utilize a prescriptive/integrative approach to treat such children, and to understand the unique challenges of children and caregivers in dealing with such complex trauma.

I begin with a definition of "complex trauma":

> The term complex trauma describes both children's exposure to multiple traumatic events, often of an invasive, interpersonal nature, and the wide-ranging, long-term impact of this exposure.
>
> These events are severe and pervasive, such as abuse or profound neglect. They usually begin early in life and can disrupt many aspects of the child's development and the very formation of a self. Since they often occur in the context of the child's relationship with a caregiver, they interfere with the child's ability to form a secure attachment bond. (National Child Traumatic Stress Network, n.d.)

As this definition makes clear, complex trauma has serious effects on the formation of attachments. In this chapter, I discuss play-based techniques that directly address complex trauma caused by loss of the biological parent(s), further broken attachments, and other subsequent abuses. I also discuss ways to work with caregivers and families to help them understand foster or residential care children's special emotional needs. The need for an integrative approach using both directive and nondirective treatment in work with these children is discussed, along with how and which expressive arts techniques can be successfully utilized to help heal the emotional holes in the hearts of these children.

CAUSES AND EFFECTS OF COMPLEX TRAUMA

The rates of complex trauma in childhood are rising. Each year approximately 5 million children experience some form of traumatic experience, with more than 2 million victims of physical and/or sexual abuse (Belluck, 2012). In addition, children may live in the terrorizing atmosphere of domestic violence, experience the impact of parental drug and alcohol abuse, and/or witness community violence (Whitty & O'Connor, 2007).

A matter of particular concern is that the number of babies suffering from opiate addictions and related symptoms at birth has tripled in the past decade (Belluck, 2012). Every hour a baby is born in the United States with symptoms of withdrawal from opiates. This amounts to roughly 13,500 babies a year (Belluck, 2012), due to the fact that about 4.5% of pregnant women use illegal drugs. All too often, the eventual fates of these babies include abuse and other forms of complex trauma, and subsequent placement in foster care or residential treatment (which may itself involve further trauma).

Neonatal Abstinence Syndrome

One result of *in utero* addiction is called "neonatal abstinence syndrome" (NAS), which is a "constellation of signs and symptoms of infant neurobehavioral dysregulation that occurs in the immediate neonatal period. The syndrome varies in both expression and intensity among infants" (Whitty & O'Connor, 2007, p. 451).

The signs and symptoms of NAS in newborn infants include difficulties with muscle tone and movement, tight muscles, tremors, and/or jitteriness. NAS can lead to difficulties in feeding, resulting in weight loss or failure to thrive. These infants and children also have difficulties with state regulation, resulting in difficulty maintaining the type of quiet, alert state that they need for feeding and other growth-promoting interactions with their caregivers (Foley, 2014; Whitty & O'Connor, 2007). They can have problems going smoothly from sleep to waking states, and often become irritable and cry. Additional difficulties and problems include overreactivity to stimuli: Atypical responses to touch, sound, movement, or visual stimulation can result in either overstimulation and poor reactivity, or "pulldown" to avoid the stimulation (Whitty & O'Connor, 2007). Infants and children with NAS also have problems with autonomic nervous system control, resulting in gagging, vomiting/diarrhea, color changes, fever, fast breathing, or hiccupping, all of which further indicate an inability to regulate their functioning smoothly (Whitty & O'Connor, 2007). Other significant neurodevelopmental problems include a short attention span, hyperactivity, and sleep disturbances at 12–34 months (Whittty & O'Connor, 2007).

Behavioral impairments (rather than physical birth defects) associated with NAS include difficulty connecting with caregivers (attachment problems) due to being resistant to cuddling or soothing; this resistance may stem from the decreased ability to respond normally to auditory or visual stimuli (Osofsky, 2004), as described above. Parental low socioeconomic status (SES), continued parental drug use, and poor parenting skills can contribute to risk conditions that could result in the additional trauma created by physical and sexual abuse (Rice & Groves, 2005). Further traumatic complications may occur as a result of eventual placement in foster care, orphanages, or residential care (Foley, 2014), as described later.

Prevalence and Symptoms of Complex Trauma

Foley (2014) has described the results of two major studies of childhood trauma, including chronic/complex trauma. The Adverse Childhood Experiences Study involved an initial nonclinical population of over 17,000 middle- to upper-SES children, 75% of whom were European American. This study found retrospectively that 28% of these children had experienced physical abuse, and that 22% had three or more trauma exposures. These experiences were correlated with subsequent mood disorders, chronic disease, early morbidity, early smoking and drinking, and early sexual activity resulting in HIV and other sexually transmitted diseases. In a second study of 14,773 children, 48% had experienced the loss of a caregiver; 47% were witnesses of domestic violence; 44% had experienced caregiver impairment (from drug use, alcohol use, and/or mental illness); and 42% had four or more traumas.

The psychological wounds resulting from multiple exceptional events that overwhelm children's capacity to cope, and shatter their trust in others and in everyday life, have a cumulative effect (Foley, 2014). These children do not have the necessary protective factors that can help to mitigate the impact of such exceptional events and the resulting complex trauma. Protective factors involving the family include availability of a primary caregiver, ties to an extended family, family routines/rituals, and overall stability. Protective factors involving the community include a safe, positive, nurturing school experience; availability of supportive adults; and cultural identity. Protective factors involving a child's own physiology include flexible temperament, secure attachment, robustness of body, and good regulatory capacity; strong cognitive, problem-solving, and verbal skills; self-esteem and positive self-image; and mastery motivation. Without many of these protective factors, these vulnerable children are likely to experience full-blown posttraumatic stress disorder (PTSD) or symptoms of PTSD, including reexperiencing symptoms, avoidance symptoms, and negative alterations in cognitions (Foley, 2014).

Reexperiencing symptoms in children over 18 months result in deficits in play (which becomes anxious, constricted, and repetitive); reactivity to triggers; changes in eating, sleeping, and elimination; avoidance symptoms, including numbing of responsiveness, withdrawal, and/or avoidance; and affectlessness, frozen state, and dissociation. There are negative alterations in cognitions, behaviors, and emotions, such as social withdrawal, hyperactivity/attention deficits, low frustration tolerance, irritability, and startle responses (Foley, 2014, Scheeringa & Zeanah, 1995). These children also may show fear of separation, anxiety about new routines, phobic-like responses, aggression, animal abuse, sexualized behaviors, and increased masturbation. Anxiety dominates over curiosity with regard to body exploration, and a child's symptom profile may mimic regulatory disorders of sensory processing. The extent and number of symptoms will vary according to individual differences, as not every traumatized child experiences PTSD (Foley, 2014).

Impact of Trauma on Brain Structure

Trauma in early childhood not only can result in psychological changes, but also can change the brain architecture. Specifically, excessive stress can change brain chemistry via the impact of cortisol. Through cortisol-related changes, trauma adversely affects an infant or child by causing abnormal organization and functioning of important neural systems in the brain (Perry, 2009). These brain changes may create problems in self-regulation, memory, ability to sustain attention, ability to form secure relationships, and the ability to learn. The timing of the trauma affects the child's emerging brain systems, and an understanding of these systems will influence the assessment process and selection of therapeutic interventions (Foley, 2014; Perry, 2009).

BROKEN ATTACHMENTS IN FOSTER AND RESIDENTIAL CARE

As a result of complex trauma (including the initial attachment trauma they have undergone), foster and residential care children tend to have a greater risk for both externalizing and internalizing problems. The children with externalizing behaviors are at particular risk for placement disruptions. Multiple placements of such children can occur over time, creating a vicious cycle of breaks in attachment that makes the children vulnerable to additional traumas and abuses.

Maltreatment of a child requires state intervention to protect the child. However, there are both intended and unintended consequences of such intervention that must be addressed. When the child is placed, this may cause the child confusion and significant emotional distress as well as grief over the loss of the parental relationship, even with parents who have been abusive and neglectful. We must consider all interventions through the "eyes of the child" (Foley, 2014) and recognize that changes in placement simultaneously mean changes in relationships: "When children are removed from their homes, they begin to experience grief over the loss of their caregiver/parent" (Foley, 2014). Two concurrent risks occur at the time a child is removed and placed into foster care or a residential treatment center: the impact of the maltreatment that caused the initial removal, and the emotional impact of separation on a child's developing attachments. Both issues can have long-term negative consequences for the child (Osofsky, 2004). Webb (2006b) and her contributors discuss these consequences at length in the book *Working with Traumatized Youth in Child Welfare.*

Children who have experienced traumatic losses are not likely to trust authority figures and adults around them, and they often become guarded and wary (Earl, 2009), making engagement in treatment a challenge. Emotional walls are put up as inner fortifications, and these defenses make it extremely difficult to gain access to these angry young persons in therapy. Arrangements for visitation with a child's biological parent(s)/family can help to calm the child's separation fears, permit the expression of feelings, help the child relate better to the foster parents or other caregivers, and give the child and foster parents/caregivers continuing opportunities to see the biological parent(s) realistically. Visitation also helps the birth parent(s)/family to face reality and to learn and practice new skills and behaviors, as well as giving clinicians a chance to assess and document the progress of the birth family (Foley, 2014). Anecdotal evidence suggests that when a first visit is held within 48 hours following placement, a birth parent may be more likely to show up for visits and more inclined to see their value (Foley, 2014). The frequency with which foster/residential care children see their parents affects the children's behavior. If they are visited once a week or once every 2 weeks, they exhibited fewer behavioral problems than children who are visited infrequently (once a month or less). These children also show less anxiety and depression than children whose parents' visits are either infrequent or nonexistent (Foley, 2014).

Testing the Limits

After an initial "honeymoon" period in treatment (and in the foster home or residence), a recently placed child often begins testing limits, looking for vulnerabilities and weak spots within the caregiving adults to see how long the adults will tolerate the child's behaviors before sending him or her away again, as all the other caregivers have done. Difficulties with affect regulation; poor identification, expression, and integration of feelings; maladaptive coping strategies; hoarding of food, poor hygiene, and/or destruction of property; low self-esteem; and undercontrol (or sometimes hypercontrol) soon begin to manifest themselves (Drewes, 2011b; Foley, 2014). These behaviors can make a foster parent, a child care worker, and even a therapist feel helpless, demoralized, emotionally exhausted, angry, frustrated, and hostile. In turn, these feelings lead to deeper feelings of inadequacy and guilt in the child.

Many foster parents, and even residential care workers, have the mistaken view that "love will conquer all." In part this may be true, but unconditional love, stability and security in the home, clear expectations, and concise directions are essential, along with nurturance of the caregiver and encouragement by the therapist to remain in control. Moreover, this is not the most comfortable environment for the child, who will resist control and clear boundaries, and will engage in control battles that may spill into the therapy sessions. It is important for the therapist to work not only individually with the child on attachment issues, but also with the caregiver.

TRAUMA TREATMENT COMPONENTS

As the preceding discussion suggests, traumatized children need trusted adults to protect them, along with a safe, predictable, and patterned environment. Consistency leads to predictability, which in turn results in security (Foley, 2014).

Within the safety of the therapy room, much like the safety of the new foster or residential home, a foster/residential child can feel secure enough to explore, identify, and make sense of thoughts, feelings, wishes, and intentions, along with discovering strengths and seeing him- or herself from a new perspective (Hughes, 2009). Therapy thus needs to be a "holding environment" that offers safety, reliability, and security in an attuned relationship.

It is therefore critical for a therapist to accept the inherent worth and dignity of a foster/residential care child with sincerity and respect, while offering a safe and genuinely supportive environment. This will be especially important when the child client begins testing the therapist's limits and resists becoming emotionally attached during treatment. The therapist needs to "pass" the child's tests by remaining firm and caring in the face of challenging behavior. As therapists, we need to show these children that caring adults can listen to them, validate their experience, and understand their feelings. In addition, we must show that a caring adult dares to deal with a frightened child through strength and perseverance (Foley, 2014).

We also need to give these children control over their physical environment, allowing them to determine how close or far they are to us, or whether they need a physical barrier (e.g., a hoodie over the head, a pillow or stuffed animal to hug). Likewise, the children should be allowed to set the pace with which they wish to engage or try to navigate the intensity of the one-to-one relationship (Earl, 2009). New development, as well as an openness to play, only occurs when a child feels safe and secure (Foley, 2014; Landreth, 2012). A child will need a therapist's help to develop freedom from self-blame, and the therapist needs to develop and believe in the self-curative power of play (Crenshaw & Hardy, 2006; Foley, 2014; Schaefer & Drewes, 2014; Webb, 2006a). In addition, the therapist may employ methods to reframe cognitive distortions; link the child's thought content with affect; help the child to construct a cohesive narrative; and, after trust has been established, guide the youth toward gradual exposure to the traumatic content and experiences. As noted earlier, the therapist must also engage in dyadic/family work with caregivers.

Indeed, the child-centered play therapy philosophy of following the child's lead and pace allows the child to feel that his or her boundaries and protective defenses are being respected. Offering invitational expressive arts and directive play-based activities within the sessions will allow the child to experience fun, while allowing sought-after control and movement at the level of the child's emotional rather than chronological age (Earl, 2009). It also gives the therapist time to understand and respect the vulnerable child's avoidant, withdrawn, or aggressive defensive behaviors, which have been developed to protect the child from perceptions of an unsafe and betraying world (Earl, 2009).

Through shared activities, the play therapist offers a form of emotional nurturance, or what Miller (2005) terms "nourishing communication." Through playfulness, acceptance, curiosity, and empathy, the foster/residential care child begins to feel nourished and to have other enhanced experiences that were lacking in infancy. The therapist helps to promote developmental progress (body, play, language, etc.) through unstructured, reflective, and developmental guidance. Modeling appropriate protective behavior, being an auxiliary ego, interpreting feelings and actions, and providing co-regulation, as well as promoting emotional support and empathic communication, all help the child link affect and experience (Foley, 2014). Play-based therapy can offer the child the necessary time, space, and choice to begin to explore the treatment relationship along with his or her personal issues. It is important to let the child know what he or she can do, as well as to help the child repair and reconnect—that is, to teach him or her how to "make up" when mistakes are made (Drewes, 2011b; Foley, 2014).

As emphasized in various chapters of the present book, working with expressive arts and play therapy allows for communication to stay within metaphors while a child explores intimate and often painful material nonverbally. The play creation can contain what has been experienced without making the child feel exposed (Drewes, 2011a; Webb, 2006a).

It is particularly critical for us as therapists to convey to foster and residential care children that we are equally interested in all aspects of their lives, not just the problems. We are not interested solely in "fixing" them; rather, we are genuinely interested in their interests, worries, strengths, challenges, and successes, as well as their past and future, with all concerns on an equal level (Drewes, 2011b). Through attunement to and matching of a child's affective state, along with a shared focus of attention, the therapeutic relationship and dialogue begin to develop.

NEED FOR AN INTEGRATIVE TREATMENT APPROACH

Because children in foster care/residential treatment have traumas that are multilayered and multidetermined, a multifaceted treatment approach is needed (Drewes, Bratton, & Schaefer, 2011). These children do not come to us with one clearly defined diagnosis, but rather several overlapping problems, due to the comorbidity of their issues (e.g., overlapping anxiety and attention problems, along with phobias and sexualized behaviors). There is no one theoretical or treatment approach that can fix all of the presenting problems such children display, or bring about therapeutic change across all of their different psychological disorders (Drewes et al., 2011).

A therapist needs to be flexible and nimble in navigating the unique demands of changing from one therapeutic stance to another, in order to meet the needs of a child and various individuals in the child's life (Drewes et al., 2011). The therapist may at one moment need to be intensely involved in deeply evocative, often very conflicted play therapy with the child, requiring attention to the child's internal struggles; at the same time, the therapist may need to set limits and to serve as an educator or mediator. The therapist may also find it necessary to engage a biological or foster parent, a school psychologist, or a classroom teacher to assess the child's functioning or offer parenting support. These roles can change rapidly, and they require the therapist to be not only prescriptive but integrative in treatment approaches, giving equal weight to the various aspects of the child's functioning as a blended and unified whole (Drewes, 2011a; Foley, 2014). In other words, the therapist needs to attend to and contain the multiple relationships among the cognitive, developmental, dynamic, interpersonal, and behavioral needs of the foster/residential care child (Drewes, 2008). An integrative approach is thus critical in working with complex trauma. Rice and Groves (2005) recommend such a multipronged integrated approach:

> Although cognitive/behavioral interventions address problematic behaviors and help the child build new skills, psychodynamic interventions are needed to help integrate traumatic memories and emotions along with buried parts of the self. At the same time, the therapist must pay close attention to family interactions, sequences of action and reaction, to root out any that maintain and reinforce symptoms. (p. 139)

Moreover, "evidence also suggests that trauma memories are imbedded in the right hemisphere of the brain, and that interventions facilitating access to and activity in the right side of the brain may be indicated. The right hemisphere of the brain is most receptive to nonverbal strategies that utilize symbolic language, creativity, and play" (Gil, 2006, p. 68). Thus there is a neurologically based need for the use of expressive arts, play, drama, body movement, yoga, and pleasurable activities within an integrative therapy. All these activities have been found to be important in helping traumatized and abused children heal, as well as create their trauma narratives (Drewes & Cavett, 2012; Gil, 2006; Perry, 2009; van der Kolk, 2005).

TREATMENT ISSUES

Issues that surface in working with foster and residential care children include grief and bereavement over the loss of their biological parents (at birth or later in their lives); difficulties with the identification, regulation, and integration of affect (particularly anger); and difficulties with forming and keeping relationships and friendships. Consequently, the treatment of choice can be dyadic therapy with a child and a foster parent/other caregiver, or family therapy. Often the treatment is individual therapy with collateral contact with the caregiver. For a younger foster care child—especially a child under the age of 10, on whose behalf the therapist is trying to build a relationship with the caregiver (and possibly the prospective adoptive parent)—there are the following therapeutic choices:

- Developmental play (Brody, 1997)
- Theraplay (Booth & Jernberg, 2010)
- Parent–child interaction therapy (McNeil & Hembree-Kigin, 2011)
- Circle of Security intervention (Powell, Cooper, Hoffman, & Marvin, 2014)
- Dyadic developmental psychotherapy (Hughes, 1997, 2009)
- Child–parent relationship therapy (Landreth & Bratton, 2005)
- Filial therapy (VanFleet, 1994)

In addition, the following treatment models can be integrated into the treatment approach for complex trauma:

- Neurosequential Model of Therapeutics (Perry, 2009)
- Trauma-focused cognitive-behavioral therapy (Cohen, Mannarino, & Deblinger, 2012; see Neubauer, Deblinger, & Sieger, Chapter 6, this volume)
- Child and adolescent Dialectical Behavior Therapy® (Miller, Rathus, & Linehan, 2007)
- Play therapy and play-based directive techniques (Drewes et al., 2011; Landreth, 2012)

Treatment may need to start with Perry's (2009) Neurosequential Model of Therapeutics. This is not a specific therapeutic technique or intervention, but rather a developmentally sensitive, neurobiologically informed approach to clinical work. It maps the neurobiological development of maltreated children, and its assessment methods identify developmental challenges and relationships that contribute to risk or resiliency.

This approach matches the nature and timing of specific therapeutic techniques to the child's developmental stage, and to the brain regions and neural networks mediating neuropsychiatric problems. Treatment starts with the lowest-level (in the brain) set of problems with functioning, and then moves sequentially up the levels of the brain as improvements are seen. Treatment for complex trauma will thus focus first on a poorly organized brainstem/diencephalon and the child's related problems with self-regulation, attention, arousal, and impulsivity; such a focus allows for the necessary development of self-regulation before therapy delves into the affectively charged material of the traumatization (Perry, 2009).

To assist a child at this level of functioning, any variety of patterned, repetitive somatosensory activities (to provide the patterned neural activation necessary for reorganization), such as music, movement, yoga (breathing), drumming, or therapeutic massage, may be utilized. Once improvement in self-regulation occurs, therapeutic work can move to more relational problems (at the limbic level), using more traditional play or arts therapies. Ultimately, once fundamental dyadic relational skills have improved, therapeutic techniques can become more verbal and insight-oriented (the cortical level), using any of the cognitive-behavioral, dyadic, psychodynamic, or play-based directive treatment approaches listed above (Perry, 2009).

After a safe environment is established in therapy, and trust begins to develop between the foster/residential care child and the therapist, use of a directive, prescriptive/integrative approach should be considered for individual therapy. This involves having the therapist take responsibility for guiding the therapy process and challenging the child to address specific concerns. An integrated model uses both directive and nondirective methods and encourages the traumatized child's competing drives for mastery and control, versus suppressing and avoiding painful and conflicted material (Drewes et al., 2011). The therapist assesses prescriptively what treatment approach and techniques should be utilized, given the client's symptoms and current concerns. As treatment progresses, the therapist may change treatment modalities (e.g., bring in dyadic work more or move more into individual work) as indicated by the needs of the child. Therefore treatment is custom-tailored to each client over time (Drewes et al., 2011).

As suggested earlier, play-based techniques and expressive arts interventions are often the most successful means of engaging a foster/residential care child and helping the child work through many issues. The way I handle an integrative/directive session is to use the first 5 minutes to "check in" on issues or homework from the last session; reports from the school, foster parent, or residential child care worker; and/or unfinished issues from the preceding session. Then the child and I spend the next 15–20 minutes on directive expressive arts and play-based techniques that address various issues facing the child. The remaining time is left for nondirective play therapy, in which the child can choose an activity or use the playroom in any way he or she wishes. The foster parent or other caregiver can be brought in during any of these time slots to join in the activities; or alternate sessions may include dyadic work with the foster parent/caregiver; or a once-monthly session may be scheduled with the foster or biological parent alone to work on parenting skills, as needed.

EXPRESSIVE ARTS AND PLAY-BASED TECHNIQUES FOR SPECIFIC ISSUES

Addressing Allegiance Issues

Allegiance is often a big topic for a child in foster or residential care, who usually has divided loyalties toward his or her current caregivers versus the biological parent(s). Often the child has ambivalence about connecting with or loving "another mother," resulting in difficulty bonding with a current caregiver or future adoptive parent (Drewes, 2011b). Loyalty to a biological parent remains, regardless of how much or little the child knows about this parent or about how the parent treated the child. Some foster clients may not want to be adopted because of their strong feelings of allegiance to their birth parents. Therefore, it is always critical that a foster parent not force a child into using the name "Mom" or "Dad" upon entering the foster home. It is also crucial that the caregiver (foster parent or residential treatment child care worker) not speak poorly of either birth parent, as the child has 50% of each birth parent's DNA! Any negative comments made about the birth parents are interpreted as though they are made about the child and become integrated into the child's sense of self, thereby further worsening what is usually already low self-esteem (Drewes, 2011b).

In addressing the loss of birth parents and the issues of divided allegiance, I explore with the children whether they ever wonder about some things: what their birth parents are like, whether they look like their birth parents, or whether their birth parents are thinking about them on their birthdays. The children's caregivers are encouraged to ask these questions too, and to make statements such as these: "Your birth parents would be proud of you, just as we are," or "I wonder if your birth mom has curly hair like you," or "I'm so glad they gave you to us!" (Drewes, 2011a; Eldridge, 1999).

Also, it is helpful to confirm with these children how confusing it must be to have two sets of parents, or mixed-up feelings on birthdays, or questions about why their birth parents placed them in foster or residential care. It is important to normalize that many foster or residential children feel they should not love "another mom." Many children feel anger at their birth mothers, wanting to punish them for abandonment while crying from the depths of their broken hearts for a reunion. I assure each of my foster children that "Your heart is big enough for two moms" (Drewes, 2011a). We work together on writing a letter to the birth parent (whether or not the child knows anything about this parent), which the child can then keep. The letter can be short or elaborate in highlighting such issues as these: "Why didn't you keep me? Is it because you didn't like me? What is your name, and what do you look like? I feel really mad because I didn't get to know you. Is there something wrong with you? Is that the reason I can't see you? Is there something wrong with me?" (Drewes, 2011a).

Dealing with Grief

Many sessions may be spent on a child's grief about the loss of the "bio-mom" or "bio-dad." Activities may include making up collages of things remembered about the birth parent, and also about things the child can enjoy about the foster parent or child care worker. Another activity is creating a "grief box" (Drewes, 2011a; Eldridge, 1999; Webb, 2006a, 2010). This is a box that can be decorated on the outside. The therapist and child can make a list of the various losses the child has had—such as the loss of the birth parents, the child's personal medical history, the birth family history, a sense of belonging, and a continuous life narrative—and put this list, or objects symbolizing items on the list, into the box.

> For example, Bethea, age 10, was encouraged to select from magazines pictures of a mother and child and a father and child to represent her birth family. In addition to these losses represented by the pictures, Bethea included in her box a Band-Aid for the loss of her full medical history because she often could not answer questions the doctor would ask about allergies and the medical history of her family. She also included a picture of a tree (to represent her lost family tree) and made a blank family tree chart for the loss of her birth family history. Other items she put into the box were a drawing or magazine photo of someone who looked sad, and a broken cord or string for the loss of a continuous life story narrative. Throughout treatment, we referred to the grief box and the various objects, and sometimes added other things to it. This box became the storage place for all the emptiness Bethea felt, and for the "hole in her heart" that was created by the loss of all these things. I became the caretaker of these heavy burdens and losses, and we kept exploring them gently and slowly throughout treatment.
>
> Throughout our work together through expressive art and play-based techniques, we explored ways to fill the hole in Bethea's heart. At various points, I would repeatedly stress how her parents did the best they could with the abilities they had at the time they were living together. Her mom's own problems got in the way of being the parent Bethea wanted her to be, so she just could not be the parent she needed her to be. I stressed to Bethea that she was lovable and was born lovable, but that, unfortunately, there was no magic that could make her parent into the one she needed and wanted so desperately (Drewes, 2011a).

Affect Identification and Regulation

Allen Schore (2003a, 2003b) writes that the most far-reaching effect of relational trauma is the loss of the ability to regulate the intensity of affect. Therefore, much of what I work on with children in foster and residential care involves building up a feelings vocabulary, helping children physically identify the locations of their feelings in their bodies, and showing them ways to integrate their feelings with better choices for problem-solving and coping skills when they are angry and upset. The Gingerbread Person Feelings Map (Drewes, 2001; Drewes & Cavett, 2012), a variation of the Color-Your-Life technique (O'Connor, 1983), uses a drawing of a gingerbread person with arms outstretched, and with eyes, nose, and smile. It can be used with teens as well as younger children, and with caregiver–child dyads. The technique is used in order to assess (1) the overall range of feelings a young client has the vocabulary to identify; (2) how aware the client is of where he or she physiologically feels emotions; and (3) how well integrated the client's emotions are. The intention of the Gingerbread Person Feelings Map is to allow for gathering of information in a nonthreatening, play-based way. It only takes a few minutes and can be used as an icebreaker in a first session, or at any time during treatment when appropriate.

Next to the shape of the gingerbread person, I make a list of the words" happy," "sad," "afraid," "angry," "love," and "worried." Then I ask the child to choose a few other feeling words to include. (I am often surprised at what children include, such as "petrified," "stupid," "anxious," "wishing I was somebody else," etc.) I write the child's word(s) underneath the standard words for emotions. This helps the child expand his or her emotional vocabulary; it also helps to give the child some control over the task, along with the feeling of being an active participant in the process. Next, I have the child choose a color for each feeling. It does not matter what colors the child picks (sometimes I get black for "happy"!). I have the child put a little line using the color chosen next to each of the feeling words, like creating a legend for a map. Then I ask the child to color the parts of the gingerbread person where he or she may physically experience each feeling listed. The child can shade each color in, scribble, or draw a shape such as a heart. I go through each feeling and have the client imagine where he or she feels each one (so no feelings are left out).

Once the activity is completed (usually after less than 5 minutes), I process the drawing with the child. I pay particular attention to where in the body anger is expressed and how this might play out in the child's world in responding to situations, and I point this out to the child. I look for how many feelings are integrated, and for how much color is used and where. I also look for discrepancies (e.g., a child may have colored in happy feelings on the face, but anger in the hands or feet or body; or may have placed a spot of color representing anger outside the figure—possibly signifying difficulty with tolerating that emotion). I process how the child may present to others as calm, but inwardly may be seething, or perhaps may be manifesting anger through hitting or restlessness in the legs. Also, I look for where the child puts love (often drawn as a heart), and whether love is "walled off" by layers of scared, hurt, or angry feelings. I explain how we each can have more than one feeling at a time within us (e.g., sometimes feeling angry and loving at the same time toward someone). And sometimes one feeling is so strong that it can hide other feelings too, thereby making us feel confused and unsure of what we are feeling.

This technique can also be used with a caregiver and teen/child together, with each working independently of the other. At the end, the caregiver and child can share their finished products and compare similarities and differences in the ways anger and other emotions are felt (Drewes, 2001). Other adaptations of this technique include using two gingerbread figures (Gil, 2006); the child colors in each figure according to the various feelings experienced when with each parent. For those children who may be uncomfortable thinking about their bodies and using a person-like shape (especially if they were sexually abused), a heart shape can be used. Heartfelt Feelings Coloring Cards strategies (Crenshaw, 2008) use preprinted cards with a drawn heart and feeling words to add colors to, in order to help children identify, label, and express their feelings about "heartfelt" issues and relationships with the important people in their lives. Similar to the Gingerbread Person Feelings Map and Color-Your-Life, the child picks colors to match various feelings listed and fills in the amount of each feeling experienced, thereby quantifying how they are feeling at the moment or a point in time. The child can also write on the card a response to a time when he or she had this feeling. Color Your Heart (Goodyear-Brown, 2010) is another variation utilizing a heart shape, which is colored in proportion to the amounts of feelings in the child's heart.

Use of Clay as a Metaphor for a Child's Life

Using a small piece of Play-Doh or "oogly" clay (*www.theooglykit.com*), which is very malleable and softens up quickly, I ask a child to close his or her eyes (or, if the child does not feel safe enough to do that, to stare off at something across the room) and, without looking or speaking, create something within 2 minutes. Once the time is up, I have the child look at the clay creation. Is it as the child had imagined it would be? Did it turn out the way the child expected? I then process with the child how the clay creation is much like his or her life. Things have happened in the child's life, many outside of his or her control: being put into foster or residential care, having parents who were unable to care for the child, being unable to magically change things, having other abuses happen, and so on. But just as the child is now able to change the creation, improve on it, make it more like how the child wants it to look, or start all over, so too the child can do that with his or her life. Some things may need to wait until the child is 18 years old or older, such as living independently or looking for the biological parents. But other things are things the child can change now—such as ways to react when he or she is angry, ways of coping, ways to begin loving and trusting other people, or ways to prevent being sent away to another home. And, just as the child can do with the clay creation at this moment, the child can decide whether to continue with what has turned out or to be an active force in making a difference in his or her life and in the lives of others (Drewes, 2011a; Drewes & Cavett, 2012).

Magical Smiles

I teach my foster/residential care clients that they have magic within themselves—something that no one can take from them, that is within them and with them all the time, and that is so magical it can make others do things. Intrigued, the children inevitably become interested. I tell them, "It's your smile. You have the most beautiful smile!" (And, truly, I have yet met anyone who cannot, sooner or later, produce a beautiful smile that makes me respond in turn with a smile!) Of course, once I say this, they respond with a bright smile! I challenge them with the "homework" of going out in the next week and smiling at three people of their choice (we talk about people they know and might try this with). The catch is that they need to look each person in the eye, so the other person knows they are looking at them. Then, when eye contact is made, they will smile and then see what happens. I immediately start the next session by checking on the homework and discussing the results of their smiles. Inevitably, even if they only tried it once, magic occurred in making another person smile back (Drewes, 2011a)!

Relaxation

To aid children with relaxation in general, and particularly to help them avoid acting out when angry, the guided relaxation exercise called Safe Place (Drewes, 2011a; James, 1989) is an effective way to teach deep breathing—which is a relaxation tool that can be used at any time. I ask children to sit with eyes closed, imagine being a movie director, and use their imaginations to make a movie. They are directed to breathe slowly in and out, and to think of a time and place when they felt safe. It could be lying in the sun at the beach, hiding under their covers, snuggling with a favorite pet, or the like. They are to zoom in the camera and film the location, taking in all that there is. Then they are to freeze the camera shot. As they continue to breathe slowly in and out, they look around and notice what they see, smell, hear, and feel, and whether or not there are any people or animals there. They are instructed to feel how safe they are and how relaxed they feel in their bodies while in their safe space. Next they give their special safe place a name, preferably one word. It is the key that will get them back to their safe place any time they wish to go. All they have to do is remember the name. The children continue to breathe in and out slowly, focusing on how relaxed and safe they feel. Then after a few minutes, they are directed to move the camera back slowly, and in another minute they will be back in the therapy room with their eyes open. The goal is to create an operant-conditioned link among the deep breathing, the experience of feeling safe, and the word chosen. Then when the children are upset or anxious, they can remember the word, and their bodies will automatically begin to relax (Drewes, 2011a).

SELF-CARE

We should never forget that the work we do in helping children with complex trauma takes a toll on us as therapists. We need to acknowledge that the work is demanding and stressful. It is critical that we get peer support or outside supervision, as well as monitoring and continuing education. I recommend finding personal self-care and stress management strategies that work, and using them regularly to prevent burnout and vicarious traumatization (Maschi & Brown, 2010; Norcross & Drewes, 2009; see also Maschi, Chapter

20, this volume). I also recommend collaborating with administrators and colleagues to create a work climate of respect and mental health (Foley, 2014).

CONCLUSION

The important key to being able to enter the worlds of foster or residential care children experiencing multiple losses, crises, and traumas is utilizing directive and integrative expressive arts and play-based techniques that are both playful and engaging, and that prescriptively meet the needs of the children's current symptoms and issues. It is also important to use such techniques to deal with underlying attachment and allegiance issues; to work on issues of loss, bereavement, and grief involving biological parents; and to assist with affect regulation and expression. Inclusion of foster parents and residential child care workers is critical in reinforcing gains and helping to generalize learned techniques for coping, while also building the bonds of attachment and helping to heal the holes in these children's hearts.

STUDY QUESTIONS

1. Discuss why using an integrative and prescriptive treatment approach for complex trauma is better than utilizing just a single treatment/theoretical approach.
2. What are the common factors between *in utero* addiction and complex trauma in early childhood, and the resulting psychological and brain architectural changes?
3. In what ways can the caregiver be supported in working with children in foster or residential care who have complex trauma and are exhibiting difficult behaviors?
4. What self-care strategies should therapists and caregivers utilize when working with behaviorally challenging traumatized children, and why?

REFERENCES

Belluck, P. (2012, April 30). Abuse of opiates soars in pregnant women. *New York Times*. Retrieved February 26, 2014, from *www.nytimes.com/2012/05/01/health/research/prescription-drug-abuse-soars-among-pregnant-women.html?_r=0*.

Booth, P., & Jernberg, A. (2010). *Theraplay: Helping parents and children build better relationships through attachment-based play* (3rd ed.). San Francisco: Jossey-Bass.

Brody, V. (1997). *The dialogue of touch: Developmental play therapy*. Northvale, NJ: Aronson.

Cohen, J., Mannarino, A., & Deblinger, E. (Eds.). (2012). *Trauma-focused CBT for children and adolescents: Treatment applications*. New York: Guilford Press.

Crenshaw, D. A. (2008). Heartfelt Feelings Coloring Cards strategies. In L. Lowenstein (Ed.), *Assessment and treatment activities for children, adolescents, and families* (pp. 80–81). Toronto: Champion Press.

Crenshaw, D. A., & Hardy, K. V. (2006). Understanding and treating the aggression of traumatized children in out-of-home care. In N. B. Webb (Ed.), *Working with traumatized youth in child welfare* (pp. 171–195). New York: Guilford Press.

Drewes, A. A. (2001). Gingerbread Person Feelings Map. In H. G. Kaduson & C. E. Schaefer (Eds.), *101 more favorite play therapy techniques* (pp. 92–97). Northvale, NJ: Aronson.

Drewes, A. A. (2008, December 22). *Cognitive behavioral play therapy with sexually abused children.* Presentation at The Astor Home for Children, Rhinebeck, NY.

Drewes, A. A. (2011a, April 29). *A skill-building workshop: Effectively blending play-based techniques with cognitive behavioral therapy for affect regulation in sexually abused and traumatized children.* Workshop presented at the annual conference of the Canadian Association for Child and Play Therapy, Guelph, Ontario, Canada.

Drewes, A. A. (2011b). Working with attachment disordered teens in foster care. *Play Therapy: Magazine of the British Association for Play Therapy, 68,* 6–9.

Drewes, A. A., Bratton, S. & Schaefer, C. E. (Eds.). (2011). *Integrative play therapy.* Hoboken, NJ: Wiley.

Drewes, A. A., & Cavett, A. (2012). Play applications and skills components. In J. Cohen, A. Mannarino, & E. Deblinger (Eds.), *Trauma-focused CBT for children and adolescents: Treatment applications* (pp. 105–124). New York: Guilford Press.

Earl, B. (2009). Exterior fortresses and interior fortification. In A. Perry (Ed.), *Teenagers and attachment: Helping adolescents engage with life and learning* (pp. 97–121). Duffield, UK: Worth.

Eldridge, S. (1999). *Twenty things adopted kids wish their adoptive parents knew.* New York: Bantam Dell.

Foley, G. (2014, May 22). *Early childhood mental health: Preparing children for success in school and life.* Training session conducted at Astor Services for Children and Families, Poughkeepsie Grand Hotel, Poughkeepsie, NY.

Gil, E. (2006). *Helping abused and traumatized children: Integrating directive and nondirective approaches.* New York: Guilford Press.

Goodyear-Brown, P. (2010). *Play therapy with traumatized children. A prescriptive approach.* Hoboken, NJ: Wiley.

Hughes, D. (1997). *Facilitating developmental attachment: The road to emotional recovery and behavioral change in foster and adopted children.* Northvale, NJ: Aronson.

Hughes, D. (2009). Principles of attachment and intersubjectivity. In A. Perry (Ed.), *Teenagers and attachment: Helping adolescents engage with life and learning* (pp. 123–140). Duffield, UK: Worth.

James, B. (1989). *Treating traumatized children.* Lexington, MA: Lexington Books.

Landreth, G. (2012). *Play therapy: The art of the relationship* (3rd ed.). New York: Routledge.

Landreth, G., & Bratton, S. (2005). *Child parent relationship therapy.* New York: Routledge.

Maschi, T., & Brown, D. (2010). Professional self-care and prevention of secondary trauma. In N. B. Webb (Ed.), *Helping bereaved children: A handbook for practitioners* (3rd ed., pp. 345–373). New York: Guilford Press.

McNeil, C., & Hembree-Kigin, T. (2011). *Parent–child interaction therapy* (2nd ed.). New York: Springer.

Miller, A., Rathus, J., & Linehan, M. M. (2007). *Dialectical behavior therapy with suicidal adolescents.* New York: Guilford Press.

Miller, P. W. (2005). *Body language: An illustrated introduction for teachers.* Muncie, IN: Patrick W. Miller & Associates.

National Child Traumatic Stress Network. (n.d.). Complex trauma. Retrieved July 15, 2014, from *www.nctsnet.org/trauma-types/complex-trauma*

Norcross, J., & Drewes, A. A. (2009). Self-care for child therapists: Leaving it at the office. In A. A. Drewes (Ed.), *Blending play therapy with cognitive behavioral therapy: Evidence-based and other effective treatments and techniques* (pp. 473–494). Hoboken, NJ: Wiley.

O'Connor, K. J. (1983). Color-Your-Life technique. In C. E. Schaefer & K. J. O'Connor (Eds.), *Handbook of play therapy* (pp. 251–258). New York: Wiley.

Osofsky, J. (Ed.). 2004. *Young children and trauma: Intervention and treatment.* New York: Guilford Press.

Perry, B. D. (2009). Examining child maltreatment through a neurodevelopmental lens: Clinical applications of the Neurosequential Model of Therapeutics. *Journal of Loss and Trauma, 14*, 240–255.

Powell, B., Cooper, G., Hoffman, K., & Marvin, B. (2014). *The Circle of Security intervention: Enhancing attachment in early parent–child relationships.* New York: Guilford Press.

Rice, F. K., & Groves, M. B. (2005). *Hope and healing: A caregiver's guide to helping young children affected by trauma.* Washington, DC: Zero to Three Press.

Schaefer, C. E., & Drewes, A. A. (2014). *The therapeutic powers of play: 20 core agents of change* (2nd ed.). Hoboken, NJ: Wiley.

Scheeringa, M. S., & Zeanah, C. H. (1995). Symptom expression and trauma variables in children under 48 months of age. *Infant Mental Health Journal, 16*(4), 259–270.

Schore, A. (2003a). *Affect dysregulation and disorders of the self.* New York: Norton.

Schore, A. (2003b). *Affect regulation and the repair of the self.* New York: Norton.

van der Kolk, B. A. (2005). Developmental trauma disorder: Towards a rational diagnosis for children with complex trauma histories. *Psychiatric Annals, 35*(5), 401–408.

VanFleet, R. (1994). Filial therapy for adoptive children and parents. In K. J. O'Connor & C. E. Schaefer (Eds.), *Handbook of play therapy: Vol. 2. Advances and innovations* (pp. 371–386). New York: Wiley.

Webb, N. B. (2006a). Selected treatment approaches for helping traumatized youth. In N. B. Webb (Ed.), *Working with traumatized youth in child welfare* (pp. 93–112). New York: Guilford Press.

Webb, N. B. (2006b). (Ed.). *Working with traumatized youth in child welfare.* New York: Guilford Press.

Webb, N. B. (2010). (Ed.). *Helping bereaved children: A handbook for practitioners* (3rd ed.). New York: Guilford Press.

Whitty, M., & O'Connor, J. (2007). Opiate dependence and pregnancy: 20-year follow-up study. *Psychiatric Bulletin, 31*, 450–453.

Chapter 8

Disruptions and Dissolution in Foster Care and Adoption

Play and Filial Therapy to Repair Attachment Relationships

ANNE L. STEWART
WILLIAM F. WHELAN

In this chapter, we set the stage for our discussion of loss and healing in foster care and adoption by first surveying the characteristics and experiences of the children/youth[1] and parents who currently populate the foster care system, as well as features of disruptions and dissolutions in care. We then explore the landscape of average, nontraumatic early development in children. Knowing what there is to lose, and what may have already been lost (or perhaps what was never acquired in the first place), when typical development has not occurred in a child's life will help us be aware of what each individual needs to gain in new attachment relationships with foster or adoptive parents. We describe the impact of relational losses and hurt for children and youth in foster care, and examine how this influences their play. We then describe the evidence-based approach we take to working with youth and families in foster care, discuss research findings from the attachment and psychotherapy literature, and conclude with a description of a case involving play and filial therapy.

Our stories of connection, separation, loss, and reunion are attachment narratives. These distinctive, most human of stories are the accounts of healthy,

[1]We endorse the United Nations Convention of the Rights of the Child definition of a "child," which covers all human beings under the age of 18. However, to remind the reader of the applicability of attachment principles for all children (indeed, for people across the lifespan), we use the terms "child," "youth," "adolescent," "teen," and "young person" jointly and interchangeably in the chapter.

average attachment development created from day-to-day life—encompassing millions of little moments of engagement, interaction, and emotional events that are humorous, warm, and joyful; sad, irritating, and puzzling; successful or unsuccessful; and fulfilling. They are especially human stories because attachment development unfolds in daily emotional events where small interactions, vocalizations, facial expressions, physical movements, demeanor, and emotive connections are the threads. The interpersonal fabric is woven bit by bit, and we are hardly aware of it until the fabric becomes visible and we realize the profundity and strength of our relationships. We realize how much we know and need each other. At times we can scarcely believe our good fortune and grace in having such connections with those closest to us—such inherently resilient and reliable relationships (i.e., attachments), in which the smallest moments can be enjoyed, and difficulties and disappointments can be endured. We learn through experience that we are not alone.

Most simply put, the story of healthy attachment development is the story of knowing that one is not alone. It is the story of knowing that one is firmly and safely connected to another person—not just thinking it or wishing it so, but knowing it through thousands of undeniable relationship exchanges and interactions. Most people, but not all people, have had such surety and confidence in one or more primary relationships, and they experience it so intrinsically that the sureness of it generally goes without saying. In childhood, a healthy, reliable, and confident relationship with a caregiver is called a "secure attachment."

FOSTER CARE AND ADOPTION SERVICES IN THE UNITED STATES

An estimated 399,546 children between the ages of 1 month and 18 years[2] were in foster care in the United States at the close of 2012 (Child Welfare Information Gateway, 2013). This number, which corresponds to the population of Cleveland, Ohio, actually reflects a substantial decrease (23.7%) from the 523,616 children and youth reported in foster care in 2002 (Adoption and Foster Care Analysis and Reporting System, 2014). Nearly half the children were in nonrelative foster family homes (47%), and more than a quarter were in relatives' homes (28%). (These proportions are similar percentages from recent years.) Placements in institutions (9%) and group homes (6%) accounted for the next most frequent placements (Child Welfare Information Gateway, 2013). National trends show that the number of children in foster care may be leveling off, but shifts are apparent in the racial and ethnic composition of the children (Adoption and Foster Care Analysis and Reporting System, 2014).

[2]Although the most frequent age limit for children in foster care is 18 years, some states permit children to remain in foster care to age 19, 20, or 21.

The decline in the number of African American youth in foster care was the most dramatic change across racial categories: This number fell by 47.1% between 2002 and 2012, and accounted for nearly three-quarters of the overall decline in numbers. (Despite the drop in this rate, however, African Americans remain in foster care at nearly twice the national average.) Over the same time period, the rates for white (the U.S. government's label for European American), Hispanic, Asian, and Native American children declined slightly and appear to be leveling off, though recently there appears to be a modest climb for whites and Native Americans. Since 2009, Native American youth have had the highest rates of representation in foster care. In contrast to the generally descending trend, children and adolescents identified with two or more races experienced significant growth, increasing from 13,857 to 22,942 from 2002 to 2012, and reflecting about 6% of the foster care population (Adoption and Foster Care Analysis and Reporting System, 2014). The preceding information reports the rates of representation in foster care, while the following list shows the percentages of children in foster care by race:

- African American: 26%
- Hispanic: 21%
- Multiracial (or other): 9%
- Undetermined: 3%
- White: 2%

Children may enter the foster care system from infancy onward, and the most recent data report the median age of children in the foster care system as 8 years, 5 months. From 2003 to 2012, the median ages of children entering the system and exiting the system showed distinct declines—from 8 years, 3 months to 6 years, 5 months, and from 10 years, 0 months to 8 years, 2 months, respectively.

The outcomes for youth exiting foster care (241,254 children in 2012) show that the majority (51%) were reunited with parents or other primary caregivers, and 21% were adopted. Ten percent of the children and adolescents exiting foster care were emancipated, while another 15% went to live with another relative or guardian (Adoption and Foster Care Analysis and Reporting System, 2014).

The decreases in numbers and placements for children in care coincide with the establishment of federal policies emphasizing family preservation and permanency for children in the child welfare system, such as the Adoption and Safe Families Act of 1997 and the Fostering Connections to Success and Increasing Adoptions Act of 2008. State child welfare system performance, through the Child and Family Services Review process, is monitored on a range of indicators, including the timeliness and permanency of reunification and the timeliness of adoption.

International adoptions and challenges with attachment have received attention in the professional publications and the popular press. The

Intercountry Adoption Service in the Bureau of Consular Affairs, U.S. Department of State, maintains records of adoptions of children from other countries by residents of the United States and adoptions of U.S. children by residents of other countries. The number of intercountry adoptions to the United States has decreased steadily and dramatically in recent years, from a high of 22,991 adoptions in 2004 to the 7,092 adoptions recorded for 2013 (Bureau of Consular Affairs, 2014). Children less than 5 years old accounted for 4,360 of the total number of children coming to the United States in 2013. This last statistic is especially relevant for play therapists interested in promoting healthy attachments through using filial and play therapy models, and consulting with agencies and prospective parents to help them be optimally prepared to welcome the children. At this writing, the countries with the highest number of children being adopted to the United States are (in descending order) China, Ethiopia, Russia, South Korea, and Ukraine. An interactive website (*http://adoption.state.gov/about_us/statistics.php*) permits visitors to explore the numbers of adoptions by county and by receiving states. The website includes guidance on decision-making processes, steps to begin the intercountry adoption process, and helpful resources.

DISRUPTION AND DISSOLUTION

For foster and adoptive parents, parenthood creates not only joy and fulfillment but considerable stress, resulting in strains on any such family's relational fabric. Inevitably, there are occasions (viz., "disruptions" or "dissolutions") when a child or adolescent does not continue to live in a foster or adoptive home, through voluntary or involuntary processes. The terms "disruption" and "dissolution" have specific meanings in the context of adoption and foster care. The Child Welfare Information Gateway (2012) has offered the following definitions:

> The term *disruption* is used to describe an adoption process that ends after the child is placed in an adoptive home and before the adoption is legally finalized, resulting in the child's return to (or entry into) foster care or placement with new adoptive parents.
>
> The term *dissolution* is generally used to describe an adoption in which the legal relationship between the adoptive parents and adoptive child is severed, either voluntarily or involuntarily, after the adoption is legally finalized. This results in the child's return to (or entry into) foster care or placement with new adoptive parents. (p. 1)

Accurate information regarding recent domestic disruption rates is not available, due to inconsistent reporting and compilation procedures. Rates for disruption from previously conducted studies typically range between 10 and 25%; higher rates are found for older children and adolescents, children with behavioral or emotional problems, or children with a preadoptive history of sexual abuse. Youth who have entered the child welfare system due to lack of supervision are more likely to experience adoption disruption. Children and teens placed with relatives have fewer disruptions reported. Reportedly, families with unrealistic expectations and a lack of social support from their relatives have higher rates of disruption. Factors associated with the agencies include insufficient information on the children; inadequate parental training and support; and lack of consistent staff to prepare the children/young persons and families.

Unfortunately, reliable data on adoption dissolution are even more difficult to obtain because the relevant records may be closed and identifying information may be modified at the time of legal adoption. Festinger and Maza (2009) devised a way to analyze data from the Adoption and Foster Care Analysis and Reporting System, and concluded that 0.5% of the children had experienced an adoption dissolution; an earlier study found a rate of 3.3% adoption dissolution (Festinger, 2002). Given the challenges of identifying the population, the factors associated with placement of children and adolescents back into the child welfare system have not been well examined. Relevant to play therapists' role in supporting youth and families, Festinger (2005) noted that adoptive families identified lack of information about available services and the cost of services as barriers.

ROLE OF PLAY THERAPISTS AND PLAY THERAPY WITH YOUTH AND FAMILIES IN FOSTER CARE

Play therapists are especially qualified to help to support children/adolescents and families during foster care and adoption placement crises. Most play therapists possess a comprehensive understanding of typical and atypical child development, a working knowledge of brain development and the impact of trauma, and a thorough understanding of attachment. A play therapist is able to work with a child, a parent, and (importantly) with a parent–child relationship in playful, meaningful, and engaging ways. Given the specialized systems of care, policies, and concerns confronted by children/teens and families in foster care and adoption, it is crucial for play therapists to acquire an in-depth and ongoing understanding of the issues, research, and resources associated with this population, in order to generate effective treatment plans.

Play is an often disregarded but essential component of a satisfying parent–child relationship. The founder of the National Institute for Play, Stuart Brown, theorizes that in typical child development, play creates the cornerstone for building all interpersonal relationships. Brown (2009) states that the unplanned and mutual delight between a child and parent creates a state of play. Brown, and others, further argue that the need to connect is evolutionarily wired to occur and is a pathway to healing across the age span

(Cozolino, 2010; Lieberman & Van Horn, 2010; Siegel, 2007, 2012). From this perspective, creating a safe and secure relationship and being engaged in play are intricately interwoven. For a play therapist engaging directly with a child (or helping to scaffold and support play between a parent and child), play is an affectively charged and dynamic experience that, as demonstrated in recent neuroscience research, increases levels of oxytocin, engendering feelings of emotional well-being and trust; activates mirror neurons, helping the therapist (or parent) accurately read and respond to the youth's feelings; and promotes neuroplasticity and the creation of new neural patterns (Cozolino, 2010). The positive affect triggered by play connects individuals with others, and the excitement sparked by play helps forge attuned and positive relationships. Thus the experience of play can produce a therapeutic encounter.

ATTACHMENT AS THE SUPPORT FOR ALL CHILDREN'S HEALTHY DEVELOPMENT

John Bowlby (1969/1982, 1988) described a child's attachment to a caregiver as a special kind of relational bond—one that has an evolutionary and biological basis, that serves to protect the child from a range of dangers and risk, and that also supports the child's experience in safely exploring the physical and social environment. Through relationship experiences in early childhood, most children develop reliable and rhythmic patterns of interaction (often in the context of playful encounters) with their parents, in which their needs for emotion regulation, soothing, refueling, and effective partnership behavior develop robustly. In this developing process, the door to a child's heart stays open so that communication of thoughts and emotions flows accurately and freely to the parent, and the parent's sensitive caregiving flows back through the door to the child. One result of this open-door pattern of emotional exchanges is that for most parents, children's emotions, thoughts, and attachment needs become relatively easy to discern. This makes parenting, which can be a hard enough job under the best of circumstances, much easier than it would otherwise be. As such, forming caregiving responses that have a good chance of helping is much easier for parents when they feel confident about reading and responding to their children's emotional worlds.

In early infancy, in the absence of significant medical or neurological problems, children come equipped with abilities to learn about their parents and begin recognizing the feel, look, voices, and facial expressions of their primary caregivers. This process develops through time and experience over the first few months of life, and usually by 3 months of age, a child is already able to discriminate between the primary caregiver and other people (Tronick, 2007). This early bonding continues and forms deep roots through physical and emotional experiences with the parent, and as long as there is not too much stress in the environment (for the child and/or the parent), the child's body begins to develop healthy, automatic, and effective patterns of relationship interactions.

Among these patterns are behavioral sequences that allow the child to make ready use of the parent for getting his or her physical and emotional needs met. As a child begins to look at and explore the parent's face and to make eye contact, the child notices that his or her eye gaze and facial expressions are mirrored and returned by the parent. The playful exchanges that ensue give the child a chance to experience and practice reading the parent's emotional signals and interacting with the parent, in ways that soon become reciprocal, synchronous, and satisfying physical and emotional exchanges (i.e., the child experiences the benefits of the parent's sensitive caregiving and is effectively co-regulated, soothed, and swept up into a dynamic and often joyful partnership). In turn, these reciprocal and attuned exchanges give the parent opportunities for reading and interpreting the child's behavior, and for responding sensitively to the child. Under circumstances of average stress, most children and parents have adequate opportunities in moments of daily interaction and caregiving to become successful (or at least successful enough) at reading and responding to each other's behaviors, and the child comes to experience the relationship as protective, predictable, loving, and life-giving. This affective security reflects a rich attachment–caregiving environment in which the child's chances for healthy development are optimized (Schore, 2005; Sroufe, Egeland, Carlson, & Collins, 2005). According to Schore and McIntosh (2011), "attachment drives brain development," and "brain growth is influenced by social forces and therefore is experience-dependent" (p. 502). These everyday attachment interactions or "conversations" communicate to infants, and can communicate to older children, that they are seen and valued by their caregivers (Lieberman & Van Horn, 2010). Play therapists use this same power—the power of attuned and responsive interactions—to demonstrate their interest in understanding young people's emotions and to build effective therapeutic relationships (Badenoch, 2008; Siegel, 2007).

One of the hallmarks of average secure attachment is that the child comes to rely on the parent for physical and emotional soothing; for co-regulation of experience, arousal, and anxiety; and for protection from physical and emotional stress. As this happens, the child's body becomes more and more at ease in the parent's presence and is able to fully engage the world in the moment, in play and exploration, without undue anxiety. In this way, the child's experience with the parent leads to greater confidence in the parent's ability to provide a safe and reliable environment of protection and support for exploration. Observing average healthy children at play is so enjoyable in part because the children appear so carefree, productive, happily engaged in activities, and proud of themselves, especially in the presence of parents. An average connection (attachment) with the parent is so strong and reliable, and the flow of emotional information is so free between them, that the average child is not generally concerned about his or her relationship with the parent, or worried about the parent's emotional state or safety. The average secure child is, most of the time, able to enjoy and engage in the experience and activities of childhood while feeling safe and supported.

In contrast, many if not most children and teens in foster care have had significant anxiety in relationships with their previous caregivers (e.g., biological parents or previous foster parents), and are typically worried about their parents' physical and emotional safety. Through experiences in their most important relationships, confidence in their parents' emotional availability and caregiving ability has been shaken—or perhaps hasn't yet developed very adequately in these young people. In this regard, many children and adolescents in foster care appear anxious and have underdeveloped abilities for emotional soothing, co-regulation of experience, and partnership behavior. In addition, they are often not used to letting grownups help them with emotions and behavior, and their central nervous systems are not able to make ready use of what the new caregivers have to offer. Play therapists can share these evidence-based findings with foster parents (and perhaps with social services and agency professionals) to help them comprehend the complicated, hard-to-understand, and sometimes bizarre behaviors, feelings, and reactions their youngsters exhibit (Crenshaw & Hardy, 2006).

EMOTIONS, BEHAVIORS, AND PLAY OF CHILDREN AND TEENS IN FOSTER CARE

In the absence of typically secure attachment development, children and teens in foster care (i.e., children who have experienced significant loss or maltreatment) tend to share a number of primary differences in their relationships and emotional patterns. Their neurologically based abilities in automatic self-soothing, partnership behavior, co-regulation of emotion and behavior, and abilities to make use of healthy adults are underdeveloped (Kim & Cicchetti, 2010; Rogosch, Cicchetti, Shields, & Toth, 1995). Given the reports of chronic family stress, environmental danger/chaos, and unpredictability in caregiving environments that often comprise these youth's preplacement histories, many foster children and adolescents have been (unwittingly) practicing patterns of overarousal, moderate to high anxiety, emotional inhibition, or dysregulation for much of their lives.

Problems that are predictable from this kind of emotionally isolated or emotionally dysregulated development include any or all of those related to deficits in self-regulation, coherent relationship interaction, and responsiveness to the environment. For example, it is not uncommon for youth entering foster care to have basic difficulties in their exploration and play behaviors. They have trouble forming and executing thematic play scenarios, and they sometimes don't appear aware of the use or function of typical toys, or at least tend not to use toys for their intended purposes. Their play behaviors are often truncated, repetitive, aggressive, unproductive, or frightening, or simply don't seem to go anywhere. Often the play behaviors of a 6-, 7-, or 8-year-old in foster care will look significantly less productive, coherent, and enjoyable than that of an average 2- or 3-year-old. In addition, foster parents often describe their foster children as being "difficult to read" (i.e., the doors to their hearts are closed; their behavior tends to be incongruent with the context and flow of moment-to-moment events). The children are also described as having trouble listening, paying attention, doing what they're told, learning from their mistakes, cooperating, being respectful, telling the truth, and repairing relationship upsets.

From a developmental and practical point of view, then, many foster children and teen's behaviors and emotions are confusing, seem to defy reason in a given circumstance, and appear intransigent because their internal development has not been integrated or coherent. One of the most important outcomes of average secure development is that children's internal experience and organization are coherent and generally fit with their experience of the caregiving environment. In other words, in a nonverbal and experiential way, their lives make sense, inside and out, most days, most of the time. This is a powerful foundation for them to stand upon when engaging people, problems, and the world. Many youth coming into the foster care system are partly or largely missing this naturally organized, integrated, and coherent internal experience. Their lives don't make sense, and it shows.

CHALLENGES AND INTERVENTION IN FOSTER CARE AND ADOPTION

Loss of important relationships, especially attachments, taps directly into a young person's anxiety and fear of being lost, rejected, and unwanted. These deep worries and fears are usually stoked when a child loses an attachment relationship, even when that relationship is unhealthy. In these circumstances, healing from a significant loss and the effects of maltreatment requires observation and awareness of the child/adolescent's internal experiences and behavior in seven broad areas of attachment development and functioning:

- The youth's needs for protection
- Sensitive and reflective caregiving
- Co-regulation of experience (along with development of internal rhythms of soothing)
- Partnership with the play therapist (and caregivers)
- Support for exploration
- Rhythms of forgiveness and reconciliation
- Coherence

Protection

Protection of children includes both physical and emotional protection. Physical protection is the part that usually comes more easily for play therapists and foster parents, and most are adept at securing the environment, monitoring the children's movements and behavior, and anticipating potential dangers (even in the playroom). Emotional protection can be more elusive for therapists and new caregivers, given that these children's automatic emotional signals regarding their relationship needs are partly (if not largely) inaccurate and difficult to read. Emotional protection includes protection from disruptive and troubling worries and memories from the youth's losses and past attachment experiences; protection from potential reactive and insensitive emotions of other people in the environment; protection from potential negative emotions and defensiveness that may get elicited in the play therapists and the caregivers; and protection from the children's or adolescents' own emotions, especially under circumstances of over arousal, anger, self-blame, and emotional dysregulation. Therefore, the play therapists and caregivers must find ways to welcome the youth's past and current dilemmas, to understand and tolerate the youth's distress, and to provide structure and meaning to it in the current context. Dismissing, derogating, and ignoring a child's past relationships and experiences, and behaving as though the past is not important and not part of the child's present, are very likely to make things worse. A common dilemma for foster parents, and sometimes for play therapists as well, is worrying that allowing and helping these youth deal with the effects of their past will somehow prolong their difficulties and or prevent the young persons from "forgetting about the past" and moving on. Instead, these children/adolescents need help in making sense of the past, acquiring a more balanced perspective, and find ways to continue loving their previous caregivers, even as they develop new attachment relationships.

Sensitive Caregiving and Co-Regulation

Sensitive caregiving is especially important for a play therapist as he or she begins developing a therapeutic relationship with a young person. Indeed, sensitivity is a process that tends to fuel relationship development. As Mary Ainsworth and her colleagues described it, sensitivity involves skill in observing a child's behavior accurately; making developmentally reasonable interpretations of the child's behavior regarding the thoughts and emotions represented; and then forming a caregiving response that will be helpful to the child in the moment (Ainsworth, Blehar, Waters, & Wall, 1978). Given that many foster children and adolescents automatically exhibit confusing emotional behavior, separating the "signals" from the "noise" is an important early step for play therapists and caregivers. Being able to recognize when these youth's behaviors are inaccurate or "noisy" in relation to their attachment needs can prevent play therapists and caregivers from becoming overly focused on misbehaviors and from being led astray from the youth's emotional needs. For example, when foster children and adolescents are upset or anxious, they often say and do things that, in effect, push away their foster parents, distract them, or hurt the parents' feelings, and make it more difficult for the parents to engage and help them at times when the youth need it the most. Instead of eliciting physical and emotional co-regulation from their new parents or play therapists, they do things that elicit confusion, punishment, or teaching and lecturing. Examples include episodes in which children and teens act as though they are not emotionally upset or anxious, don't need their parents' help, want to be alone, or want to get away. Other examples of common attachment "noise" and inaccurate communication include patterns of lying, stealing, aggression, disrespectful or provocative vocal tone and verbalizations, and secretive behavior. From a developmental point of view, these patterns typically arise in the absence of sensitive, reliable, and co-regulating partnership behavior with a reflective caregiver. In this way, such behaviors are often echoes of the past and reflect long-standing unhealthy patterns that have been activated, rather than intentional behaviors related to current events in their new relationships.

The Experience of Felt Partnership and Support for Interaction

Another attachment need important throughout development is the experience of felt partnership with a sensitive, benevolent, and reflective caregiver. In this sense, although "partnership" includes both the emotional and practical connotations of the term, its most important meaning for foster youth may have to do with the experience of palpable and reliable companionship. A secure caregiver or play therapist lets the young person know that the two of them are "in it" together. At times the caregiver or therapist leads and organizes relationship interactions so that the child/adolescent can feel their togetherness and can begin to learn through experience that, most of all, the parent or therapist wants to be with the youth. This tends to free the young person from anxiety and makes it more likely that the youth will (somehow) express what is in his or her heart and mind. It also helps release the youth from fears of failure and of disappointing the caregiver or being rejected. The experience of being in each other's presence is its own reward, without necessarily including any other agenda, and helps the child/adolescent learn that this new relationship is more important than his or her performance or compliance; those abilities will come with time. A danger for many foster and adoptive parents comes from their worry about the future and feelings of responsibility (and pressure) to "fix," correct, or educate these youth. When this happens, they may inadvertently focus too much on the young persons' competence and performance in doing things correctly, in following rules, and in doing chores and schoolwork. An overfocus on competence and learning can result in distracting a caregiver from the relationship itself and from a youth's more basic attachment needs (e.g., for a partner who is an active, personal helper and booster, and not simply a task master and rule enforcer). Nonetheless, competence, cooperation, learning and achievement are more likely outcomes in the context of average co-regulation and secure partnership behavior.

Among others, a simple and enjoyable approach for helping a child/adolescent experience the palpable (and healing) effects of co-regulation and partnership behavior can be found in narrating some of the child's experiences through the day while imbuing them with structure and meaning. This process involves finding opportunities to sit as an "angel" on the young person's shoulder—helping the youth become aware of what is happening to and around him or her, and making some simple statements about what it means for the adult and youth as partners in this moment of discovery, joy, sadness, or anxiety. As the child/adolescent becomes close to the adult as an interaction partner, he or she will have the opportunity to witness the adult's physical and emotional responses, thoughts, and behaviors in real time to a shared event. With any luck, and over time, the young person will be swept up in the caregiver's life and begin to experience the physical and emotional world in new ways that are more realistic and healthy than his or her previous experiences have been. This experience of intimate partnership is part of the process of change and healing.

For example, a child who has perhaps never witnessed (i.e., vicariously experienced) a caregiver successfully navigate emotional upset or disappointment at an unanticipated turn of events now has a chance to do so. The child can share the parent's experience, the rise of emotion, the disappointment, and the physical and emotional feel of the parent's staying balanced and regulated throughout to resolution of the event and return to normal baseline (homeostasis). The child also absorbs the experience through the parent's tone of voice and gets to hear the parent narrate the event, his or her emotions, and the meaning for both of them. In such an experience, the child's body can learn that the ups and downs of daily life need not become destabilizing, but rather can be navigated with strength, confidence, and even humor. Repeated practice with the parent in these kinds of situations can help build neurological subroutines of soothing and co-regulation within the child. By another name, this is one form of healing.

Rhythms of Forgiveness and Reconciliation

In average secure development, patterns of forgiveness and reconciliation typically emerge out of experience in attachment–caregiving interactions. Given that occasional emotional and relationship upsets are normal parts of average family life, most children/adolescents have many opportunities to gain experience in navigating small relationship upsets, with parents leading the way. Through such experiences, the children/adolescents learn that upsets are not dangerous or threatening, that emotions will be soothed, and that parents will lead the way in "making up" so their relationships are repaired and set right again.

Coherence

As foster parents and play therapists lead and shape reliable and sensitive interactions with a child/adolescent, they are also creating a new experiential narrative that makes sense to the youth. Often missing from foster children's earlier (i.e., preplacement) development is adequate practice in reality-based interactions, including intimate experience with adults' emotions that are modulated, congruent with situational context, and helpful in regulating children's emotion and relationship experience. As foster parents and play therapists accurately observe children's attachment patterns, they can become more sensitive and effective in leading the young persons into emotional partnership experiences, co-regulating the youth's behavior, and providing them with predictable emotional responses in caregiving.

EVIDENCE-BASED PRACTICE FOR USING PLAY THERAPY AND ATTACHMENT-BASED APPROACHES FOR YOUTH IN FOSTER CARE

The American Psychological Association's (2006) definition for "evidence-based practice" is the "integration of the best available research with clinical expertise in the context of patient characteristics, culture, and preferences" (p. 273). Integrating the "best available research" means that play therapists must be familiar with current scientific results regarding intervention techniques, diagnostically determined disorders, and clinical problems. Although the field of play therapy does not yet have sufficient empirical support from studies using randomized trials with control groups, it does have a sound foundation demonstrating its effectiveness with a number of emotional and behavioral issues and populations, in studies with quasi-experimental designs, correlational designs, and pre- and posttest methodologies (see Bratton, Ray, Rhine, & Jones, 2005; Ray, 2015). There are book chapters and articles discussing clinical and research support for the use of play therapy with children in foster care (Bratton, Carne-Holt, & Ceballos, 2011; Clausen, Ruff, Von Wiederhold, & Heineman, 2012). Additional support for the use of play therapy and filial therapy is obtained by examining their effectiveness in addressing symptoms presented by children in foster care, including depressed mood, anger, and disruptions in relationships. Attachment-informed interventions that incorporate play as a mechanism for healing or for enhancing the quality of the parent–child relationship include Theraplay (Booth & Jernberg, 2010), child–parent relationship therapy (Bratton, Opiola, & Dafoe, 2015), and flexible sequential play therapy (Goodyear-Brown, 2010).

The importance of integrating "clinical expertise" to inform best practices for children/adolescents and families in foster care and adoption covers a wide range of skills, strategies, techniques, and resources. To promote positive therapeutic outcomes for these young people and families, play therapists should (1) display the ability to establish and maintain a strong therapeutic alliance with the youth and caregivers; (2) possess knowledge of attachment theory, relevant findings from neuroscience, and mechanisms of co-regulation of emotion; (3) demonstrate knowledge of the impact of trauma and effective trauma interventions; (4) exhibit consultation skills with child welfare agencies and schools; (5) have knowledge of parent–child and family-based interventions; and (6) demonstrate an awareness of systemwide child protective policies and programs, as well as specific foster care and adoption intervention programs and resources (Coakley & Berrick, 2008; Goodyear-Brown, 2010; Stewart & Green, 2015; Webb, 2011). It is crucial for therapists to incorporate a thorough assessment as they build conceptualizations to guide and evaluate their interventions (Nader, Chapter 2, this volume; Webb, 2011).

Integrating "patient characteristics, culture, and preferences" into treatment for clients in the foster care system is crucial. An initial and enduring task in play therapy is to create a strong therapeutic alliance with a child/adolescent who has not experienced the powerful security of protection and comfort from a caring adult. Successful play therapists understand the importance of engaging in a responsive and attuned manner. A play therapist creates a meaningful treatment plan that incorporates the child/adolescent's age, developmental status, medical and educational history, presenting symptoms, and other problems. The interactions of culture, gender, and familial factors and stressors (e.g., ethnicity/race, socioeconomic status, religion, disability status, family structure, employment status) with the impact of the institutional and environmental contexts (e.g., prior trauma and current safety, health care disparities, and access to care) all must be considered in completing an inclusive intake and formulating a relevant case conceptualization.

THE CASE OF TYLER, AGE 7

This case example is a composite based on our shared clinical experience.

Tyler did not look up when I entered the waiting room. His sturdy 7-year-old frame was slouched over but filled with tension (and, I guessed, apprehension). He was seated beside and slightly leaning against his foster mother, Ms. Elkins. I filed away a memory of that scene, thinking it was a hopeful sign that he was able to lean on his foster mother after being placed in the home for just 6 months. After Ms. Elkins told him that she would be waiting for him, followed by "See you later, alligator," and a playful fist bump, Tyler reluctantly separated from her and dragged his way down the hallway to the playroom.

As usual, I met with Mr. and Ms. Elkins prior to beginning play therapy with their foster child. The Elkinses, who had been foster parents for three previous children, shared their knowledge of Tyler's history, as well as their current concerns. Tyler's developmental history was limited by a complete lack of medical and educational care until his removal from his birth home at age 4, following a complaint from a neighbor. The foster parents said that according to the department of social services records, Tyler had sustained extreme neglect and chronic physical and sexual abuse by his birth parents, who were both addicted to methamphetamine and alcohol. An agreement to terminate parental rights was obtained, and, due largely to the documentation of the severe physical injuries Tyler had sustained, both parents were prosecuted and incarcerated. The Elkinses were clearly upset about this horrific history, but demonstrated a high level of acceptance of Tyler, commenting positively about the resilience and strength that had enabled him to withstand such harm.

Mr. and Ms. Elkins shared that the placement with them was Tyler's fifth foster home in less than 3 years. They noted that the other disruptions were due to his explosive and aggressive behavior, including hitting, biting, cursing, and violent threats against the foster parents and other family members. Similar reports about episodes of aggressive and frightening behavior had been forwarded from his teachers. Importantly, however, comments about Tyler's likeability and his ability to get along with peers (albeit sporadically) were also noted in the reports from school. Due to his behavioral difficulties and questions about his academic abilities, Tyler was scheduled to complete a comprehensive psychoeducational evaluation to determine his eligibility for services. The Elkinses reported that they found Tyler's behavior challenging, but that they also saw a little boy, in their words, "overwhelmed with worry and so hungry, so ready for love and attention."

Therapist's Reflection

After meeting with the Elkinses, I reflected on the information they had shared. The foster parents had already shown a remarkable ability to take Tyler's perspective and to set limits on his behaviors without escalating coercive interactions. They accomplished this primarily by anticipating stressful situations and staying close by to help Tyler navigate both everyday and novel tasks, accompanied by authentic (not overly bright) expressions of delight, and punctuated by a routine that had become a fun ritual—their celebratory fist bump. They described this way of parenting as still new to them and called it their "coaching for co-regulation" approach. The couple had participated in an attachment-based parent education class for foster parents prior to Tyler's placement; both parents said that the information from the class had been vital in helping them understand Tyler's provocative behaviors (such as name calling or balling up his fists) differently, by calling it "noise." They said they now understood how quickly children with traumatic and neglectful histories could become dysregulated and respond by behaving in ways that did not allow their needs for nurturance to be met. The parents were discovering ways to maintain their expectations for behavior, and realized how important it was for them to remain calm and close by when Tyler was overwhelmed and unable to more forward adaptively on his own. They believed that the "coaching for co-regulation" strategy was helping to protect Tyler from further disorganized and hurtful behavior when his own emotions were just too big and intense for him. They readily acknowledged that Tyler's strong reactions often did not match the event to which he was responding, and that it took him much longer to calm down than they expected; however, they reported that over the past 6 months, his outbursts had gradually become less frequent and less extreme.

Collateral Contacts and Review of the Literature

Outcomes for children in foster care are improved with coordinated care, so I contacted Tyler's teacher and school counselor to hear their ideas about him. Both expressed concern about his aggressive behaviors, and particularly about how much more upset he seemed to get when they tried to help him problem-solve a different way to react. They also noted how enjoyable he could be when he was involved in hands-on learning (e.g., activity-based science lessons).

I then met with the teacher and counselor to share information about an attachment-based and trauma-informed approach to address Tyler's misbehavior (Siegel, 2007; Steele & Malchiodi, 2012). Although the expectations for his behavior remained the same, the teacher, counselor, and I generated strategies to use with Tyler after misconduct. For example, the school's typical strategy was to place the student in a short time out, hold a teacher–student discussion regarding causes/reasons for the problem, and then compose a plan to prevent future misbehavior. Given Tyler's history of neglect and harmful parenting, and his tendency toward rapid dysregulation, it was clear that he would not be soothed or learn how to become better regulated by being placed in time out. Furthermore, the staff members realized that he would not be able even briefly to discuss his misbehavior or problem-solve alternatives while he was so upset, and they agreed to discontinue the usual approach to behavior problems. Instead, they integrated information from an attachment perspective and devised a way to stay close by him and help him become calm (much as the foster parents did). The school counselor developed and practiced a variety of playful cognitive-behavioral techniques to use for this purpose with Tyler at school. For example, when he was distressed, he could show (not even have to say) his level of upset by pointing to a color on a paint chip sample.

Consultation with Tyler's developmental pediatrician included a discussion about a possible trial of medication for anxiety. A review of the literature showed that preadoptive risk factors such as prenatal drug exposure, male gender, a history of male sexual abuse, and multiple out-of-home placements were linked to acting-out behaviors, which in turn were associated with post-adoptive disruptions (Goldman & Ryan, 2011). Unfortunately, Tyler's records showed that he had all these adverse events in his brief history. However, the literature also showed the affirmative influence of caregiver acceptance, commitment, and positive attributions about the child. These responses could contribute to creating protective relationships and environments that would promote healing. One study found that in a circular way, positive appraisals from caregivers helped children re-author their own negative appraisals of themselves (and others) in moment-to-moment interactions (Ackerman & Dozier, 2005).

Play Therapy and Filial Therapy Sessions

Tyler toured the playroom, methodically picking up and examining the toys, games, and sandtray figures, but keeping his back to me. He stood for a while in front of the guns and knives; he then reached into the shelf, abruptly selected a deck of cards, turned to me, and asked, "Wanna play?" For the next 3 weeks, Tyler played a variety of card games, such as War, Uno, and his own changeable version of Rummy, always making sure that he won each game. He was very precise in his direction of how each game was to be played and became quickly upset if there was any deviation. Initially, Tyler only offered comments on my poor choices or bad luck, and on his superior skills and talent at the game. Then he began to add expressions of sympathy that I was always losing. During this time, I offered comments about how great it was to be in charge sometimes, that it felt good to win, and how important it was to him that things turn out just the way he wished in the game.

In the fourth session and thereafter, Tyler became focused on using toy cars and the sandtray in the sessions. As with the card games, Tyler's initial play with the cars and with human figures in the sandtray was rigid and controlling; he created precise scripts and prescribed specific actions for me to fulfill. The play was filled with cars crashing or figures getting hurt or killed, often trying to get through impossible dilemmas with no solution. This was much like his early life experiences with his own birth parents, it seemed. Gradually, however, rescues became a part of the play, followed by repairs of the damage and injuries. Lastly—and this was a joy to see—this little soul became a genuine partner in play and would follow plots and disruptions introduced by me. Tyler created roads in the sand for our cars to go on grand adventures together. We confronted and successfully navigated dangers and hardships, accepting and providing help to each other along the journey.

Every third session of play therapy, a parent consultation was conducted. The Elkinses reported that Tyler continued to act in ways that "pushed away" their support. They persevered, trying not to be distracted by his provocative behavioral "noise," and instead to respond sensitively to his needs for support and nurturance. We discussed a wide variety of ways to develop Tyler's ability to be soothed and his capacity to self-soothe. The strategies included practicing deep breathing (in moments of distress and during regular bedtime family meditation time), reading stories with therapeutic messages, and taking tai chi lessons with his foster father.

A series of 12 biweekly filial therapy sessions were held to supplement the play therapy sessions. Each filial session included a sequence of brief, engaging playful activities from the Theraplay model (Booth & Jernberg, 2010) and family expressive arts or sandtray activities. These activities provided opportunities to practice co-regulation of Tyler's emotions (excitement, disappointment, frustration, etc.), as well as to engage in pleasurable exploration and partnership behaviors. We also discussed the vital importance of not behaving in frightening ways, such as yelling or hitting. With Tyler, the Elkinses put together a number of "memory books" to create a narrative of his life with his birth family, his previous foster families, and their time together. The stories addressed his questions and confusion about his biological parents, and helped ease his worries that he might be separated from the Elkins household (as he had been from all the earlier ones).

After 11 months, Tyler's aggressive behaviors had decreased substantially. For termination, a particularly challenging event for children in foster care, I held a final celebration with him and his foster parents. Due to the rarified meaning of separations and loss in Tyler's life, we spent a few weeks preparing for the session. In addition, we extended the time between sessions to 3 weeks for the final three meetings. At the termination session, the Elkinses and Tyler played their favorite activities from the filial sessions—and, as Tyler had requested, we had a cake topped with cars to represent him, Mr. and Ms. Elkins, and me.

The Elkinses and I also had a termination session where we discussed Tyler's progress, their own trials, and anticipated challenges ahead. The success of the treatment was due in large part to Mr. and Ms. Elkins's ability to create a strong therapeutic alliance with me and to be sensitive to Tyler's emotional needs. The Elkinses did not permit Tyler to push them away with "noisy" misbehavior and aggression; rather, they found ways to stay in proximity to Tyler and to meet his needs for co-regulation and connection. They remained curious about and committed to understanding him and taking his perspective; this commitment provided him with protection from overwhelming emotions and helped him find ways to become calm and be soothed. In addition to helping Tyler explore the affective realm, the Elkins actively engaged Tyler in an exploration of their neighborhood and community—all in the context of their caring relationship with him.

Day by day, the Elkins household, the school, and the play therapy sessions provided environments that helped Tyler develop more normative regulatory capacities. The sessions emphasized the role of rituals and clear expectations for behavior, and—most importantly in this context—warm, attuned, and responsive relationships. In each setting, caring adults established routines with meaning (e.g., bedtime routines, mediation, fist bumps) and initiated repairs and apologies when feelings were hurt and threatening acts occurred. Over time, Tyler started to relax into the message—from the Elkinses, his community, and the world—that "We are here for you."

CONCLUSION

Using the explanatory power of an attachment-based approach to intervention for children/adolescents and families in foster care enhances the youth's opportunity for building internal coherence and improving affect regulation. We wish for all foster children/adolescents a life where their emotions and relationships make sense. Providing protection, co-regulation, and relationship security and coherence can go a long way toward healing the effects of loss and maltreatment, and can set a child on a healthy developmental trajectory.

STUDY QUESTIONS

1. Review the information describing the characteristics of children (ages, ethnicities, placements, etc.) in the foster care system. What information surprised you and why? Think about the source of your surprise: Is it a lack of experience, misinformation, or biases regarding children in the foster care system, or were you surprised for other reasons? How might these beliefs influence your role with families, colleagues, and the public?
2. Reflect on your knowledge and/or experience with children and families in foster care. What do you believe would help prevent disruptions or dissolutions?
3. Consider the process of co-regulating a child's emotions, thinking, and behavior. What are some ways you can do this in play therapy, using your tone of voice, statements, and affect?
4. Imagine narrating your own thoughts and emotions regarding partnership experiences with a child in the playroom. What would you say to help the child feel your emotional partnership? What would you say to help the child discover that you are beginning to accurately see and understand him or her?

REFERENCES

Ackerman, J., & Dozier, M. T. (2005). The influence of foster parent investment on children's representations of self and attachment figures. *Applied Developmental Psychology, 26*, 507–520.

Adoption and Foster Care Analysis and Reporting System. (2014). *Recent demographic trends in foster care, Data Brief 2013-1*. Washington, DC: U.S. Department of Health and Human Services, Administration for Children and Families. Retrieved from *www.acf.hhs.gov/sites/default/files/cb/data_brief_foster_care_trends1.pdf.*

Ainsworth, M. D. S., Blehar, M. C., Waters, E., & Wall, S. (1978). *Patterns of attachment: Psychological study of the Strange Situation*. Hillsdale, NJ: Erlbaum.

American Psychological Association, Task Force on Evidence-Based Practice. (2006). Evidence-based practice in psychology. *American Psychologist, 61*, 271–285.

Badenoch, B. (2008). *Being a brain-wise therapist: A practical guide to interpersonal neurobiology*. New York: Norton.

Booth, P., & Jernberg, A. (2010). *Theraplay: Helping parents and children build better relationships through attachment-based play* (3rd ed.). San Francisco: Jossey-Bass.

Bowlby, J. (1982). *Attachment and loss: Vol. 1. Attachment*. New York: Basic Books. (Original work published 1969)

Bowlby, J. (1988). *A secure base: Parent–child attachment and healthy human development*. New York: Basic Books.

Bratton, S., Carnes-Holt, K., & Ceballos, P. (2011). An integrative humanistic play therapy approach to treating adopted children with a history of attachment disruptions. In A. A. Drewes, S. C. Bratton, & C. E. Schaefer (Eds.), *Integrative play therapy* (pp. 341–370). Hoboken, NJ: Wiley.

Bratton, S. C., Opiola, K., & Dafoe, E. (2015). Child–parent relationship therapy (CPRT): A 10-session filial therapy model. In D. A. Crenshaw & A. L. Stewart (Eds.), *Play therapy: A comprehensive guide to theory and practice* (pp. 129–140). New York: Guilford Press.

Bratton, S., Ray, D., Rhine, T., & Jones, L. (2005). The efficacy of play therapy with children: A meta-analytic review of the outcome research. *Professional Psychology: Research and Practice, 36*(4), 376–390.

Brown, S. (2009). *Play: How it shapes the brain, opens the imagination, and invigorates the soul.* New York: Penguin.

Bureau of Consular Affairs, U.S. Department of State. (2014). Intercountry adoption: Statistics. Retrieved from *http://adoption.state.gov/about_us/statistics.php.*

Child Welfare Information Gateway. (2012). *Adoption disruption and dissolution.* Washington, DC: U.S. Department of Health and Human Services, Children's Bureau.

Child Welfare Information Gateway. (2013). *Foster care statistics 2012.* Washington, DC: U.S. Department of Health and Human Services, Children's Bureau. Retrieved from *www.childwelfare.gov/pubs/factsheets/foster.pdf.*

Clausen, J. M., Ruff, S. C., Von Wiederhold, W., & Heineman, T. V. (2012). For as long as it takes: Relationship-based play therapy for children in foster care. *Psychoanalytic Social Work, 19*, 43–53.

Coakley, J. F., & Berrick, J. D. (2008). Research review: In a rush to permanency: Preventing adoption disruption. *Child and Family Social Work, 13*, 101–112.

Cozolino, L. (2010). *The neuroscience of psychotherapy: Healing the social brain* (2nd ed.). New York: Norton.

Crenshaw, D. A. & Hardy, K. V. (2006). Understanding and treating the aggression of traumatized children in out-of-home care. In N. B. Webb (Ed.), *Working with traumatized youth in child welfare* (pp. 171–195). New York: Guilford Press.

Festinger, T. (2002). After adoption: Dissolution or permanence? *Child Welfare, 81*(3), 515–533.

Festinger, T. (2005). Adoption disruption: Rates, correlates, and service needs. In G. P. Mallon & P. M. Hess (Eds.), *Child welfare for the 21st century: A handbook of practices, policies, and programs* (2nd ed., pp. 452–468). New York: Columbia University Press.

Festinger, T., & Maza, P. (2009). Displacement or post-adoption placement?: A research note. *Journal of Public Child Welfare, 3*, 275–286.

Goldman, G., & Ryan, S. (2011). Direct and modifying influences of selected risk factors on children's pre-adoption functioning and post-adoption adjustment. *Children and Youth Services Review, 33*, 291–300.

Goodyear-Brown, P. (2010). *Play therapy with traumatized children: A prescriptive approach.* Hoboken, NJ: Wiley.

Kim, J., & Cicchetti, D. (2010). Longitudinal pathways linking child maltreatment, emotion regulation, peer relations, and psychopathology. *Journal of Child Psychology and Psychiatry, 51*(6), 706–716.

Lieberman, A., & Van Horn, P. (2010). *Psychotherapy with infants and young children.* New York: Guilford Press.

Ray, D. C. (2015). Research in play therapy: Empirical support for practice. In D. A. Crenshaw & A. L. Stewart (Eds.), *Play therapy: A comprehensive guide to theory and practice* (pp. 467–482). New York: Guilford Press.

Rogosch, F. A., Cicchetti, D., Shields, A., & Toth, S. L. (1995). Parenting dysfunction in child maltreatment. In M. H. Bornstein (Ed.), *Handbook of parenting* (Vol. 4, pp. 127–159). Mahwah, NJ: Erlbaum.

Schore, A. N. (2005). Back to basics: Attachment, affect regulation, and the developing right brain: Linking developmental neuroscience to pediatrics. *Pediatrics in Review, 26*, 204–211.

Schore, A. N., & McIntosh, J. (2011). Family law and the neuroscience of attachment, Part 1. *Family Court Review, 49*(3), 501–512.

Siegel, D. J. (2007). *The mindful brain: Reflection and attunement in the cultivation of well-being.* New York: Norton.

Siegel, D. J. (2012). *The developing mind: How relationships and the brain interact to shape who we are* (2nd ed.). New York: Guilford Press.

Sroufe, L. A., Egeland, B., Carlson, E., & Collins, W. A. (2005). *The development of the person: The Minnesota Study of Risk and Adaptation from Birth to Adulthood.* New York: Guilford Press.

Steele, W., & Malchiodi, C. A. (2012). *Trauma-informed practices with children and adolescents.* New York: Routledge.

Stewart, A. L., & Green, E. (2015). Integrated approaches to play therapy. In E. Green & A. Myrick (Eds.), *No child left forgotten.* Lanham, MD: Rowman & Littlefield.

Tronick, E. (2007). *The neurobehavioral and social-emotional development of infants and children.* New York: Norton.

Webb, N. B. (2011). *Social work practice with children* (3rd ed.). New York: Guilford Press.

Chapter 9

The Traumatic Aftermath of Parental Abandonment, Separation, and Divorce

Play and Family Therapy to Deal with Ongoing Crises

PAMELA DYSON

"I wish someone would invent a machine that would make my parents be nice to each other."
"I don't know if my parents are going to get divorced or stay separated forever."
"The worst day of my life was when my mom and dad told me they were getting a divorce."

These are typical statements made by children experiencing separation and divorce, who are often caught in the middle of warring parents. Uncertainty regarding what is presently happening and what might happen in the future can produce anxiety in such children. They often feel responsible for the parental breakup and fear abandonment by the noncustodial parent. This chapter addresses the impact of parental separation and divorce on children; it then explores how play therapy, facilitated by a sensitive, knowledgeable therapist, can support a child through the crisis of divorce.

DIVORCE TRENDS

Of the 253 million people over 15 years of age living in the United States, approximately 2.2% are separated and 11.1% are divorced. A substantial number of these persons' households include children under the age of 18 (U.S.

Census Bureau, 2012). In the year 2000, the national divorce rate stood at 4.0 per 1,000 persons. By 2008–2009, it had declined to the rate of 3.5 per 1,000 persons. It rebounded to 3.6 per 1,000 persons in 2010–2011 (National Center for Health Statistics, 2013). The reasons behind these fluctuating divorce rates are uncertain, but the economy may have played a role. From December 2007 to June 2009, the United States faced an 18-month economic recession (National Bureau of Economic Research, 2010). Loss of employment, declining home values, legal fees, costs of maintaining two households, and additional child care may limit couples' financial resources and make divorce more costly, or contribute to couples' postponing or even forgoing divorce. On the other hand, a recession may contribute to significant financial and emotional stress for married couples that can lead to marital unhappiness and divorce (Cohen, 2014).

LIVING ARRANGEMENTS FOLLOWING DIVORCE

Divorce decrees include provisions for legal custody, or decision-making responsibility for children. They also include provisions for physical custody, which outline with whom minor children will live and for how long at a time. During most of the 20th century, children lived with their mothers in a sole-physical-custody arrangement after divorce because mothers were viewed as better caregivers for children. Fathers visited their children on the weekends and holidays. In recent years, however, significant changes have occurred in children's living arrangements after a divorce. The percentage of mothers granted sole physical custody declined from 80% in 1986 to 42% in 2008. The number of fathers with sole physical custody during that time period declined from 11 to 9%. Shared, or joint, physical custody among parents increased dramatically, from 5 to 27% (Cancian, Meyer, Brown, & Cook, 2014). Many states are adopting custody policies that include the involvement of both parents, based on what is deemed to be in the best interests of children.

With more and more children dividing their time between their parents, they must deal with transitions between two households on a regular basis. The frequency of such transitions can be stressful for children. The rules of each household and the parenting style of each parent require children to adapt to each situation. They have to remember what clothes, toys, and other items should be with them in each household.

Children must also adapt to losing the ability to communicate at will with the absent parent (Kelly & Emery, 2003). One child I saw said, "Sometimes when I'm with my dad, I have something I want to tell my mom. It's hard to only be able to talk to your mom on the phone when you wish you could talk to her in person." Each time children leave one parent for the other, they may experience the emotional loss of the parent they are leaving, even if they will only be separated for a day (Saposnek, 1998). Another child said, "I miss my mom when I'm with my dad, and when I go to my mom's house I miss my dad." Advances in technology have provided divorced parents and children with additional ways of staying in touch. Skype, FaceTime, email, and text messaging all give a parent the ability to connect with children when the children are with the other parent. However, a parent who has a conflicting or hostile relationship with his or her ex-partner may not welcome having the children communicate with the absent parent during their time together. This means that although the technology exists for long-distance communication, the children may not be able to use it without risking disapproval or alienation of the resident parent.

THE IMPACT OF DIVORCE ON CHILDREN

The amount of time that a child spends with a parent, and their shared living arrangements, are likely to shape the quality of the parent–child attachment. The parent (either the father or the mother) with whom the child primarily resides is extremely likely to be the one with whom the child feels more secure. The timing of parental divorce can also have an impact on attachment. One study found that when divorce occurred during early childhood, people reported more parental attachment insecurity than did people who were older when their parents divorced (Fraley & Hefferman, 2013).

The majority of children experience a range of feelings during the early stages of separation and divorce. When parents announce they are going to separate, most children respond with anger, apprehensiveness, and opposition to the divorce. They may also experience sadness over the loss of the family structure, anxiety about who will take care of them, fear of abandonment by their parents, and guilt over feeling responsible for the parental breakup. Their responses will be influenced by their age and their developmental stage (Wallerstein & Kelly, 1996).

The developmental process involves a series of tasks a child needs to master in order to function within the world. Each stage of development brings with it new tasks, and each task provides the foundation for the ones that follow. A child's reaction to the conflict between divorcing parents may interrupt this normal developmental progress (Davies, 2011). Therapists should provide education to divorcing parents regarding developmental milestones, so that parents can approach their children with empathy and understanding, and will be better equipped to respond appropriately (McGuire & McGuire, 2001).

Opinions on the long-term effects of divorce on children are divided because much of the research comes to very different conclusions. The 25-year longitudinal study begun by Judith Wallerstein in the 1970s concluded that the effects of divorce on a significant minority of children lingered into adulthood and included anxiety, depression, fear of failure, and fear of commitment (Wallerstein, Lewis, & Blakeslee, 2000). E. Mavis Hetherington's three decades of research found that 25% of children from divorced families, compared to 10% of children from nondivorced families, had serious social, emotional, or psychological problems. However, the great majority of children of divorce showed little long-term damage, and, as adults, were functioning as well as their peers from intact families (Hetherington & Kelly, 2002). Nevertheless, even the 25% statistic represents a substantial number of children affected by divorce who could benefit from therapeutic interventions.

PLAY THERAPY WITH CHILDREN OF DIVORCE

Child Custody and Consent to Treat

A therapist working with a child of divorced parents will need informed consent from the appropriate legal guardian giving permission for the child to be in therapy. It must not be presumed that the person who wants to bring the child for therapy has custodial rights (Landreth, 2012). The therapist needs to request a copy of the most recent court order addressing who has the authority to give consent for treatment. It is important for therapists to carefully review the legal documents that pertain to children of divorce before proceeding with treatment, and to stay up to date on statutes regarding these minors in the state in which they practice (Hartsell & Bernstein, 2013). Complaints against therapists are often filed with state licensing boards by disgruntled parents in divorce and custody cases. The process of having a complaint removed can be financially and emotionally draining to a therapist.

Some divorced parents may have a hidden agenda when seeking therapy for their children: They may be seeking professional support to use in legal proceedings regarding custody. Therapists may be able to prevent these types of situations from arising by having parents sign an agreement during the intake session that the role of the therapist is to provide therapy only, and not to provide custody evaluations or to make recommendations to the court. Such an agreement is not legally binding, but it does give a therapist a strong basis for a motion for a protective order if helping a child was the purpose of the therapy, rather than assisting with a lawsuit (McGuire & McGuire, 2001).

Involving Parents in the Therapeutic Process

It is beneficial to the entire family if a child's symptoms are viewed from and dealt with in the context of the family system. Divorce greatly disrupts the family system, and children and parents alike have to make adjustments that can be challenging (McGuire & McGuire, 2001). It is also beneficial to be knowledgeable of and sensitive to the systemic nature of parental disputes (Saposnek, 1998) when providing therapeutic services to divorced families. The likelihood that child therapy will be successful is enhanced when both parents agree on the nature of the treatment that will be implemented (Hartsell & Bernstein, 2013). My policy is to meet with both parents, preferably together, before I meet with their child. I do not include the child in this session because I want the parents to be able to speak freely without upsetting the child. During this initial consultation, all required paperwork is completed, and I explain the therapeutic process. I recommend to the parents that they alternate bringing their child to therapy sessions, as doing so communicates to the child that both parents are committed to the process. I obtain a detailed family history, and I give each parent an opportunity to share information about him- or herself and the child. I answer their questions and validate their concerns.

This kind of arrangement is the ideal. However, when a divorce is very hostile, it may not be advisable to see the parents together. They may be too invested in arguing and making their own points. In that case, plans should be made to see the parents separately and to include them both in follow-up reports about the child. In some such cases, the parents may not even agree to the idea of therapy. When there is serious division about this decision and about other matters concerning the child, the court may appoint a guardian *ad litem*, whose job it is to represent the best interests of the child.

Divorcing parents are under tremendous stress and experiencing a myriad of emotions, which they often express while meeting with me. I acknowledge the feelings they are expressing, and I try to convey empathy and help them feel heard and understood. I am cautious not to align myself with one parent or the other, however, and I avoid being caught in the middle of their disputes, as this can add to the conflict and cause more emotional distress for their child. A strategy I utilize to keep parents' disputes from escalating during the session is requesting that they bring along a photo of their child. When interactions between the parents become tense, I point to the photo as a gentle reminder of the reason why we are meeting.

Play Therapy Interventions

Play therapy is a therapeutic intervention that can be used to understand a child's inner world, and that can greatly relieve and benefit a child experiencing the types of distress caused by separation and divorce. As emphasized throughout this book, children have trouble talking about their feelings, but will communicate through play what they are unable to communicate verbally (see also Landreth, 2012). For instance, children may not be able to provide details about their worries, but their play will suggest a disguised indication of their worries. If a child's development has been disrupted by divorce, play therapy can help the child get back on track and move from maladaptive behavior to more developmentally appropriate behavior (Davies, 2011).

The toys and materials in my play therapy room are selected from these categories: (1) toys for imitating real life, such as a dollhouse with furniture and a doll family, small vehicles, a telephone, a cash register, and play food and dishes; (2) toys for aggressive release, such as wild animals, toy soldiers, aggressive animal puppets, a dart gun, and handcuffs; and (3) toys for creative expression, such as paper, crayons, markers, paint, blunt scissors, Play-Doh, transparent tape, and a sandtray (Landreth, 2012; Webb & Baggerly, Chapter 3, this volume). A playroom should be culturally sensitive and include such toys as dolls with different skin tones, ethnic play foods, and other toys that symbolize a child's own experiences. My experience in working with children who make frequent transitions between two households suggests that they benefit from having two dollhouses in the playroom. Children will often play out their experiences of going back and forth from one home to the other. Providing bride and groom dolls that are not joined together can be used by children to depict the family situation before and after the divorce, or the addition of a stepparent to the family by remarriage.

When working with children of divorce, I utilize a combination of directive and nondirective play therapy treatment approaches. Children of divorce have little control over the changes in their lives, and nondirective play therapy allows them to lead their own play at their own pace and developmental level, giving them the feeling of being in control. On the other hand, directive play therapy interventions help a child develop coping skills specific to the needs of children of divorce. (See Webb & Baggerly, Chapter 3, this volume, for further discussion of directive and nondirective play therapy.)

My play therapy sessions for children are 45 minutes in length. The first four sessions are nondirective: I allow the child to explore the play therapy room and develop a trusting relationship with me. During these four sessions, I am assessing the child to determine whether he or she would benefit from a continuation of nondirective play therapy, or whether 15 minutes at the beginning of each session with a directive intervention addressing divorce would be a better fit. This integrative approach is tailored to the needs of each child and can be adapted as therapy progresses (Schaefer, 2011; Shelby & Felix, 2005).

After four sessions, I meet with the parents without the child present to discuss my therapeutic observations of their child. I ask the parents to share how their child is doing at home and at school, and I offer parenting tips they can use to support their child during this challenging time. We decide together whether I will have four more individual sessions with the child, or whether each parent will be included during a portion of the play therapy sessions to work on enhancing the parent–child relationship. Children who are brought to therapy amid a divorce usually reach a point where they have adjusted to the divorce and are functioning well at home and school, and therapy is no longer necessary. Instead of abruptly ending the therapy, however, and risking stirring up feelings of abandonment, I make it a practice to gradually taper children off therapy. We may go from weekly sessions to once every other week and then one session a month. Several families I have worked with have chosen to bring their child to see me once every 2 months for what I refer to as "maintenance sessions," which are similar to taking a child to the pediatrician for a well-child check. I tell parents that I will be available to them in the future if the need for therapy arises.

This intermittent model of therapy provides interventions when a child is having difficulties, terminates when problems are resolved, and offers the therapist's services to the family if future therapy is necessary (Davies, 2011). Change and growth are inevitable and ongoing in all families, but especially in divorced families. A parent may be planning to marry again, or a remarried parent and stepparent may be expecting a new baby. Moreover, when a child grows older and crosses into a new developmental stage, the child usually begins revisiting the divorce from a more abstract perspective. At a later point, perhaps 1–2 years after termination, the child may be brought back to see me to work through reactions to these changes. The relationship between me and the child is already in place, and the playroom is a familiar, safe place for the child. Because of our previous work together, parents are generally confident that problems will once again be resolved.

CASE EXAMPLES

The cases described in this chapter are composites of several cases. Details have been changed so that no case corresponds to any actual client.

The Case of John, Age 9

John, age 9, was referred to me by his parents, Richard and Lisa, 4 months after they had separated. He had two older half-siblings residing with their father, who was Lisa's ex-husband from a prior divorce. Richard and Lisa stated that when they first told John they were separating, he responded angrily by hitting and kicking them and telling them his life was ruined. He had always been a cooperative child, but since the separation, he was refusing to cooperate and complete chores when with either parent. Prior to the separation, he had also been functioning well at school, but his teacher was now reporting that he was distracted, unmotivated, and not meeting his academic potential. When Richard and Lisa tried to talk to John about his feelings, he would tell them that everything was fine and that "I don't want to talk about it." Richard and Lisa contacted the school counselor and requested he speak to John regarding his feelings about the separation. The school counselor also reported that John didn't want to talk about the separation, and suggested the parents schedule a consultation with me to determine whether play therapy would be an appropriate intervention.

During our consultation, Lisa expressed her concerns about John: "He gets so frustrated lately. He will hit or pinch me when I ask him to do his homework or chores. I talk to him and reassure him that it's OK to be angry, but it's not OK to hurt me. He will cry and apologize, and for the next few days he will be his old self. Then something will upset him and he will fly off the handle again." As she wiped tears from her eyes, I validated that her response was appropriate, and encouraged her to continue responding to John in that manner. Richard shared that he had similar experiences when John was with him. Both parents stated that before they separated, they frequently argued in front of John; he would get between the two of them and try to push them apart, yelling at them to stop. Richard was concerned about the impact this might have had on John. I validated his concern and inquired whether this was still happening. They admitted that it still occasionally happened, even though they had agreed not to argue in front of John any more. I suggested that when they had something to discuss, it would be a good idea to schedule a time and place to talk where John would not be exposed to the conversation.

During the consultation, Richard and Lisa decided that they would like John to have play therapy sessions with me to deal with the impact of the separation and impending divorce. After completing all the necessary paperwork, I gave them suggestions on how to prepare John for coming to see me, and I encouraged them to show him the video tour of my office and playroom that I have on my website. The next week, I started seeing John for weekly play therapy sessions. During his first four nondirective play therapy sessions, John began a series of stories with a theme of conflict between two worlds.

Session 1

During his first play therapy session, John immediately went over to the sandtray, smoothed the surface with his hands, and used his index finger to draw a line down the middle of the tray. "These are two worlds, and they each have special power," he said. I nodded to convey understanding, and he asked if he could put toys in the sand; I replied, "In here, you can choose how you would like to play with the toys." He reinforced each world by placing toy soldiers, army tanks, and other vehicles around the parameter of each world. I commented that it looked like the two worlds were fighting. "Yeah," he replied. "They fight all the time about who has the most power." As our session came to an end, I announced, "John, we have 5 more minutes left in our playtime today, and then it will be time to go back to the waiting room where your dad is." He replied, "When Dad comes over to pick me up, he and Mom fight sometimes. I try to get them to stop, but it doesn't work, so I go to my room and play video games when they start yelling." I commented, "It sounds like you have figured out a way to not hear the arguing." John shrugged his shoulders and added, "Yeah, but I can still hear them, so sometimes I pull my hoodie up and put my hands on my ears."

Session 2

As he had done in the previous session, John created two warring worlds in the sandtray. A wizard came along and spied on the two worlds. The wizard had a weapon in each hand that had special powers. He shared the powers with one of the worlds, but would not allow the other world to have any. The wizard laughed when the world without any powers asked if it could have some.

Session 3

John's theme of two warring worlds was again played out in the sandtray. One world was evil, and the other was good. They were fighting with one another about who had more power. A monster who had special superpowers came between the two worlds, telling them that he was the boss and had more power than they did, and they had to listen to what he said. Near the end of the session, he quietly said, "When Mom and Dad separated, they told me that they were going to have a time out to think about what they want to do. But it feels like I'm the one in time out." I replied, "When you're with one parent, you really miss the other one."

Session 4

John repeated the theme of two worlds, but this time instead of using the sandtray he drew the worlds on the dry-erase board. One world had the power of bravery and overtook the other world. Near the end of the session, John said to me, "I'm not talking to you very much because I don't trust you yet." I replied, "Sounds like people are telling you to talk to me." "Yeah, Mom and Dad and Mr. Thompson [the school counselor] keep telling me that I should talk to you about my feelings." I nodded my head to convey understanding and said, "You're the only one who knows when you will be ready to talk to me. Would you like me to talk to your parents about that? I will be meeting with them next week." He said that he would; he added, "Can you also tell my dad that I don't like broccoli?"

In his initial work, John's anxiety over the ongoing conflict between his parents emerged in the play theme of competition between two powerful worlds. When a wizard or monster would enter the play, it was symbolic of John's need to be the boss sometimes and have all the power. I decided that John would benefit most from continuing with this nondirective play therapy.

Parent Session

The following week, I met with Richard and Lisa. They stated that John had told them he wasn't talking to me, and they were wondering whether the therapy was beneficial. I explained that it takes time to develop a relationship with a child, and asked them if they were telling John to talk to me. Richard replied, "Of course we are. That's why he's coming here." I told them I felt that John was hesitant to talk to me because that was what everyone was telling him to do. Lisa asked what they should say to him, and I replied, "Tell him that you're sorry for telling him to talk to me, and that you trust he will know when he's ready." I also reassured them that even when John wasn't verbally communicating, he was still communicating through his play. Together, we decided that I would have four more play therapy sessions with John.

Session 5

John used the sandtray to continue the theme of two warring worlds. They were once again fighting over who had the most power. A soldier came along, who I felt represented John, carrying a gun. He told the worlds that he was in charge, and they had to follow the rules of being respectful and getting along.

Session 6

After John drew a line down the middle of the sandtray depicting the two warring worlds, the same soldier from the previous session came along. He waved his gun, reminding the worlds to be respectful and get along. He also told the worlds that they had a new rule to follow: They needed to listen to what kids were saying.

Session 7

John once again drew the two worlds on the dry-erase board, divided by a thick, straight line. They started to fight, but remembered the rules of being respectful and getting along, so the fighting stopped. John erased the line he had drawn between the two worlds and said, "When they don't fight, it's like they're one world." He smiled and added, "My mom is moving to a new house near my dad's apartment. I can walk between them if there's an emergency." I replied, "You're happy that they will be close to each other."

Session 8

John came into the playroom saying that he wanted to start where he left off last time with the two worlds. Instead of using the sandtray or the dry-erase board, however, he used puppets. He put a frog puppet on his left hand and a wolf puppet on his right, and said, "The wolf and the frog used to argue a lot, but now they're friends and they help each other." He handed me a king puppet and told me to put it on my hand. I asked, "What do you want me to say?" He replied, "That you're proud they worked things out."

In these four sessions, John was still playing out the theme of competition between two worlds, but the conflict was beginning to subside and the worlds were learning how to cooperate and get along.

Parent Session

Richard and Lisa reported that John was doing well in school: He was paying attention, his grades had improved, and his teacher had suggested testing him for the gifted program. They also stated that he was less oppositional in both their homes and seemed happier. They were particularly pleased to tell me that they were working hard not to fight in front of John. Since John had made so much progress, Richard and Lisa felt that he no longer needed play therapy. I agreed that John had made significant progress, but suggested they consider four more play therapy sessions to maintain that progress. They were unconvinced that more therapy was necessary. I shared that it's best for children to have a gradual rather than abrupt ending to therapy, and that I hoped they would allow me to have two final play therapy sessions with John spread out over the next month. They agreed, and I gave them suggestions on how to prepare John for termination.

Session 9

The ninth session was scheduled for 2 weeks after I met with Richard and Lisa. John flung open the door of the playroom and said, "It feels like 20 years since I've been here." I replied, "You really like coming to the playroom. I need you to know that we have today and then one more playtime together, and then that will be all for now." He nodded his head and said, "Yeah, Mom and Dad told me." As he had done previously, he went to the sandtray and created two worlds. They were still warring, but the conflict had less intensity than in earlier sessions.

Session 10

The day of John's final session arrived. He silently entered the playroom and went to the sandtray, not making eye contact with me. As he had done in previous sessions, he used his finger to draw a line down the center of the sandtray, creating two worlds. He said, "The worlds have figured out how to get along. They don't have to use their evil power anymore." He moved from the sandtray to the art table and picked up a piece of a paper, a marker, and scissors. After several minutes of silently drawing and cutting, he handed me what he had made, saying, "This is a phone for you. And this is a phone for me." I replied, "You made that just for me." He went back to the sandtray, motioned with his hand for me to join him, and said, "Bring your phone." He picked up two small sand shovels and handed one to me. I said, "Show me what you want me to do," and he replied, "We need to bury them just like this." I buried my phone in the same manner he was burying his. After a minute he told me to stop. He waved his hands over the sandtray in a circular motion and said, "Now the phones have magical power." He carefully dug them out of the sand and handed mine back to me. I responded, "You figured out a way for us to stay in touch." John nodded his head and smiled at me. I announced, "John, we have 5 more minutes left in our playtime today, and then that will be all for now." John replied, "I remember that this is our last time today." He spent the final 5 minutes running his hand through the sandtray until I announced our session was over. He quickly left the playroom and headed to the waiting room, where Lisa was waiting for him. She thanked me for my help, said goodbye, and urged John to do the same. He did not respond, so I quietly told Lisa that John and I had said goodbye in the playroom. They left my office hand in hand.

Over the course of 10 sessions, John worked through his feelings about his parents' divorce by playing out warring worlds and helping them find resolutions to problems. Nondirective play therapy gave him a feeling of control, which helped alleviate the anxiety and feelings of helplessness he was experiencing because of the divorce.

The Case of Emilie, Age 5

Five-year-old Emilie's parents had separated and filed for divorce when she was 3. She lived with her mother, and her father visited sporadically, until the divorce was final a year later. Her mother was then awarded sole legal and physical custody, and her father was given no visitation rights. He remarried and moved across the country with his new wife shortly after the divorce. Over the course of the past year, Emilie's mother, who had a history of clinical depression, had begun to have a difficult time caring for her daughter and would often leave her for extended periods of time in the care of her maternal grandmother, Sharon. When Emilie's mother moved out of state with her boyfriend, Sharon petitioned the court and was granted guardianship of Emilie.

In the past 6 months, Emilie had been exhibiting regressive behaviors that were very concerning to Sharon. She took her granddaughter to the pediatrician, who ruled out any physical reasons for the behaviors. He suggested that Sharon contact me for a consultation. When we met, I asked Sharon to tell me about the behaviors Emilie was exhibiting. Without hesitating, she said, "She sucks her thumb, occasionally wets the bed, and wants to play with toys she hasn't played with since she was a preschooler. She has nightmares several times a week, where she wakes crying and crawls into bed with me. Lately she has been asking me a lot of questions about her parents. She wants to know if she was a bad girl, and if that's why her mother and father left. She also asks me if I am going to leave. I change the subject or tell her she's just being silly. Surely she knows I love her and won't leave. Sometimes I wonder if she's saying that just to get attention."

After I learned more about Emilie's family history, I explained to Sharon that Emilie's behaviors were probably rooted in fears of being abandoned. Like many caregivers, Sharon lacked patience and understanding, and was dismissive toward Emilie instead of comforting and reassuring. Sharon continued, "I need to vent. I love Emilie and am glad I am able to take care of her. But this is not what I signed up for. I already raised my children. I just want to be a grandma and not a mom. I am disappointed and angry that my daughter is unable to be a mother to Emilie."

I was grateful that Sharon felt comfortable enough with me to share this deep concern. I validated her feelings, reassuring her that many caregivers in her situation feel the same way. I wondered whether she might benefit from participating in a support group of other grandparents raising their grandchildren, and I provided her with the contact information for a local group. I also suggested four play therapy sessions with Emilie for me to assess her, and then I would meet again with Sharon to decide about future treatment. I anticipated involving Sharon in future play therapy sessions.

Session 1

Emilie walked around the playroom, exploring the toys and play materials. She went over to the shelf containing miniature animals and picked up a horse, which she placed in the middle of the sandtray. She then picked up a larger horse and placed it in a corner of the sandtray. The smaller horse started moving toward the larger one, saying, "Mommy? Where are you? Mommy! Wait for me!" The two horses came together. They hugged while the smaller horse said, "I love you! Don't go, Mommy!" The larger horse pulled away from the smaller one and went to the opposite corner of the sandtray. I responded, "The baby horse is scared. She wants her mommy." Emilie responded, "She's going away. She's never coming back. Mommy, please come back!"

Session 2

Emilie played in the sandtray and repeated the theme she played out in the first session. This time, though, instead of horses, she used two princess dolls, which she called the "mommy princess" and the "baby princess." They were playing at the park, and when their playtime was over, the mommy princess began to walk away. The baby princess called out, "I love you, Mommy! Don't leave me, Mommy!" The mommy princess ignored the baby princess and walked away.

Emilie's feelings of abandonment and distress were clearly visible in her play. I felt that it would be beneficial to include Sharon in the sessions, so I put aside my original treatment plan of four individual play therapy sessions with just Emilie. When I contacted Sharon with my recommendation, she was reluctant. After I reassured her that I would be providing support and encouragement during the sessions, and that being together would be fun for both her and Emilie, she agreed.

Session 3

As the three of us entered the playroom, I told Sharon that we would allow Emilie to lead the play. I told her to watch me for cues on what she needed to do and say. As I had anticipated, Emilie again played out the theme of abandonment. This time, she placed two bears in the sandtray. The baby bear walked over to the mommy bear and gave her a hug. The mommy bear said, "I don't want to hug you. I'm going away!" The baby bear began to cry, saying, "Mommy, Mommy, don't go away." I picked up a third bear, handed it to

Sharon, and said, "The grandma bear is here. Don't cry, baby bear." Sharon picked up on what I was suggesting; she placed the grandma bear near the baby bear and said, "Grandma bear loves you and will take care of you. I'm not going away." The baby bear replied, "I love you too, Grandma. Don't leave me. Stay with me forever."

Caregiver Session

I told Sharon that children like Emilie, who have been abandoned by not one but both parents, have a fear of being abandoned again. Emilie needed continual reassurance that the abandonment was not her fault and that she would be cared for. I encouraged Sharon to take Emilie to a toy store to select an animal family that the two of them could play with at home. I suggested she direct the interaction of the animals so that the grandma animal was in charge and taking care of the baby animal. I requested she play with Emilie in this way each day for at least 15 minutes, perhaps at bedtime, and then come back next week for another family play session. Sharon was very receptive to this suggestion. I also asked her if she had any old photos of Emilie and her parents from when the family was still intact, and, if so, whether she could make copies of them and bring them to the next session. She said she would be happy to do that.

Session 4

Emilie and Sharon arrived for the next session, with Emilie pulling Sharon by the hand and saying, "Come on, Grandma, let's go play." Emilie went to the dollhouse and, with Sharon's help, began putting furniture and people in the rooms of the house. The interaction between them was playful and loving. When we had 15 minutes left in the playtime, I asked Sharon if she had remembered to bring along the family pictures. She took them out of her purse, and we laid them on a table. I asked Sharon and Emilie if they could tell me who was in the pictures and what they were doing. As they shared with me the details of each photo, I put them into a small, inexpensive photo album I had purchased specifically for this intervention. I then said, "Emilie, these pictures tell the story of your family. Nobody else in the world has a story like this one." Sharon added, "Miss Pam, would you take a picture of us so we can add it to the story?" I said that this was a wonderful idea, and as Sharon handed me her iPhone, they posed in the middle of the playroom.

Session 5 and Later Sessions

The session scheduled for the next week had to be canceled due to inclement weather. Sharon phoned me to update me on things at home: "Emilie loves her book! We've added more photos of the two of us, and she sleeps with it under her pillow. She hasn't had a nightmare in a week, nor has she wet the bed. She still asks me if I am going to leave, but doesn't ask as often as she used to. We still play with the animals each night at bedtime, and I think I look forward to it as much as she does!"

I continued to see Emilie and Sharon together in family play therapy twice a month for the next 4 months. At that point, Emilie's regressive behaviors had nearly disappeared, and she was much less fearful that Sharon would abandon her. In addition, Sharon was more empathic and understanding of Emilie's needs, and more confident in her ability to fulfill them. Therefore, therapy was terminated.

CONCLUSION

There are many issues to consider in working with children of divorce. Viewing these children from a developmental perspective is crucial because they can experience a wide variety of reactions to separation and divorce that can disrupt their developmental progress and impair their ability to function well at home and at school. New play therapists often wonder what child behaviors are developmentally appropriate and which ones are atypical. Play therapists should seek knowledge and understanding by reading books on child development. This knowledge also needs to be communicated to parents, so that they can better understand their children and be supportive as their children adjust to the changes in the family structure brought about by the separation and divorce.

Children generally fare best when they have the emotional support and ongoing involvement of both parents. Meeting with parents on a regular basis to discuss therapeutic progress will keep the parents involved and invested in the process. Including the parents in play therapy sessions gives the therapist an opportunity to assess the dynamics of each parent–child relationship, and to model and practice supportive parenting strategies that will encourage a positive parent–child relationship.

Working with a child whose parents are involved in legal child custody proceedings poses potential risks for therapists. Professional liability insurance should be acquired, and the policy holder needs to be contacted immediately if a complaint is filed against a therapist's license or if the therapist receives a subpoena to appear in court or to release treatment notes. Therapists need to be familiar with the laws of their state regarding minors, and to consult with an attorney who specializes in mental health law if clarification is needed. Professional supervision and consultation with mental health professionals who understand the complexity of working with divorcing families can be beneficial as well.

Play therapy for children of divorce does not have to be limited to agency and private practice settings. Counselors in school settings can offer short-term individual or group therapy for students whose reactions to parental separation and divorce are impeding their academic success. Group therapy is an especially appropriate intervention for school-age children because peer relationships are so important at this development stage. Children whose peers are also in divorce situations feel less isolated and alone in their experiences. A child in a school-based group therapy setting shared that he couldn't take his dog along when he visited his dad because his father lived in an apartment that didn't allow pets. Another child replied that he had the same problem, and soon the two of them were discussing how they kept photos of their dogs in their suitcases when they were making transitions between households.

An empathic, highly trained play therapist who is knowledgeable about family dynamics can be a valuable resource to parents by providing them with the skills needed for emotionally supporting their children through the challenges of divorce. For children who are experiencing ongoing conflict between parents regarding divorce and custody, play therapy can provide a safe place to express their feelings and make sense of their world. They can learn coping skills, discover their own strengths and resiliency, and come to accept the fact that they are not responsible for the divorce.

STUDY QUESTIONS

1. Why is it important for therapists to look at children of divorcing parents from a developmental perspective?
2. Discuss the advantages and disadvantages of including parents in play therapy sessions with their children.
3. A parent requests play therapy for his young daughter. Upon reviewing the paperwork, the therapist learns that the parent is actually the stepfather. How should the therapist proceed?

REFERENCES

Cancian, M., Meyer, D. R., Brown, P. R., & Cook, S. T. (2014). Who gets custody now?: Dramatic changes in children's living arrangements after divorce. *Demography, 35*, 147–157.

Cohen, P. N. (2014). Recession and divorce in the United States, 2008–2011. *Population Research and Policy Review.* Retrieved April 10, 2014, from *http://link.springer.com/article/10.1007/s11113-014-9323-z.*

Davies, D. (2011). *Child development: A practitioner's guide* (3rd ed.) New York: Guilford Press.

Fraley, R. C., & Hefferman, M. E. (2013) Attachment and parental divorce: A test of the diffusion and sensitive period hypotheses. *Personality and Social Psychology Bulletin, 39*(9), 1199–1213.

Hartsell, T. L., & Bernstein, B. E. (2013). *The portable lawyer for mental health professionals* (3rd ed.). Hoboken, NJ: Wiley.

Hetherington, E. M., & Kelly, J. (2002). *For better or for worse: Divorce reconsidered.* New York: Norton.

Kelly, J. B., & Emery, R., E. (2003). Children's adjustment following divorce: Risk and resilience perspectives. *Family Relations, 52*(4), 352–362.

Landreth, G. L. (2012). *Play therapy: The art of the relationship* (3rd ed.). New York: Routledge.

McGuire, D. K., & McGuire, D. E. (2001). *Linking parents to play therapy.* New York: Routledge.

National Bureau of Economic Research. (2010). Statement from the business cycle dating committee. Retrieved April 16, 2014, from *www. nber.org/cycles/sept2010.html.*

National Center for Health Statistics. (2013). National marriage and divorce rate trends. Retrieved April 16, 2014, from *www.cdc.gov/nchs/nvss/marriage_divorce_tables.htm.*

Saposnek, D. T. (1998). *Mediating child custody disputes* (rev. ed.). San Francisco: Jossey-Bass.

Schaefer, C. E. (Ed.). (2011). *Foundations of play therapy* (2nd ed.). Hoboken, NJ: Wiley.

Shelby, J. S., & Felix, E. D. (2005). Posttraumatic play therapy: The need for an integrated model of directive and nondirective approaches. In L. A. Reddy, T. M. Files-Hall, & C. E. Schaefer (Eds.), *Empirically based play interventions for children* (pp. 79–103). Washington, DC: American Psychological Association.

U.S. Census Bureau. (2012). Selected population profile in the United States. Retrieved June 2, 2014, from *http://factfinder2.census.gov/faces/tableservices/jsf/pages/productview.xhtml?pid=ACS_12_1YR_S0201&prodType=table.*

Wallerstein, J. S., & Kelly, J. B. (1996). *Surviving the breakup: How children and parents cope with divorce.* New York: Basic Books.

Wallerstein, J. S., Lewis, J. M., & Blakeslee, S. (2000). *The unexpected legacy of divorce: The twenty-five year landmark study.* New York: Hyperion.

Chapter 10

After a Parent's Death

Group, Family, and Individual Therapy to Help Children and Adolescents

DONNA L. SCHUURMAN
JANA DeCRISTOFARO

THEORETICAL FRAMEWORK

In 1940, British developmental psychologist John Bowlby incensed his psychoanalytic colleagues through propositions that he later developed into his theory of attachment (see Bowlby, 1969/1982, 1973, 1980, 1988). One basic tenet of this theory is that separation anxiety in children results from adverse family experiences, such as real or threatened abandonment or rejection, illness, or death. Adaptations of his theories and writings form the foundation of much current scholarship and practice with children, including the realm of grief and loss.

More recent research on the brain and neuroscience provides additional insight, though not necessarily different conclusions, into Bowlby's pioneering work. For example, child psychiatrist Daniel Siegel's research into how the brain works (see Siegel, 2012) suggests that "From the moment we're born, our most important relationships fire into being the neural circuits of the brain that allow us to understand and empathize with others and feel their feelings" (Wylie, 2004, p. 30).

In 1988, Siegel attended a talk by Mary Main, one of the pioneers in attachment theory, on her work in "coherent narrative."

> Main's research indicated that the way parents told their own stories—how they made sense of their past lives, or didn't—was the most powerful predictor (85 percent accuracy) of whether their own children would be

> securely attached to them . . . it wasn't *what* happened to them as children, but *how* they came to make sense of what happened to them that predicted their emotional integration as adults and what kind of parents they'd be. (Wylie, 2004, p. 34)

In other words, *making meaning* of one's childhood, regardless of what actual events transpired, corresponded positively with "emotional integration" and better parenting.

Siegel's applications of Bowlby's and Main's underlying principles have opened new vistas for understanding the impact of our early experiences on the brain, as well as on future feelings and behaviors. Perhaps the most significant relevancy is his belief that the most important element in the therapeutic relationship (whether therapy or support) is a simple concept from a young woman he was seeing in therapy. She "was suffering from unresolved grief and guilt at the loss of a parent. Eventually, she got better, and when she was ready to leave, Siegel asked her what had been most helpful about her treatment. She thought for a minute and then said, 'When I'm with you, I feel *felt*'" (Wylie, 2004, p. 33).

Our role—whether as play therapists or counselors, grief support practitioners or psychologists—is helping the children, adolescents, and families we serve to *make meaning* through *feeling felt*. It's that simple, and that complex.

In this chapter, we provide an overview of the four principles of grief that guide how we view and approach grief at The Dougy Center, an organization that provides support for grieving children/teens and their families, and training for professionals who help them. We also outline common and developmentally appropriate grief responses for children and adolescents dealing with the death of a parent. The chapter concludes with a series of interventions that are applicable in group, individual, and family therapeutic settings.

THE DOUGY CENTER MODEL

The Dougy Center's peer support group model arose in 1982 out of the need to provide a safe environment where grieving children and families could come together and share their experiences—to make meaning, and to feel felt. The founder, Beverly Chappell, a former nurse and the wife of a pediatrician, recognized society's inability to provide adequate support for grieving children and families. The Center's model is based on four principles of grief, which inform the program structure and our interactions and responses to the children, teens, young adults, and adults who access our services.

Four Principles of Grief

The first principle of our program is a view of grief as a natural reaction to death. Grief is often labeled as a set of behaviors and experiences that need to be alleviated or changed in some way. We believe that grief is the expected, and healthy, response to having someone die. Rather than "treat" or "fix" children and their families, our peer support groups help participants learn to integrate the loss into their lives. Participants in our program talk about—and play out—the impact of death on them emotionally, behaviorally, physically, cognitively, and spiritually. These discussions work to normalize their reactions and decrease the fear that people in grief are crazy, sick, or damaged in some way.

Increasingly in the field of death and bereavement, grief and grievers are labeled with terms such as "pathological," "complicated," "traumatic," "prolonged," and "persistent," as if their responses are somehow abnormal and in need of curing. The Center's participant youth have experienced the tragic deaths of parents, siblings, and friends from every imaginable accident and disease, as well as through horrific murders and suicides, some of which they have witnessed. Rather than labeling their responses as "pathological" or as signs of "acting out," we choose to view their behaviors as attempts to cope. Some of these attempts may be harmful to the children/adolescents or others and require additional therapeutic or medical attention, but an "acting-out" response to, for example, watching your father shoot and kill your mother and then himself is not pathological. Rather, it is normal for a young person in such circumstances to have nightmares, and perhaps to express internal pain by becoming aggressive toward others. In other words, neither the grief nor the response is pathological.

Our second principle is that within each person is the natural capacity to heal. When they are provided with a safe and confidential environment, grieving children/adolescents can learn from each other and offer mutual support based on their personal experiences. Young people can talk to one another about how to deal with school, family, and friends after a death. From these exchanges, the youth and adults can gather new ideas for integrating loss into their lives. This is not to suggest that time heals all wounds or that professional intervention is never warranted. Rather, it speaks to the belief that with healing conditions that include opportunities for expression and feeling understood, we all have the capacity to heal.

In addition to telling and hearing stories, many grieving youth benefit from alternative means for expression (Chilcote, 2007; Hilliard, 2007; Malchiodi, 2008). To address this, we provide opportunities in the areas of art, dramatic play, music, and "big-energy" work. Whereas some children and adolescents are eager to tell their stories and to share experiences with others in a verbal fashion, others prefer more physical avenues to process their reactions. Some are simply too young to have a verbal vocabulary to express their feelings. Our belief that everyone has the capacity to discover what they need in times of grief guides our nondirective model, which allows individuals to choose what they do while at The Dougy Center. We train staff members and volunteer group facilitators to reflect what the young people do and say, rather than to interpret or lead conversations and play. In this way, children and adolescents are encouraged to find what works for them, both at The Dougy Center and in their personal grief processes. Selecting their activities and means of expression aids them in restoring the lost sense of control that accompanies deaths they could not prevent.

Our third principle is that the duration and intensity of grief are unique to each individual. How each person experiences grief will depend on a number of factors, but these factors cannot solely be used to predict his or her reactions. Age, relationship, existing challenges and strengths, the nature of the death, and the grieving person's framework for creating meaning all have an impact on what grief looks and feels like. Our nondirective peer support groups work to acknowledge that each person is different, and that there are many ways to respond during times of grief. Within a family, a teenage son may want to keep pictures of his dad who died around the house, while his sister may want them taken down and stored out of sight. In another, the surviving parent may want to talk with his children about their mother, while the children prefer to talk to their friends. The peer support group helps families understand that each member's wishes are valid, and that there are ways to mutually respect those differing needs. The teen in the first example above may learn from another participant that he can ask to hang pictures of his dad in his room, so that his sister doesn't have to be around them all of the time. The dad in the second example can talk about his wife with his peer support group, and can thus learn that his children are not the only ones available to listen.

Within this third principle is the understanding that grief is not something youth and their families have to "get over." Grief is a mutable experience that changes over time and exists on a spectrum from very intense to very manageable. We believe that grief is not a linear phenomenon that moves from stage to stage; rather, it is something experienced in waves. As children grow and reach developmental milestones, they may reexperience their grief in new ways because they are equipped with new cognitive capacities and comprehension to process the death and the impact it continues to have on their lives. This conceptualization of grief as ongoing drives our commitment to offering open-ended peer support groups as opposed to time-limited sessions. Individuals choose when they want to join a group and when they are ready to end their involvement with our program.

Our fourth principle—that caring and acceptance assist in the healing process—is based on the belief that mainstream North American society avoids talking about or accepting the inevitability of death and does a poor job of equipping people to support the bereaved. In the school setting, students encounter pressure to concentrate and complete assignments, with no acknowledgment of the ways in which grief can hinder their ability to concentrate. The structure and routine at home are often disrupted after a death, which in turn impairs a youth's capacity to focus and to complete homework. In the work setting, surviving parents may lack support not only for their grief, but also for the additional responsibilities of being single parents.

These four principles are the foundation for our peer support groups and inform how we respond to and interact with grieving children and teens. The groups provide an environment where grieving young people and their family members share, verbally and nonverbally, the challenges they face. These challenges include expectations, both internal and external, that grieving individuals struggle to meet. Whether internal or external, expectations for grief arise from a mix of social, cultural, interpersonal, and intrapersonal factors. Examples include pressure to take on additional household chores, caregiving for younger siblings, a need to be strong through not showing emotion, desire to protect adults from being sad or upset, and a wish to be seen as normal. Changing roles and responsibilities are common topics in our support groups. Our program provides a wide variety of creative expression rooms that children can utilize to play or act out these shifts in their lives. The literature shows that "attachment relationships that offer children experiences that provide them with emotional connection and safety, both in the home and in the community, may be able to confer resilience and more flexible modes of adaptation in the face of adversity" (Siegel, 2012, p. 83). As a result, our staff members and volunteer facilitators rely on the essential skill of reflective communication, in order to create a warm and caring atmosphere that makes children and adolescents feel safe enough to express these challenges.

In the adult groups, which run concurrently with the children's groups, caregivers are able to talk about the challenges and opportunities they face in parenting their grieving children. The ongoing nature of our program means that the groups have a wide range in terms of length of time since the death. When an adult or child/teen comes to a group for the first time, he or she may encounter people who are 1 month, 6 months, or 4-plus years away from the time of the deaths they have experienced. Established members are able to offer both hope and understanding to the more recent members. In their separate groups, children, adolescents, and caregivers are invited to tell stories about the persons who died. Sometimes these stories directly relate to death itself and how participants found out or what they saw and felt at the time. Other stories focus on memories that the participants have about their lives with the persons who died. People dealing with grief often use stories to help make sense of and connect the pieces of their lives before and after the deaths. Being able to share stories with each other helps participants to connect through the common experience of piecing their histories together (Siegel, 2012).

The previous paragraphs outline the four principles that are foundational to the peer support group model used at The Dougy Center. Our program strives to create a supportive environment where bereaved youth and their families can find connection, a sense of belonging, and healthy outlets for feelings and reactions associated with grief. These principles are informed by what we know from the literature, as well as by our collective experience of how children and teens grieve and the ways in which their developmental stage impacts the process. The Dougy Center's model has been adapted and replicated in hundreds of sites throughout the United States and other countries. For more information on programs and locations, see the National Alliance for Grieving Children website (*www.childrengrieve.org*).

Goals

Some of the goals of our work, which are applicable whether we are seeing grieving children/adolescents individually or in groups, include the following:

1. Help the grieving youth restore a diminished or damaged sense of control. ("The world is out of control, or at least out of *my* control.")
2. Normalize their experience. ("I'm not crazy; there are other kids like me who feel what I do. I'm going to be OK.")
3. Provide social support and let them know that others care. ("I'm not alone. There are people who care.")
4. Let them know that their feelings matter.
5. Provide outlets for their feelings, whether they can verbally articulate them or not.
6. Help them to keep their connections with the persons who died—to remember.
7. Support them in seeing their own progress, and provide them with the opportunity to help others.

Group Meetings

Our ongoing groups meet in 90-minute sessions held every other week throughout the year, with a brief summer break. The conditions for participation include adherence to a small number of safety rules. We have successfully integrated youth we were initially told were not appropriate for a group setting. What we have found is that through permitting them to guide their own play and their own activities, within our safety guidelines, even children and teens with histories of acting out (again, we regard "acting out" as *coping behaviors*) can successfully participate in the groups.

Individual Therapy

Although The Dougy Center's basic model is a group model, which we believe assists in normalization and socialization, the principles, methods, and activities can be integrated into individual therapy as well. We recognize that some children, teens, and adults do not wish to be in a group setting, for various reasons; these may include being shy, preferring more individualized attention, or being overwhelmed by other people's stories. In addition, individual or family therapy may be indicated either instead of or in conjunction with a support group—particularly if families are struggling with additional major issues (such as substance abuse or domestic violence), or if behavioral issues interfere with youth's ability to maintain safety for themselves and others.

Family Therapy

Because death affects everyone in a family, we believe that family involvement in support or therapy is more helpful than treatment of a specified "problem" individual. The work of researchers like Irwin Sandler, Tim Ayers, Phyllis Silverman, Nancy Boyd Webb, and William Worden unequivocally points to the influence of the health of the surviving parent on a bereaved child (Lutzke, Ayers, Sandler, & Barr, 1997; Silverman, 1999; Worden, 1996). Coping with the death of a spouse and the challenges of single parenting under the strains of bereavement, along with additional changes in income, self-image, and a host of other changes following the death, may strain even the best parent's energy and understanding. Children are deeply affected by how the adults around them cope in times of tragedy, and therefore including the family in therapy or support is paramount.

Children and adolescents grieve within a family context and within the expectations, assumptions, and beliefs in this context about what grief should and shouldn't look like. As Silverman (1999, p. 25) states, "Parents may worry that their children are not more expressive. Yet children see themselves as quite expressive, given their age and stage of development. . . . Thus, it is not easy for parents to connect to their children's grief." Family therapy that focuses on helping all members identify and express what they find helpful in grief can help to mitigate the pain of feeling misunderstood or misperceiving the intentions behind the behaviors of others.

THE NATURE OF CHILDREN'S AND ADOLESCENTS' GRIEF AND UNDERSTANDING OF DEATH

In this section of the chapter, we provide an overview of the common elements involved in children's and adolescent's grief, and we describe how our program works to respond to varying developmental needs.

Young Children Are Concrete in Their Responses

If the person who died was a consistent presence in a baby's life, the infant will have a sense of someone missing. The infant grieves because a formerly stable environment is suddenly in disarray. Young children often do not initially respond to hearing that someone has "died," because they do not understand the words used by the adults. Many adults become concerned when children have no reaction or visible grief. It is important to remember that a young child's perception is concrete, short-ranged, and based on what is being felt in the moment.

Research conducted by Freud and Burlingham (1947) in the early 1940s was the first attempt to document the effects of grief on children younger than 4. This study found that the loss of a primary caregiver, whether by death or separation, profoundly affected an infant's emotional state. Although young children do not fully comprehend the meaning of death, they understand and can feel "gone-ness" (Webb, 2010). Because they have difficulty thinking in abstract concepts and language, words such as "dying" or "died" need to be explained and described concretely. For example, an adult may say, "Daddy's heart stopped working so his whole body stopped working. He died. When you die, you can't breathe or sleep or eat or poop or laugh, or anything."

It is important to give simple and honest descriptions and explanations. Children who hear that "Mommy's in heaven" may respond, "I know! When's she coming back?"

> One grandmother, wishing to help her 3-year-old grandson understand that his daddy was dead, took him to visit the cemetery where his dad was buried. The next day the child reported to his preschool classmates, "I went to heaven and saw my daddy!" When the other children expressed disbelief, saying, "You can't go to heaven! You're not dead!" he responded, "Yes, I can. I went to heaven! It's right down the street from IKEA." This child was unable to distinguish between heaven as a place where the adults in his life told him his daddy went, and the physical location of his father's body.

As children mature, they begin to understand abstract thought and will develop a new comprehension of death, including the following three concepts (Norris-Shortle, Young, & Williams, 1993):

1. Nonfunctionality: Death means the cessation of all life functions (eating, sleeping, breathing, pooping).
2. Irreversibility: Death is permanent. A dead person cannot come back to life.
3. Universality: Eventually, everything and everyone will die.

Children's and Adolescents' Understanding of Cause and Effect Changes with Development

Children's understanding of cause and effect changes according to their level of development and reasoning. Children in the preoperational stage of development rely first on transductive reasoning (specific to specific) to explain a chain of events: "The thunder made Mommy's phone ring." As they grow, they turn more to deductive reasoning (specific to general): "A dog bit me; all dogs are mean." They also begin to use inductive reasoning (general to specific): "Dogs have four legs; Harry [a cat] has four legs; so Harry is a dog."

In grief, these developmental characteristics can translate into worry, misattribution, and confusion when it comes to how and why people die.

If someone has died in a hospital, children may think that hospitals are for dying. If someone has died in his or her sleep, children might be afraid to go to sleep. If one person has died, "Someone [or everyone] else will die," or "I will die." As they age, they assimilate new truths as additional experiences disprove their reasoning. This process can be assisted by adults in their lives who listen carefully to their concerns and help to clear up misinformation. A common example is telling children that "Grandma died because she was really sick," which can lead to anxiety the next time the children or persons they care about are sick. Identifying and naming the illness can help to reassure children: "Grandma had a disease called leukemia; it is very different from having a cold or the stomach flu. You can't catch it from someone else." Even adolescents, despite their increasing cognitive capacity for understanding death, can be confused about how a person died ("I know my dad died in a car crash, but what actually happened to his body?" or "What if my skipping school stressed my mom out and gave her the aneurysm?"). It's helpful to ask adolescents whether they have questions about the death, and to offer information or reassurance when it is needed and appropriate.

Children Are Repetitive in Their Grief

Children learn by repetition and repeatedly asking questions. Repetitive play is common and normal for young children; it can be seen as an attempt to bring a modicum of control and predictability to a world that may feel frightening (Evans et al., 1997). This is especially true for children who are grieving. Repetitive themes and actions in their play are part of the searching inherent in grief. Their questions indicate their thoughts and feelings of confusion and uncertainty. It is most helpful to listen and support their searching by answering patiently and repetitively. Parents should be instructed to listen and support their children's searching by doing exactly this. They may have to tell the story of a death over and over again, as the children learn gradually and slowly grasp the truth.

Children and Teens Are Physical in Their Grief

In the 1500s, French Renaissance thinker Michel de Montaigne stated, "It should be noted that children at play are not playing about; their games should be seen as their most serious-minded activity" (*www.brainyquote.com/quotes/quotes/m/micheldemo166546.html*). Young children respond emphatically with their bodies to their feelings, emotions, and thoughts. Grieving is a physical experience for all ages, and most especially for younger children. Although older children are more capable of verbal expression, their activity may continue to be a significant way of communicating feelings, emotions, and thoughts. Their movements and play speak as their language of grieving as much as their words. Reflecting their physical and verbal expressions is a way of understanding and supporting their communication. Thus they will feel that they are being heard and respected, and they may continue to communicate.

Young people will play out various scenarios from their experiences, often taking on roles that enable them to change the outcome of the situation. We consistently see this in our hospital room playroom, where children adopt the roles of doctor, nurse, patient, and family member. Shifting the course of past events during reenactment play allows children to explore their questions about death and dying. For instance, by taking on the doctor role and coming up with a new cure for cancer, children get to try out different narratives and exert an element of control over the course of events. This chance to orchestrate new experiences can lead to reassuring experiences of safety and stability (Malchiodi, 2008).

Children and Adolescents Grieve Cyclically

Grief moves in cycles throughout childhood and as an individual ages. At each new developmental level, the individual will reintegrate important events by using recently acquired cognitive processes. For instance, an infant girl whose mother dies will become absorbed in the death again when her language skills develop and she can verbally express feelings and thoughts. She may reexperience the grief again as an adolescent, using her capacity for abstract thought. The cyclical nature of grieving can be stirred by acknowledged or unacknowledged calendar events such as birthdays, holidays, the anniversary of the death, or other special days associated with the parent who died. Children and teens seem to do best when adults remind them of these dates and suggest options for how to acknowledge those days.

> Eight-year-old Sarah had difficulty sleeping and an increase in nightmares as the first anniversary of her mother's death approached. Her father asked Sarah how she would like to spend that day, and she replied, "Mommy loved orange, so everyone should wear orange, and we should eat orange food!" Sarah and her father then drew a picture together of what they would look like wearing orange clothes, and made a list of foods to eat and cook that day. While Sarah continued to need extra hugs and reassurance in the days leading up to the anniversary, she was able to sleep through the night, and she tacked the picture she and her dad drew up on the wall above her bed as a comforting reminder that they had a plan.

Children and Adolescents Need Choices

Death is a disruption in a young person's life that can be disorienting, confusing, and frightening. Formerly predictable daily routines suddenly become unclear and confusing, and life can feel out of control. One way to help children/teens reestablish a sense of control over the events in their lives is to give them choices. These choices can be directly related to the loss (e.g., what role a youth might like to play in a memorial service, or even whether the youth wants to attend the service or where he or she wants to sit). They can also be incorporated into daily life (e.g., "We have two cereals. Which would you like for breakfast?"). Other situations where it can be helpful to ask children/adolescents what they prefer include going to the hospital, viewing the body, and planning the funeral or memorial service (music, food, etc.).

Children and teens appreciate being offered pictures and possessions of the person who died. Family members should allow them to have clothing, memorabilia, and photos. Clinicians should also encourage adult family members to ask them if they would like to be involved in the process of sorting through the belongings of the person who died.

Young People Grieve as Part of a Family

When a family member dies, it affects the way the entire family functions. All the relationships within the family shift as the surviving members adjust to changes in the family structure. Children and teens often grieve not only for the person who died, but also for the loss of the environment and structure they experienced prior to the death. It is helpful if family members are encouraged to grieve in their own ways, with support for individual differences. Children/teens seem to do better when they know that other people are affected by the death. This can help them feel less isolated. Offering them the option to stay in or leave any gathering will facilitate their sense of inclusion, empowerment, and permission to accept their own feelings and thoughts related to the loss.

Children and Teens Experience a Range of Emotions and Feelings

Children's and adolescents' feelings are avenues for them to learn how grief and loss affect them on emotional, physical, cognitive, and spiritual levels. Through attentiveness to and acceptance of their feelings and emotions, they can reach new understandings about the circumstances of the death, the nature of the relationship lost, and the new realities of life without the person. They gradually become acquainted with their own unique grief processes.

Fear and Anxiety

Two of the most common feelings after a loss for children and teens are fear and anxiety: fear about past events, and anxiety about the future. They wonder: "What happened? Who will die next? How will we live without the dead person? Will I ever feel better? Will other family members die? Who will take care of me? Where will I go if I die? Why did it happen to me? Will I die?" If youth receive attention and nurturing during this stressful time, they will recover a sense of the basic dependability of life and of their own personal resiliency. Listening to and validating their difficult feelings and emotions can assist with this process.

Fear and anxiety can be manifested differently, depending on the person. Some children act younger or regress. They want the reassurance, care, and attention they received when they were younger. Some adolescents become overachievers in an attempt to contradict their own feelings of helplessness. They may do everything "right," even to the extent of parenting a surviving parent or siblings. Some young people exhibit exaggerated displays of power to counteract their fears. This may take the form of superhero manifestations, or may surface as disruptive behavior, explosive anger and/or belligerence. Some youth may withdraw, becoming very quiet, almost frozen in fear.

> Ten-year-old Ethan's father died from a heart attack on his way home from work. A few weeks after the death, Ethan developed resistance to going to his after-school music program. His mother was confused by his refusal because Ethan loved playing instruments and would perform songs for her every night before dinner. Thinking that Ethan was having trouble with an after-school classmate, his mom first acknowledged his resistance and then asked him some questions. Ethan told her that he didn't like watching her pull up to the sidewalk to pick him up from music because it reminded him of the day his dad died: "You told me he was dead when I got in the car after music school, and now I'm afraid if I go to music, you'll pick me up with more bad news!" Together, Ethan and his mom devised options for decreasing the dread he felt when she came to pick him up. For 2 weeks, he would ride home with his friend Lisa and her mom. Then he would try out getting picked up by his mom, but only if she came inside to get him, so he didn't have to watch her drive up to the school. Four weeks after the conversation, Ethan felt comfortable enough to look out the window next to the front door as his mom parked. Then one day, his mom drove up to find Ethan standing on the sidewalk with the other kids, smiling, waving, and yelling, "Over here, Mom!" Allowing Ethan the opportunity to talk about his fear and then work together with his mother to come up with a plan helped him feel safe, supported, and understood.

Guilt and Regret

Guilt and regret may stem from an intentional or unintentional act that contributed to the death. (For example, 11-year-old Tobias started a fire in which his baby brother died.) Guilt may also manifest from a false belief that something a child did or failed to do somehow caused the death. This is most commonly heard from children who have experienced a suicide, but it is not exclusive to that mode of death. (Six-year-old Kaitlyn shared with her group, "If only I'd stayed home that night instead of going to my cousin's house, I could have stopped my dad from hanging himself.") When adults choose to withhold information about the death, children may start to think they must have contributed in some way to the death. This can lead children to attempt to make sense out of what is happening in their surroundings, and to do so by filling in the gaps with their own imagined explanations—often with a sense of personal responsibility for what has taken place.

Anger and Frustration

There are different kinds of anger expressed in grieving. There may be unresolved issues between the young person and the person who died, or the deceased may have been abusive or neglectful to the child/adolescent. An adolescent's anger may also be a protest against the unfairness of the death. Anger can sometimes be a front for fear, manifesting in an outward display of personal power. A teen may communicate through anger that "I am strong enough to control life with my force." Children and adolescents sometimes become rebellious or resistant as a way to counteract the vulnerability of their other feelings and emotions.

Sorrow/Sadness

Sorrow can be an expression of a young person's emotions and feelings of vulnerability as he or she continues to live without the security of the person who died. The child may be sad over the loss of predictability and certainty, in addition to missing the person who died.

Relief

Relief frequently gets left out of conversations about grief. Youth who feel some element of relief when a parent dies are vulnerable to shame and embarrassment about this reaction. Listening to a child say that she's glad her mom died because her mom's drinking led to so many fights and instability often inspires adults to respond with statements like "Don't feel that way; you know your mom loved you," or "It's wrong to say bad things about someone who died." It is more helpful in such cases to listen and reflect children's expressions of emotion, and to give them room to come to their own conclusions. In this example, a more helpful response would be "You feel relieved that your mom died. Her drinking led to lots of fights." This opens the door for the child to go further with her own thought processes. She might respond with "Yep. It was awful," or "Yeah, it is nicer at home now, but I do still miss my mom. Sometimes she was nice," or "It's weird. Sometimes I feel better with her gone, and other times I'm mad I don't have a mom, even a mean one."

The preceding discussion illustrates just some of the possible emotions a child or adolescent may feel after a family member dies. Moreover, as children grow older, they may begin to distinguish between the emotions they keep to themselves and the ones they feel they can reveal to others. Figure 10.1 is a drawing depicting a 14-year-old girl's distinction between these two types of emotions.

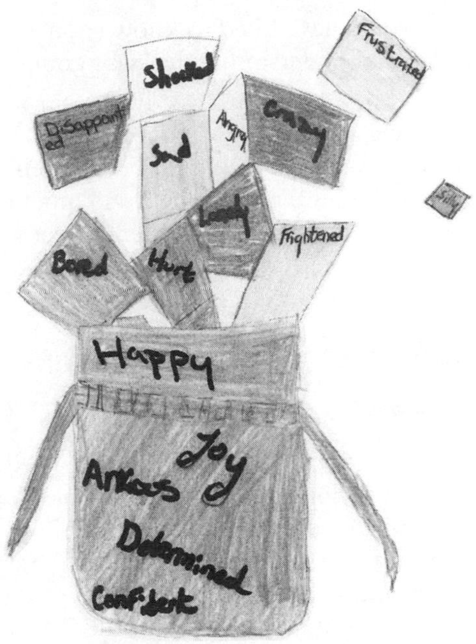

FIGURE 10.1. "Inside" and "outside" feelings: Drawing by a 14-year-old girl, whose mother died from ovarian cancer, of the feelings she keeps to herself (the items that go inside the pouch) and those she shows others (the labels on the outside of the pouch).

The following discussion among a group of children between the ages of 6 and 12 illustrates the variety of emotions that grieving children may experience after the death of a parent:

FACILITATOR: What are some of the feelings you had, or still have, after the person died?

HANNAH: I was *so* mad!

FACILITATOR: You were *so* mad. Who else felt mad?

ZACHARY: Well, I was kinda mad at the doctor for not fixing my mom, but mostly I'm just sad.

FACILITATOR: You felt a combination—mostly sad, but a little mad at the doctor.

LIZA: My dad's doctor cried, so I didn't get mad at him. I was just really confused because I didn't understand what happened. Every other time we went to the hospital, my dad got better.

FACILITATOR: Mad, sad, and confused. It didn't make sense to you that your dad didn't get better this time.

LIZA: Yeah. I wish my mom had told me sooner.

FACILITATOR: You would have liked to know sooner. Did anyone else feel confused or not understand what was going on?

WILLIAM: Not me. I knew my mom was dying; our friend Grace told me when she came over that morning. I mean, I knew, but I sort of didn't want to, you know? It's weird. I didn't tell anyone, but I was a little happy too because it was always so quiet at my house when my mom was sick. Now I can have friends over and play games and run around.

DEVELOPMENTAL CONSIDERATIONS

Groups Based on Ages and Experiences

The literature acknowledges that children are influenced by their developmental age, as well as by previous experiences and by how they make sense of what has happened (Norris-Shortle et al., 1993; Silverman, 1999; Webb, 2010; Worden, 1996). On the basis of this literature, the groups in our program are divided by age and in some cases by type of death. Our "Littles" groups are for children between the ages of 3 and 5. The next age range is children from 6 to 12 years. Within this age range, there are groups specifically for children who have experienced a death due to chronic illness, sudden death (e.g., plane crash, car crash, heart attack), suicide, and violent death. We also offer "Middlers" groups for those ages 11–14, teen groups for those ages 13–18, and young adult groups for those ages 19–35. During each of our child and teen groups, there are concurrent peer support groups for the adults and caregivers.

Varying Responses to Loss

In the last century, researchers have moved from viewing grief as a passive experience to seeing it as an active response to loss—one that results in a reordering of priorities. This reordering moves the bereaved to make choices about how to grieve, engage with life, and make meaning out of the experience (Attig, 1991). Based on this view, we offer children opportunities to actively engage with their physical and emotional responses to loss. Figure 10.2 reflects this type of active engagement; this drawing by a 9-year-old boy whose mother was run over by a car depicts the boy's symbols of life and death.

We add a note of caution about using a developmental lens in work with grieving children: Although it can be helpful to put children's emotional, cognitive, and behavioral responses into a developmental context, it is less helpful to use them as rigid categorizations to assess whether a child is grieving "well" or "right." Even adults, with full capacities for abstract thinking, may find themselves having the same questions as their toddlers ("Why?" and "Why me?") and similar protestations ("No! This can't be happening!").

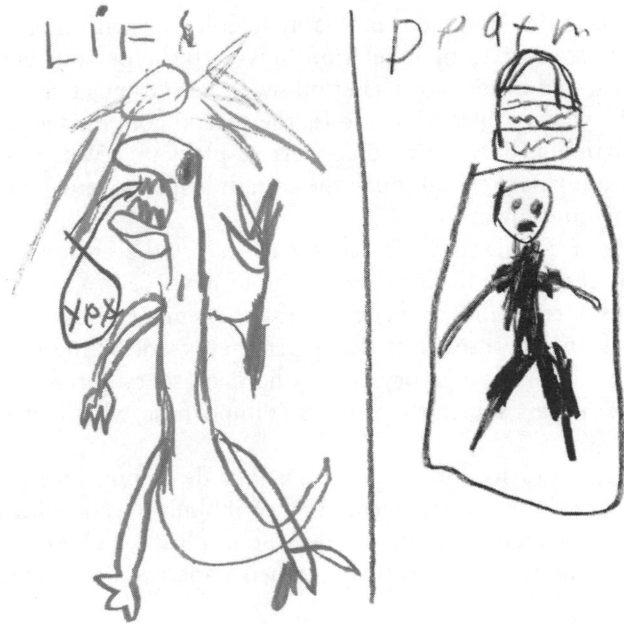

FIGURE 10.2. Symbols of life and death drawn by a 9-year-old boy whose mother was hit and killed by a car. Life is a lizard dance party; death is a human figure in a coffin.

ACTIVITIES TO USE WITH GRIEVING CHILDREN AND TEENS

There are a variety of activities to use for working with grieving children in individual, family, and group settings. In this section, we describe activities in a peer support program, but these can be adapted to other therapeutic contexts as well.

Ritual Storytelling

Researchers Norton and Gino (2014) found that "engaging in rituals mitigates grief by restoring the feelings of control that are impaired" when someone dies (p. 272). The rituals they studied were self-defined and encompassed diverse activities from across cultural and religious traditions, as well as personalized ones designed by participants. This wide spectrum of rituals supports the claim that the effectiveness depends more on the act of engaging in a ritual than on the particulars of the ritual itself. Building rituals into practice with grieving children is an important method, for it can help to decrease distressing emotions and even build positive ones that come to be associated with the ritual itself. The rituals studied by Norton and Gino actually enabled their participants to regain a sense of control, regardless of whether or not they believed in the effectiveness of the ritual.

Grieving children and teens are likely to come up with their own unique rituals that are specific to their relationships with the persons who died. For instance, 8-year-old Emma wraps her pillow in her father's t-shirt every night before bed; 12-year-old Brandon carries the special coin his mother gave him for his 4th birthday to every band concert he plays in. "Whenever I get nervous, I reach in my pocket and touch the coin. It helps me remember how calm I would feel around my mom."

In groups at The Dougy Center, we use a ritual storytelling activity as an avenue for children and teens to engage in new ways with their loss stories. We invite participants to write or draw a memory about the death, and then do something to transform the paper they used. While many children and teens will choose a memory that is hard or scary for them, some will pick happy memories. Which they pick isn't important; what matters is letting them choose.

Options for transforming their paper include ripping it into pieces and putting it in a bowl of water, burning it, scribbling over it with markers or other crayons, or burying it in the ground. Some children choose to say something or make a noise as they transform their paper as a way of marking the transition.

Label Your Feelings

Grieving children and adolescents may struggle with identifying and understanding the various emotions they experience. (Arvidson et al., 2011). The activity we call Label Your Feelings assists youth to name their feelings, as well as to describe where and how they are affected. First, we ask the participants to identify different feelings—both ones they associate with grief and those they experience at any time (happiness, sadness, anger, confusion, "being different," etc.). Then we hand out sheets of blank labels, and we invite the youth to write down whichever emotions they relate to and place the stickers on the places in their bodies where they experience the feelings. This activity enables participants to increase self-awareness of their emotional responses and to acknowledge how those emotions affect them on a physical level. When the activity is done in a group or with a therapist, the participants also have the opportunity to learn how their emotional landscapes are similar to or different from those of other people who are also dealing with grief. Throughout this activity, having caring adults (in this case, trained volunteers and staff members) reflect the words, facial expressions, and body movements of the participants helps them "use creative methods to transform fear, worry, anger, and sadness, helping them identify their own healing responses through sensory experiences" (Malchiodi, 2008, p. 36). The drawing shown in Figure 10.3 is an extension of the Label Your Feelings activity: It depicts the emotions experienced in various parts of her body by an 8-year-old girl whose father died in a plane crash.

Neutralizing Negative Memories

Memories are what those who are grieving have left. Many of these memories come with laughter and sometimes tears of joy. Others can bring great sadness, regret, and intense physical responses. When remembering difficult memories, people tend to focus on the emotions they experienced (sadness, embarrassment, fear, etc.). Recent discoveries in the realm of memory recall offer a way to help dispel the emotional charge of the worst memories. Denkova, Dolcos, and Dolcos (2015) found that by simply turning the focus away from the emotions and putting it instead into remembering contextual details (such as the weather, what they were wearing, and who was with them), people were able to reduce the intensity of the emotions associated with these memories. This process of "distracting" during the recollection process engages the area of the brain related to emotional regulation (the ventromedial prefrontal cortex), thus mediating the emotional impact of negative memories. Placing difficult memories within a nonemotional context provides an alternative to the two main ways people tend to deal with challenging memories: suppression and reappraisal. Suppression has been shown not only to be an ineffective strategy for decreasing subjective emotional distress, but to invoke a sympathetic nervous system response. Suppression has also been found to "produce a rebound of unwanted thoughts during post-suppression periods" (Campbell-Sills, Barlow, Brown, & Hoffman, 2006, p. 1260).

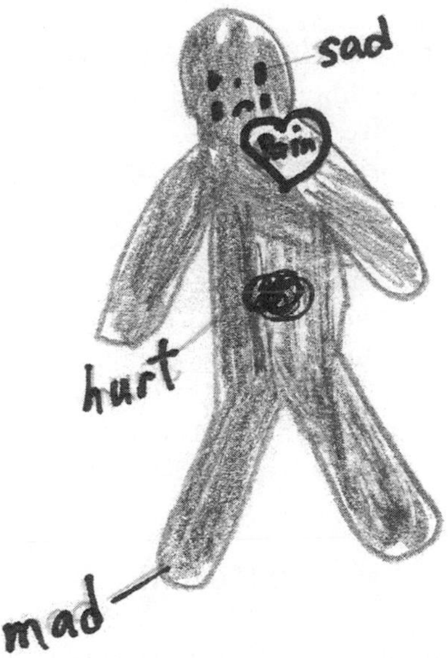

FIGURE 10.3. "Emotions in my body": A picture of the Label Your Feelings activity, drawn by an 8-year-old girl whose father died in a plane crash.

Reappraisal—the process of cognitively restructuring an event to find a "silver lining"—has been documented to be effective in down-regulating emotion without leading to an increase in sympathetic nervous system response, but it also requires energy and skills that may be in short supply for someone in the midst of grief (Denkova et al., 2015; Gross, 2002). Based on these research findings, we have created an activity to help young people process hard memories. We ask them to bring to mind a situation related to their grief that is hard for them to think about, and then to list anything they can recall about the situation that wasn't related to their emotions. A 9-year-old boy named Jacob wrote about the last day he saw his mother at the hospital. He recalled the color of the walls ("White!"); the Superman t-shirt he wore; Nancy, the nurse who always had lollipops in her pocket; and the pizza he ate for lunch that day. This approach helps people understand that they have choices when it comes to images or thoughts that have the potential to overwhelm them with distressing emotions.

Support Chain

When children and teens lose parents or other primary caregivers, they commonly have fears and worries about who will take care of their day-to-day needs. The Support Chain activity is designed to address the need for a variety of options when it comes to activities that help them feel cared for and safe. Work in the realm of trauma demonstrates that individuals are better able to calm themselves when they receive both emotional attunement and assistance with skills for self-regulation (Bornstein, 2014). This activity encourages participants to think creatively about various options for support, and to trust that they can calm themselves as well as call on others for help. The young people are provided with strips of construction paper and asked to think of activities, people, or anything else that provides comfort. On each piece of paper, they write an activity ("listening to music," "getting a hug," "squeezing my teddy bear") on one side, and a person or thing they can go to for that activity ("myself," "my grandma," "George, my teddy bear") on the other. After all the ideas they can think of are written down, the strips can be looped and stapled to make a chain. Children and teens can be invited to hang these chains somewhere in their homes, so that when they feel overwhelmed, they have visual reminders of options for ways to find support and reassurance.

CONCLUSION

In our experience, the foundation of working with children/teens and grief is engaging them at some level in the concept of process—whether that process is verbal, physical, or creative. We work to engage them enough that they are able to find one or many ways to move within their experience of grief. This engagement may be generated by an individual therapist, within the context of a family therapy, or by other participants in a peer support group. A child who comes to a session or to group to see and play with her "friends" is a child who feels comfortable in an environment that is grief-focused. Although these young people come to our offices and our programs to play and have fun, they do so in a context that is grounded in the concept of loss.

In our program, we teach volunteers the skills of awareness, reflection, conversation, and group cohesion in an effort to help them learn best how to create alliances with the children, adolescents, and adults who attend our groups. These same skills are useful in the many settings where we helping professionals work with grieving youth. They also allow us to create a context in which children and adolescents can direct their own meaning-making process after a death.

STUDY QUESTIONS

1. Think through The Dougy Center's peer support group model for bereavement. Which elements from the program could you adapt to use in individual or family therapy? What would those adaptations look like?
2. Given that everyone grieves in his or her own way, how would you help a family navigate the conflict and misunderstanding that can arise when members are trying to support one another?
3. In thinking through your personal experiences with grief, what did you learn from family and friends about "right" and "wrong" ways to grieve? How do you think your past experiences may affect your work with grieving children?
4. After reading about the ways children and adolescents may feel guilt and regret after a parent's death, how would you respond if this came up in your work with grieving youth?

REFERENCES

Arvidson, J., Kinniburgh, K., Howard, K., Spinazzola, J., Strothers, H., et al. (2011). Treatment of complex trauma in young children: Developmental and cultural considerations in application of the ARC intervention model. *Journal of Child and Adolescent Trauma, 4*, 34–51.

Attig, T. (1991). The importance of conceiving of grief as an active process. *Death Studies, 15*(4), 385–393.

Bornstein, D. (2014). Teaching children to calm themselves. Retrieved May 9, 2014, from *http://opinionator.blogs.nytimes.com/2014/03/19/first-learn-how-to-calm-down/#more-152440*

Bowlby, J. (1973). *Attachment and loss: Vol. 2. Separation: Anxiety and anger.* New York: Basic Books.

Bowlby, J. (1980). *Attachment and loss: Vol. 3. Loss: Sadness and depression.* New York: Basic Books.

Bowlby, J. (1982). *Attachment and loss: Vol. 1. Attachment.* New York: Basic Books. (Original work published 1969)

Bowlby, J. (1988). *A secure base: Parent–child attachment and healthy human development.* New York: Basic Books.

Campbell-Sills, L., Barlow, D. H., Brown, T. A., & Hofmann, S. G. (2006). Effects of suppression and acceptance on emotional responses of individuals with anxiety and mood disorders. *Behaviour Research and Therapy, 44*(9), 1251–1263.

Chilcote, R. L. (2007). Art therapy with child tsunami survivors in Sri Lanka. *Art Therapy: Journal of the American Art Therapy Association, 24*(4), 156–162.

Denkova, E., Dolcos, S., & Dolcos, F. (2015). Neural correlates of "distracting" from emotion during autobiographical recollection. *Social Cognitive and Affective Neuroscience, 10*(2), 219–230.

Evans, D. W., Leckman, J. F., Carter, A., Reznick, J. S., Henshaw, D., King, R. A., et al. (1997). Ritual, habit, and perfectionism: The prevalence and development of compulsive-like behavior in normal young children. *Child Development, 68*(1), 58–68.

Freud, A., & Burlingham, D. (1947). *Infants without families: The case for and against residential nurseries.* New York: International Universities Press.

Gross, J. J. (2002). Emotion regulation: Affective, cognitive, and social consequences. *Psychophysiology, 39*(3), 281–291.

Hilliard, R. E. (2007). The effects of Orff-based music therapy and social work groups on childhood grief symptoms and behaviors. *Journal of Music Therapy, 44*(2), 123–128.

Lutzke, J. R., Ayers, T. S., Sandler, I. N., & Barr, A. (1997). Risks and interventions for the parentally bereaved child. In S. A. Wolchik & I. N. Sandler (Eds.), *Handbook of children's coping* (pp. 215–243). New York: Plenum Press.

Malchiodi, C. A. (2008). Effective practice with traumatized children: Ethics, evidence, and cultural sensitivity. In C. A. Malchiodi (Ed.), *Creative interventions with traumatized children* (pp. 22–43). New York: Guilford Press.

Norris-Shortle, C., & Young, P. A. (1993). Understanding death and grief for children three and younger. *Social Work, 38*(6). 736–742.

Norton, M. I., & Gino, F. (2013). Rituals alleviate grieving for loved ones, lovers, and lotteries. *Journal of Experimental Psychology: General, 143*(1), 266–272.

Siegel, D. J. (2012). *The developing mind: How relationships and the brain interact to shape who we are* (2nd ed.). New York: Guilford Press.

Silverman, P. R. (1999). *Never too young to know: Death in children's lives.* New York: Oxford University Press.

Webb, N. B. (2010). (Ed.). *Helping bereaved children: A handbook for practitioners* (3rd ed.). New York: Guilford Press.

Worden, J. W. (1996). *Children and grief: When a parent dies.* New York: Guilford Press.

Wylie, M. S. (2004, September–October). Mindsight. *Psychotherapy Networker*, pp. 29–39.

SUGGESTED READING

Books for Children

Ages 3–6

Brown, L. K., & Brown, M. (1996). *When dinosaurs die: A guide to understanding death.* Boston: Little, Brown.

Silverman, J. (1999). *Help me say goodbye: Activities for helping kids cope when a special person dies.* Silver Spring, MD: Fairview Press.

Thomas, P. (2001). *I miss you: A first look at death.* Hauppauge, NY: Barrons Educational Series.

Ages 7–10

Eldon, A. (2002). *Angel catcher for kids: A journal to help you remember the person you love who died.* San Francisco: Chronicle Books.

Goldman, L. (1998). *Bart speaks out: Breaking the silence on suicide.* Los Angeles: Western Psychological Services.

Romain, T. (1999). *What on earth do you do when someone dies?* Minneapolis, MN: Free Spirit.

Ages 10–13

Cosby, B. (2000). *The day I saw my father cry.* New York: Scholastic.

Dennison, A. (2003). *Our dad died: The true story of three kids whose lives changed.* Minneapolis, MN: Free Spirit.

Dower, L. (2001). *I will remember you: What to do when someone you love dies.* New York: Scholastic.

Books for Professionals and Other Adults to Help Grieving Children

Dougy Center. (2000). *35 ways to help a grieving child.* Portland, OR: Author.

Dougy Center. (2005). *Memories matter: An activities manual for grieving children.* Portland, OR: Author.

Schaefer, D., Lyons, C., & Perez, D. (2002). *How do we tell the children?: A step-by-step guide for helping children two to teen when someone dies.* New York: Newmarket Press.

Wolfelt, A. (1996). *Healing the bereaved child: Grief gardening, growth through grief and other touchstones for caregivers.* Fort Collins, CO: Companion Press.

Chapter 11

The Crisis of Parental Deployment in Military Service

JOSEPH R. HERZOG
R. BLAINE EVERSON
JENNIFER TAYLOR

Since the turn of the 21st century, all branches of the U.S. military have experienced increased involvement in a variety of conflicts. These conflicts have increased the amount of time service members spend away from their families as a result of more frequent and longer deployments. Less well known is the fact that these deployments take place in times of peace, as well as in war. In today's military, it is not uncommon for a father, mother, or both parents in a family to deploy. This deployment may be of short duration (such as for a training mission), or for a longer period (such as for sea duty, peacekeeping missions, unaccompanied tours [those without family members], or extended tours in combat zones). Parental separation can have a profound impact on the family in general and on children/adolescents in particular. The family member(s) in the military may view the deployment as business as usual, but children experience this separation as loss of daily contact with their parent(s). This loss is compounded by the potentially dangerous duty in which the parent(s) may be engaged.

The family lives of soldiers, sailors, or air personnel involve numerous associated stressors and strains, including frequent relocations and lengthy separations that create incongruency between work and family life (Albano, 1994; Everson, Herzog, Figley, & Whitworth, 2014). Furthermore, a military family often consists of members from various regions of the world and/or different ethnic backgrounds, and one or both parents may have had previous marriages or relationships.

This chapter provides an overview of a family-systems-based approach with children/adolescents in military families. We begin by discussing pertinent issues for families with children and adolescents within the military context. In particular, we discuss the family, child, and adolescent stressors specifically associated with the deployment cycle, as well as the occurrence of combat-related trauma in service members and secondary traumatic stress in their family members. Next, an evolving dynamic model for play therapy is discussed by developmental stages and phases of treatment. Finally, we review two cases that illustrate this approach to play therapy with children in military families.

ISSUES FOR FAMILIES AND CHILDREN WITHIN THE MILITARY CONTEXT

Effects of Service on Military Personnel Themselves

Military service renders armed forces personnel more susceptible to a variety of health concerns, including cardiovascular disorders, endocrinological dysfunction, neoplasms, mental illnesses, and substance-related problems (Bray et al., 2003). Among the mental illnesses for which military personnel are at risk, posttraumatic stress disorder (PTSD) in combat troops has been a focus of particular concern for several decades. Evidence from one study suggests that PTSD may be more prevalent among U.S. ground forces serving in Iraq and Afghanistan than previously thought (Hoge et al., 2004). This sample of inpatients, who had experienced a wide range of injuries from combat, reported problems associated with the three major PTSD symptom sets of intrusion, hyperarousal, and affective constriction. Hoge and colleagues (2004) further suggested that as many as one in six soldiers (17%) were suffering symptoms of this disorder. More recent evidence suggests that members of the U.S. military's ground forces may suffer from a variety of depressive and anxiety-related symptoms due to combat exposure, as well as from "moral injury" related to experiences of a horrific nature (death, destruction, etc.) within a combat theater (Nash & Litz, 2013). The emotional and behavioral aspects of combat stress and moral injury constitute a less visible problem for the military than do formal diagnoses of PTSD, but a more pervasive set of challenges for service members and their families.

Deployment-Related Stress and Problems for Families

No other stressor assails the coping abilities of military personnel, spouses/partners, and families like the separations created as a result of frequent deployments (Black, 1993; Everson et al., 2014). Regardless of a deployed person's experience, the emotional impact of the separation on parents and their children represents a significant and profound loss for all family members. The involvement in either combat or peacekeeping missions causes considerable stress for family members who remain behind. Separation from significant attachment relationships and the resulting anxiety caused by military deployments often disrupt the daily functioning of children and family members, and create the need for intervention by helping professionals. The increase in length and number of deployments associated with the U.S. military involvement in both Afghanistan and Iraq has caused excessive strain on family members and the various community relationships in which they are involved (Bowen, Mancini, Martin, Ware, & Nelson, 2003). A number of indicators point to a link between the separations caused by wartime deployments and an increase in the emotional difficulties experienced by military families, including the breakup of marriages and families (Ruger, Wilson, & Waldrop, 2002). We discuss the effects of the deployment cycle on the family system more fully in a later section.

The Specific Effects of Parental Separation on Children/Adolescents

The effect of parental absence on children/adolescents has been an important area of study in the military family research literature. Most of the research to date has been on father absence, although there has been growing interest in mother absence. Father absence has been found to be negatively related to children's behavioral adjustment and academic performance, as well as to increased levels of anxiety and depression (Hiew, 1992; Jensen, Grogan, Xenakis, & Bain, 1989). Children/adolescents of deployed parents are at risk for increased psychiatric hospitalization rates (Levai & Kaplan, 1995); increased aggression and dependency have also been found in later-born sons, and decreased quantitative ability in daughters (Hillenbrand, 1976). Kelley (1994) found that even routine missions were disruptive to military families to some degree, especially for families with young school-age children. She identified the period just before deployment as the most stressful for children. Children/adolescents who experienced a peacekeeping deployment had some behavioral problems that decreased over time, whereas the problematic behavior of war-separated children did not improve over time. Furthermore, although total *number* of deployments did not increase anxious and depressive symptoms in children/adolescents, the *length* of deployment had the opposite effect (Jensen et al., 1989).

As the number of mothers in the armed forces increases, research concerning the effects of mother absence has also increased. The finding that children's and adolescents' psychosocial functioning is equally affected, regardless of whether they are separated from mothers or fathers (Applewhite & Mays, 1996), suggests that much of the literature on father absence may be relevant for mother absence as well. As in the research on father absence, children of deployed Navy mothers have been found to have higher levels of internalizing behaviors (e.g., fearfulness and sadness) than do their civilian counterparts

(Kelley et al., 2001). These children and adolescents also exhibit higher rates of externalizing behaviors (including aggressiveness and noncompliance). Pierce, Vinokur, and Buck (1998) found that children separated from their mothers during wartime deployments often experienced adjustment problems; these problems worsened with the degree of disruption in a child's life and with a mother's failure to provide stable child care during the deployment. These effects, however, disappeared 2 years later.

Additional Stressors for Military Families

Geographic Mobility

A common feature of military family life is geographic mobility. This mobility may occur within the continental United States, as well as in farther-flung U.S. states and possessions (Alaska, Hawaii, Guam, etc.) and across the world (Germany, Japan, etc.). Military families may move as often as once every 2–3 years. This can be difficult for military children/adolescents, who may repeatedly experience the loss of friends, change of schools, and separation from extended family members.

Generally, length of residence is associated with better peer relations and less loneliness for children/adolescents (Kelley, Finkel, & Ashby, 2003). Family relationships in general and relationships with mothers in particular play an important role in mediating the effects of relocation (Kelley et al., 2003; Pittman & Bowen, 1994). The quality of parent–child relations is the most important factor in children's adjustment (Pittman & Bowen, 1994). Positive relationships with mothers are related to a reduction in feelings of loneliness and fears of negative evaluation. Depression in mothers is associated with anxious and depressed behaviors in children, who also display more aggression and noncompliance (Kelley et al., 2003).

Race/Ethnicity and Family Composition

Military families may include all races and ethnicities, and sometimes they are mixed in their composition. For example, it is not unusual to have a family in treatment in which the father is African American, the mother is German with biological children from an earlier relationship, and the children of the present relationship are of mixed African American and German heritage. Foreign-born military spouses/partners may have limited English skills, further complicating their adjustment and that of their children. Everson, Darling, and Herzog (2012) found that minority female Army spouses experienced more parenting stress during long-term combat-related deployments than their European American counterparts, due primarily to perceived lack of support and lower sense of coherence. Cultural and blended-family issues can be major factors in practice with these families and should be initially acknowledged.

Other Issues

Further matters to consider in working with military families include sexual harassment, limited financial resources, and single parenthood. Female military personnel may experience sexual abuse/harassment on the job, and this can have an impact on their children (Mathewson, 2011). This sexual harassment may compound past sexual abuse, awakening this issue within a family. Junior enlisted families also often do not have the financial resources to buffer the stressors they experience. For instance, they may not have reliable transportation, and many military installations are located in rural areas with no public transportation. On-post housing may be in short supply, forcing these families into substandard off-post housing. Finally, increasing numbers of military personnel are single parents, and the effects of this on their children must be considered, especially in combination with the other issues mentioned here.

Effects of the Deployment Cycle on the Family System

The average length of deployment associated with military service in the U.S. Army or the U.S. Marines in Iraq and Afghanistan has ranged from 12 to 15 months. This represents an increase over previous peacekeeping missions of 6 months to the Balkans and Kuwait during the late 1990s. From a family systems perspective, the deployment cycle represents a change and a challenge to the structural integrity of a family system.

After the deployed service member departs, the family system must adjust to this loss. As part of this adjustment process, family members often experience a variety of physical disruptions (e.g., lack of sleep, loss of appetite, anxiety, malaise) and emotional maladies (e.g., sadness, irritability, dysphoria) during the first few months of a long-term deployment (Everson, Herzog, & Haigler, 2011). Often during this time, families will seek assistance for any number of symptoms associated with the strain of deployment. As a deployment lengthens, a family tends to adjust to the stressors and strains associated with functioning without the service member, eventually achieving a new homeostasis. This adjustment may be achieved with professional assistance and/or through the family's extrasystemic involvements, such as religious affiliation, military unit support, or the school system.

Later, the prospective return of the service member creates a new set of strains as the family prepares for the upcoming changes in its functioning. The waiting spouse/partner (traditionally a wife, but increasingly often a husband) may experience ambivalence in balancing the anticipated loss of autonomy with the joy of reconstituting the family. Children may respond to the return of the service member with many different emotions, depending on their developmental stage and any existing emotional difficulties. The family members often experience a "honeymoon phase" after the return of the service member, varying in length and intensity; yet after a lengthy absence, the return often presents the family system with a new set of challenges, as the family and the service member attempt to readjust and realign their roles within the system.

When the service member has experienced physical or emotional trauma associated with combat exposure (wounds, PTSD, combat stress, etc.), this trauma may be experienced by the family system in a reactive manner (Figley, 1998a; Nash & Litz, 2013). The spouse/partner experiences role strain as he or she takes on the burden of caring for the ailing service member, potentially reducing her (or his) caregiving capacity for any children within the household. This strain increases the children's anxiety, creating new symptoms or exacerbating existing symptoms from previously unresolved stresses. This set of circumstances causes further role strain in the cycle, due to increased demands from various family members. Over the course of multiple deployments, stresses may pile up and remain unresolved, thereby creating a backlog of difficulties within the family system (McCubbin, Thompson, & McCubbin, 2001).

Secondary Trauma: Implications for Children and Families

Many soldiers returning from Afghanistan and Iraq have trauma symptoms related to their war experiences, as noted earlier. Soldiers with PTSD are often withdrawn and avoidant; may experience flashbacks, exaggerated startle responses, and even fugue states; and may also be prone to intermittent rage. These symptoms can have a profound effect upon other family members. Spouses/partners and children in families of military personnel with PTSD are susceptible to developing secondary traumatic stress symptoms (Herzog, Everson, & Whitworth, 2011; Herzog, Scott, Lewis, & Everson, 2013).

The origins of secondary trauma theory were described in reports on clinical practice with Holocaust survivors and their families (see Danieli, 1998) in the late 1960s. A seeming conspiracy of silence prevented Holocaust survivors from integrating their traumatic experiences, due to the failure of others (including therapists) to listen to and believe their traumatic accounts. Danieli (1998) found that the children of these survivors seemed to have absorbed their parents' Holocaust experiences and displayed psychological symptoms that appeared to be connected with those experiences. Secondary trauma theory further evolved from the reports dealing with military families. Rosenheck and Nathan's (1985) clinical experience with children of Vietnam veterans led them to coin the term "secondary traumatization," which they defined as "the relationship between the fathers' war experiences and subsequent stress disorder and their children's problems" (p. 538).

Figley (1998b) has developed and defined many of the concepts related to the definition of secondary trauma. According to Figley, such trauma includes "the experience of tension and distress directly related to the demands of living with and caring for displays of the symptoms of post-traumatic stress disorder," as well as "the natural and consequent behaviors and emotions resulting from knowledge about a stressful event experienced by a significant other" (p. 7). Over time, secondary traumatic stress can lead to emotional exhaustion and burnout. In a family, this burnout results in "the breakdown of the family members' collective commitment to each other and a refusal to work together in harmony as a function of some crisis or traumatic event or series of crises of crises or events that leave members emotionally exhausted and disillusioned" (Figley, 1998b, p. 7).

Secondary trauma symptoms have been considered to be similar to but less intense than PTSD symptoms; they include avoidance, intrusion, and arousal (Motta, Joseph, Rose, Suozzi, & Leiderman, 1997). Figley (1998a) suggests that these symptoms include "visual images (e.g. flashbacks), sleeping problems, depression, and other symptoms that are a direct result of visualizing the victim's traumatic experiences, exposure to the symptoms of the victim, or both" (p. 20). Indeed, children of parents with PTSD have been found to have significantly more somatic complaints, social problems, attention problems, and aggression than the children of parents with substance abuse have (Dan, 1996).

Due to the high levels of trauma experienced by military personnel in Afghanistan and Iraq, and the resultant levels of PTSD, therapists will be called upon to treat members of these families. Although the military is now making every effort to identify personnel with PTSD, many members of the military continue to feel that a stigma is attached to mental health treatment. Often family members of traumatized military personnel take the initiative in seeking treatment. Children in these families may present in therapy with symptoms that mimic PTSD, as well as with anxiety and depressive symptoms. These symptoms are directly related to the trauma symptoms of their parents. Play therapy is a useful approach in the treatment of children/adolescents within these traumatized families.

SYSTEMIC PLAY THERAPY WITH CHILDREN/ADOLESCENTS IN MILITARY FAMILIES

The systemic approach to play therapy views children, adolescents, and their families as members of a dynamic, ever-developing system, capable of constant adjustment and adaptation within their larger social contexts. The following three goals apply to play therapy with a child of a military family who is in crisis:

1. Reduce the child's symptoms.
2. Include the parent(s) in the child/adolescent's therapy, in order to help her, him, or them understand the child/adolescent's difficulties and to encourage parental interaction with the child.
3. Employ psychoeducational interventions to assist the child/adolescent with life changes related to the parent's deployment.

The therapist begins by seeking to engage the child/adolescent (and family) in a therapeutic setting and a secure environment in order to relieve the youth's symptoms. Because these symptoms are often related to the military parent's stressful service-related experiences, it is important from a systemic perspective that this parent be present if at all possible (and certainly that the other parent be present). Parents are also included in sessions to create positive understanding of the therapeutic interventions and to model play as an interactional component of the parent–child/adolescent relationship. In short, not only are parents crucial to the assessment process, but they should remain in as many sessions as are necessary to complete the planned course of treatment. Finally, play is utilized in a proactive way to help reduce anxiety over anticipated or actual life events and changes, such as relocation, deployment, or reunification. This multifocal model, adapted from Webb's tripartite approach (see Webb, Chapter 1, this volume), provides a framework for understanding the impact of a crisis situation in interaction with personal and familial factors influencing the crisis response, as well as the extrasystemic support factors determining the nature of the familial (mal)adaptations. Ultimately, the use of play as a therapeutic tool allows for a corrective emotional experience, bringing the child/adolescent's daily functioning into synchrony with his or her appropriate developmental age and with systemic expectations (Smith, 2011).

A child/adolescent's cognitive, emotional, and social developmental stage influences the young person's perception about his or her role within the family system. The play therapist takes account of the child/adolescent's developmental stage and responds to him or her according to a particular theoretical and practice framework. O'Connor (1991) presents several different models of play therapy, but space does not permit us to discuss all of these here. We use an approach that attempts to integrate family systems methods with crisis intervention play therapy, while always relying on developmental factors to guide the treatment. We believe that this systemic, contextual model is appropriate for children and adolescents in military families. The developmental stage of the child/adolescent determines the particular methods of play used, with family dynamics and larger systemic factors providing the context for assessing the symptoms, treating the problems, and working on relapse prevention (Smith, 2011).

PHASES OF PLAY THERAPY FOR MILITARY CHILDREN AND TEENS

A number of factors determine the approach to play therapy for children/adolescents of families within the military. The cycle of a service member's departures, separations, and returns due to deployments creates a difficult set of circumstances for all family members (Daley, 1999; Hardaway, 2004); these issues are compounded if the service member returns from duty physically injured or psychologically traumatized by the experience. Furthermore, the adjustment upon return may be disrupted by problems that may have transpired at home while the service member was deployed (Figley, 1998a). Taking a multifocal systemic view of the child/adolescent and the family is thus imperative for the clinician who is beginning a therapeutic relationship with the youth.

Assessment

The first phase of treatment involves assessing the child/adolescent for symptoms, and the family for systemic problems that may be associated with the child/adolescent's current problems. Sleep and appetite disturbances, bad dreams, negativistic fantasies, crying spells, irritability (related to anxiety), agitation, fearfulness, reemergence of bedwetting, and hypersensitivity to interaction are common among children/adolescents across various developmental stages (O'Connor, 1991). Steinberg (1998) has argued that such symptoms may stem from a child/adolescent's experience of secondary traumatic stress. According to Steinberg (1998), several risk factors for secondary traumatic stress should be considered; these include the child/adolescent's gender and birth order (an oldest female child may be particularly susceptible), the existence of previous symptomatology, and a lack of familial social integration (i.e., lack of religious or other community involvement). If the child/adolescent has preexisting emotional or behavioral problems, such as symptoms of attention-deficit/hyperactivity disorder or oppositional defiant disorder, these may be compounded by the stress associated with the deployment cycle and may actually mask deeper symptoms of depression or anxiety, which should be assessed thoroughly and carefully.

Multigenerational genograms (McGoldrick, Gerson, & Petry, 2008) have been used to assess families upon entry into family therapy, and these are especially important in teasing out the extent to which systemic difficulties may be influencing a child/adolescent's symptoms. Initial treatment planning should be completed by the end of this assessment period. This phase of treatment usually lasts one to three sessions, and the introduction of play within the family sessions is a part of this phase of treatment.

Joining

The second phase of treatment involves joining with the child/adolescent and the family. This phase builds upon the trust and rapport that have been established in the assessment phase. This process usually lasts between three and five sessions, as the child/adolescent and family members grow more comfortable with the therapist and the therapeutic process. If family members have reservations about play therapy and/or trepidation about its effectiveness, the therapist needs to reduce their resistance to play's inclusion in the ongoing therapy. It is important to build the therapeutic alliance before the next phase of treatment begins (Sori, 2006). The end of this phase involves an agreement about the essence of the problem (or problems) and all of its systemic aspects.

Maintenance

The next phase of therapy involves the maintenance of the already existing therapeutic relationship. This is the longest stage of treatment, lasting from 5 to 15 sessions; it often involves engaging in play therapy with the child/adolescent, seeing the entire family for family therapy, and combining the two approaches in single sessions from time to time. It is often prudent to involve a sibling in the play therapy and/or family therapy sessions. Continuing to cultivate the deepening therapeutic relationship is most important; however, problem solving and the use of directives for changing behaviors among members of the system are also important. Fostering problem-solving behavior improves coping and helps to buffer the family members from ongoing stressors in their daily lives, while therapeutic directives and first-order feedback are used to bring about change in the system (Berg-Cross, 2000). One of the primary expectations of this approach is that "triangulation" will occur between the family and the therapist, and that the therapist can use this dynamic as a tool for facilitating change within the family system.

Closure

The final phase of therapy involves reaching closure with the child/adolescent and the family in the process of terminating the case. During this final phase of the relationship, it is important to check progress, begin the end of therapy with appropriate processes, and make sure that relapse prevention procedures have been put into place. This phase of therapy usually lasts from two to three sessions. The therapist must use intuition and sensitivity to the family's circumstances in determining when the time is right for ending a particular course of treatment. Central to this approach is the understanding that the therapeutic relationship means different things to the various people involved in the therapeutic process. In essence, therapy may never be "over," and clients may return at different stages of the family life cycle as problems reemerge. It is not uncommon in a practice with military families for these families to return even after they have moved away from one installation to another. With this approach, it is always best to maintain an "open-door" policy.

CASE EXAMPLES

The Case of Mateo, Age 11

The client, Mateo, was an 11-year-old Latino male who relocated with his family from a northern state after his father accepted a transfer to another base. The new station was in the southeastern United States. Mateo "loved" his old home and "hated" his new one. He was experiencing a very difficult adjustment to the move, with problems making friends at the new school despite superb functioning in his old school. The initial reason for referral was the poor adjustment to this move. Mateo had two siblings, one of whom (a younger sister) had very complex medical problems and a lot of pain. Over time, he was becoming more angry and aggressive toward his siblings (hitting them and being mean to them); he also refused to do his schoolwork and was generally uncooperative.

Mateo's mother disclosed that the boy's father had been deployed for over half of his son's life. The father was described as a "pretty good guy," but his last deployment in Afghanistan was "rough"; he didn't talk about it with the family, but he had seen "bad stuff." After he came back, he was extremely violent and explosive at times—hitting holes in walls, screaming at the family, and talking down to his wife/children. Overall, he had been very aggressive, and the children were afraid of him. This had been going on for the past few months. The client's father had also had an affair with another officer. The parents were planning to divorce, but had stayed together up to this point because of their daughter's medical issues. Mateo's mother had received counseling regarding protecting the children from their father, and now he was not allowed to be unsupervised with any of the children. Mateo's mother had a very strong personality and intervened if her husband became angry for any reason; she also did not allow the father to make any decisions regarding the children's care, and he was not involved in their school.

At the time of the most recent visit, Mateo's mother reported that her husband was preparing for another deployment in 12 weeks, for probably 9 months or more. A complicating factor was that Mateo's therapist (Jennifer Taylor, the "I" in what follows) was married to a military member who had just received orders, and she and her spouse would soon be moving. Mateo's mother was worried that her son was going to feel doubly abandoned, due to his therapist's moving and his father's deploying at about the same time.

Content of Session	*Rationale/Analysis*
THERAPIST: Hey, how are you?	
MATEO: Ugh (*head down, walking to office*).	Mateo is angry with me for missing the appointment last week. (I didn't tell him I was going to be gone.)
THERAPIST: I missed you last week when I was out of town.	Attempted to apologize and emphasize his value in my schedule.
MATEO: (*No response.*)	
THERAPIST: So what would you like to do or talk about today?	
MATEO: (*Fumbles through box of soldiers and superheroes, but does not respond.*)	
THERAPIST: (*Silence.*)	I give him some space to reestablish rapport after the missed week.

Mateo: (*Continues picking up things and putting back in drawer, finds stretchy snake, and turns toward therapist.*)

Therapist: (*Shrieks and pretends to be afraid of snake.*)

My actions allow Mateo to get revenge on me and to release his anger at me for "not showing up" (as his father often does).

Mateo: (*Laughs, turns back away from therapist, and then repeats action several times.*)

Therapist: (*Picks up feet off floor.*) I'm afraid of snakes.

Mateo: (*Laughs and continues action repeatedly.*)

Therapist: I am afraid of that one, and I don't know what to do!

Mateo: You have to fight him. He is the boss.

The boss represents his father, who explodes violently for no reason. Mateo is afraid of him.

Therapist: I don't know how to fight him. I'm scared to fight him.

Mateo: I'll show you how to fight the boss! (*Starts punching and hitting toy alligator, which is not the boss. Throws alligator on the floor and stomps on it, slams it with elbow, etc.*) See, he's dead.

Mateo is expressing anger at his father, which he is unable to do in real life.

Therapist: Wow, I feel so much safer now that the boss is dead.

Mateo: Now it's your turn to fight the boss. (*Starts to pick it back up, but then starts hitting and stomping on it again.*)

Therapist: Even when the boss is dead, you still want to hit it.

Mateo: Yeah . . . he deserves it. Now it's your turn, but you need some help. (*Gives therapist dinosaur, police officer, tractor.*)

THERAPIST: Oh thanks, I love having help! I'm scared to fight the boss by myself.

MATEO: (*Takes alligator, and uses it to attack all of the helpers, one by one.*)

Mateo is acting out his emotion at being all alone and having help taken away.

THERAPIST: Oh, no, my helpers are being attacked! The boss is so strong and powerful! What am I going to do now?

I emphasize the helpers' helplessness and the boss's power.

MATEO: The boss wins! All of your people are dead. (*Acts victorious as the boss.*)

Mateo's past helpers have not stopped the violence from his dad. He is afraid of abandonment and of being left to fight his dad without anyone intervening.

THERAPIST: I am all alone again. I have no one to help me against the boss (*sad face, looks down*).

I show Mateo's feelings of being alone and helpless. (Mateo has often reported, "No one can help," or "It will never change.")

MATEO: Here, this guy can help you (*gives therapist Power Ranger*) and this one (*gives police officer back*).

THERAPIST: I'm so relieved to have help again. I feel better already.

MATEO: If your guy falls into the lava pit, he dies.

THERAPIST: Oh, I know. I hope that doesn't happen.

MATEO: (*Makes alligator attack helpers again, and they each fall into "lava pit," one by one.*) That guy's dead . . . that one's dead, too. (*Brings out ballerina and makes her start fighting.*)

The ballerina appears to represent Mateo's mother, who is a strong figure for him, but who also has some history of anger and failure to protect Mateo from his father's outbursts. Mateo has mixed feelings about his mother: He blames her for the missed appointment last week (taking out helper), but he also recognizes that she has done a lot of work recently to stop the father from being violent with Mateo (no alone time; setting rules and enforcing them).

THERAPIST: Now there is someone new attacking me.

MATEO: This is the ballerina. She is the real boss, and she is the most powerful. (*Makes ballerina fight the helpers and put them all into the "lava pit."*)

THERAPIST: The ballerina is very strong and powerful. She took away all of my help.

MATEO: She can also fight the boss. (*Takes ballerina and uses her to attack alligator; spins her around and has her poke with toes.*)

This is evidence that the mother is being more protective of Mateo in the home against the father.

THERAPIST: I see she is very powerful. I feel better when she is around to fight the boss.

MATEO: Yes, the boss is afraid of her.

This suggests that the father is listening to the mother, despite his anger issues.

MATEO: (*Ends fight and lies on his back on the floor.*) You should read the Brother Band Chronicles.

Mateo makes a transition to a new topic, about a book series he is reading for school. (His schoolwork is a big issue.)

THERAPIST: What is it about?

MATEO: I'm not telling you . . . you have to read it.

THERAPIST: Hmm, I don't know where to find it.

MATEO: Barnes and Noble. I read the first one in 3 hours. It's 400 pages.

THERAPIST: You are a fast reader. It will take me forever to read 400 pages.

MATEO: You must be a slow reader like my dad. It took him a whole year to finish a book that was only 300 pages.

Mateo wishes that he had a better relationship with his father, and is sad (although somewhat mocking) regarding their differences.

THERAPIST: You are much smarter than your dad. Maybe you can

bring the book on your next visit, and I can start reading it?	
MATEO: You want me to bring it to you?	Mateo is surprised that someone is interested in his life.
THERAPIST: Sure, I'll read the book. What are you going to do as part of this deal?	
MATEO: I will eat a tree.	Mateo has difficulty with reciprocity in relationships; he wants to be in charge all the time.
THERAPIST: That sounds disgusting.	
MATEO: I am a centaur, and I eat metal trees like the one on the wall. (*Points to art on the wall.*)	
THERAPIST: Well, that doesn't sound like work. That's like me saying I will eat a lot of cookies.	
MATEO: Centaurs don't eat cookies.	
THERAPIST: They like trees the way I like cookies, so it's not going to work for a centaur. What kind of work is the centaur going to do?	
MATEO: Eat a sprinkler. He's lazy.	Mateo describes himself as lazy because, despite being tested as gifted (he skipped a grade in his old school), he is currently refusing to complete schoolwork.
THERAPIST: The centaur is not lazy. He can read very fast when he wants to. What is he willing to do this week?	I attempt to use the metaphor of the centaur to address/motivate Mateo, but he deflects the attempt and it fails.
MATEO: Don't mock me . . . I'm not doing anything.	
THERAPIST: How about you? Think about what the centaur is willing to do, and we can talk about it again next week when you bring the book for me?	
MATEO: You're not going to read it.	Mateo again expects to be disappointed in a relationship, but is willing to take a chance.

THERAPIST: I will read it, and then we can talk about it.

MATEO: OK, fine. I'll bring it.

THERAPIST: Oh, I forgot next Friday is a holiday. Do you want to skip next week, or should we add an appointment on Thursday?

MATEO: Thursday.

Mateo articulates the value of therapy by requesting the appointment.

THERAPIST: OK, I'll tell your mom. See you next week.

MATEO: Fine.

Mateo's anger improved over the next 3 weeks, as he was now involved in a social group on base every day and making friends (finally). His mother also scheduled him for several camps during the upcoming summer vacation, to keep him busy.

I learned that Mateo's mother had a history of abuse and sexual abuse as a child. She also admitted to her own anger problems and problems with being supernurturing (although she had sacrificed her entire career for her children). I worked with her and Mateo's sick sibling regarding their relationship (the sick child thought that the mother hated her), and I did filial play therapy with them with much success. The mother was very cooperative and followed recommendations.

The Case of Alisha, Age 2¾

Background on Referral

My agency received a call inquiring whether we saw children as young as 2. I (Joseph R. Herzog, the therapist in this case) assured the office manager that indeed we could see the child. I spoke with the child's mother before the first session. She reported that her husband, an Army sergeant, was away from home on an extended peacekeeping mission, and that she was concerned that her 33-month-old daughter, Alisha, was very depressed. She stated that Alisha often seemed sad, cried easily, and frequently awoke at night asking for her father. She also said that prior to the separation, neither she nor her husband had had any concerns about their daughter's physical or emotional development. Based on my previous experience with military families experiencing these kinds of difficult and prolonged separations, my concern as I went into this session with Alisha and her mother was that Alisha might be reflecting her mother's upset as well as her own.

Parent–Child Play Therapy Session

When Alisha and her mother arrived for their appointment, I began by explaining my position in the agency, my educational background, and the limits of confidentiality. I then gathered information about Alisha and her family. They had been living in this community for about a year, and this was their second Army duty station. Alisha was the couple's only child. Alisha's father had enlisted in the Army and intended to make the military a career. Prior to this deployment, Alisha's father had been away from home for only one brief training mission. This was the first and only lengthy absence for either Alisha or her mother. The child had been told that her father was away at work and wouldn't be coming home for a while. For the past 2 months, while on this peacekeeping mission, the father had been maintaining contact with his wife and daughter through regular letters and occasional phone calls.

My interview with Alisha and her mother took place in a playroom with a variety of toys, and Alisha was immediately attracted to a table with large Legos blocks. After gathering the background information from Alisha's mother, I got down on the floor with Alisha; she readily accepted my presence and my participation in play with the blocks. A few minutes into the play, I built an airplane from the Legos and said, "Is this an airplane like the one your daddy flew away on?" (I knew from my earlier conversation with her mother that Alisha had been brought to the airport to see her father off at the beginning of the deployment.)

Alisha immediately stopped her play and put her head down on the table. A moment later, she quickly withdrew from the play table to the couch where her mother was sitting, and crawled up and onto her mother's lap. It was clear that she was no longer interested in play. It was also clear that my statement was just as upsetting for the mother (there were tears in her eyes as well), and that Alisha was holding on to her mother in what was seemingly an experience of mutual comfort. I said I could see that they both were sad, and that they must miss their father/husband.

At this moment I realized that my original speculation concerning Alisha's symptoms was probably correct. I also realized now that Alisha was responding to her mother's sadness as well, and that the mother's own sadness might be making it difficult for her to provide the type of parenting needed at this stressful time in this young child's life.

Comments on the Session, and Description of Further Interventions

When I constructed the airplane, I was initiating a directive play approach because I wanted to assess Alisha's reaction to the toy plane. I also wanted her to know that I was aware that her father had left. Some therapists might consider that my actions were upsetting to the child and caused her to withdraw from me. I took the risk because I knew that the mother was present and available to comfort the child.

Further interventions in this case focused on providing guidance and supportive counseling for Alisha's mother, to meet her own emotional needs associated with her husband's absence. Pointing out to her how her daughter was responding to her obvious sadness and worry, rather than being able to use her as a source of comfort and support, allowed the mother to see the importance of dealing with her own emotional needs first. In addition to a period of brief supportive intervention, I was able to encourage her to get involved in a support group for unit spouses on the military installation. She also joined a local church, where she found a number of other young mothers who were very supportive. At my suggestion, Alisha's father recorded himself reading one of Alisha's favorite bedtime stories, and he sent home pictures of himself overseas. He also made more frequent phone calls that included time for Alisha to hear her dad's voice. Over the course of the separation, Alisha responded to her mother's renewed resilience and continued her normal development.

The key therapeutic interventions in this case were acknowledging Alisha's and her mother's depressive symptoms, working with Alisha's mother in brief treatment to express and better understand her own feelings, and connecting Alisha's mother with military and community support systems. I also offered the mother some useful suggestions for helping her daughter and husband maintain their relationship during this absence.

CONCLUSION

This chapter has emphasized the therapeutic opportunities and challenges of play therapy with military children/adolescents and families. We have illustrated the importance of understanding families within the context of an inflexible institution like the U.S. military that creates its own stressors, such as relocation, deployment, and reunification. These stressors affect not only a deployed parent, but his or her spouse/partner and children, and must be considered in any therapeutic interaction using a systems-based approach.

As we continue into the 21st century, the world has become increasingly complex and dangerous. Children/adolescents whose parents are repeatedly placed in harm's way through military service must live not only with the reality of parental separation, but also with the possibility of parental injury or death. Practitioners must be adept at using a variety of methods and approaches to helping these families before, during, and after deployments. We hope that this systems-based model of play therapy will provide those who utilize it with the tools necessary to help improve well-being and quality of life for those military families they treat.

STUDY QUESTIONS

1. The therapist took a directive role in the case of Alisha. What are the pros and cons of confronting a child with reminders of a traumatic memory (such as the airplane that took her father away)? How else could the therapist have intervened with Alisha?

2. The therapist used a nondirective approach in the case of Mateo. Evaluate the effectiveness of this approach in comparison to a more directive technique. Are there other possible interpretations of the child's use of symbols and metaphors during this session? How could you use the information gained from this play session to plan a parent consultation session with the mother and/or father to help repair the parent–child relationship?

REFERENCES

Albano, S. (1994). Military recognition of family concerns: Revolutionary War to 1993. *Armed Forces and Society, 20*, 283–302.

Applewhite, L., & Mays, R. (1996). Parent–child separation: A comparison of maternally and paternally separated children in military families. *Child and Adolescent Social Work Journal, 13*(1), 23–39.

Berg-Cross, L. (2000). *Basic concepts in family therapy: An introductory text* (2nd ed.). New York: Haworth Press.

Black, W. G., Jr. (1993). Military-induced family separation: A stress reduction intervention. *Social Work, 38*(3), 273–280.

Bowen, G., Mancini, J., Martin, J., Ware, W., & Nelson, J. (2003). Promoting the adaptation of military families: An empirical test of a community practice model. *Family Relations, 52*, 33–52.

Bray, R. M., Hourani, L. L., Rae, K. L., Dever, J. A., Brown, J. M., Vincus, A. A., et al. (2003). *2002 Department of Defense survey of health related behaviors among military personnel: Final report.* Research Triangle Park, NC: RTI International.

Daley, J. G. (1999). Understanding the military as an ethnic identity. In J. Daley (Ed.), *Social work practice in the military* (pp. 291–303). New York: Haworth Press.

Dan, E. (1996). Secondary traumatization in the offspring of Vietnam veterans with posttraumatic stress disorder. *Dissertation Abstracts International, 56*, 12B. (UMI No. 9610835)

Danieli, Y. (1998). Introduction. In Y. Danieli (Ed.), *International handbook of multigenerational legacies of trauma* (pp. 1–17). New York: Plenum Press.

Everson, R. B., Darling, C. A. & Herzog, J. R. (2012). Understanding parenting stress among U.S. Army spouses during combat related deployments: The role of sense of coherence. *Child and Family Social Work, 18*, 168–178.

Everson, R. B., Herzog, J. R., Figley, C. R., & Whitworth, J. (2014). A multivariate model for assessing the impact of combat-related deployments on U.S. Army spouses. *Journal of Human Behavior in the Social Environment, 24*(4), 1–16.

Everson, R. B., Herzog, J. R., & Haigler, L. A. (2011). Seeing systems: An introduction to systemic approaches with military families. In R. B. Everson & C. R. Figley

(Eds.), *Families under fire: Systemic therapy with military families* (pp. 79–96). New York: Routledge.

Figley, C. R. (1998a). Burnout as systemic traumatic stress: A model for helping traumatized family members. In C. R. Figley (Ed.), *Burnout in families: The systemic costs of caring* (pp. 15–28). Boca Raton, FL: CRC Press.

Figley, C. R. (1998b). Introduction. In C. R. Figley (Ed.), *Burnout in families: The systemic costs of caring* (pp. 1–13). Boca Raton, FL: CRC Press.

Hardaway, T. (2004). Treatment of psychological trauma in children of military families. In N. B. Webb (Ed.), *Mass trauma and violence: Helping families and children cope* (pp. 259–282). New York: Guilford Press.

Herzog, J. R., Everson, R. B., & Whitworth, J. (2011). Do secondary trauma symptoms in spouses of combat-exposed National Guard soldiers mediate impacts of soldiers' trauma exposure on their children? *Journal of Child and Adolescent Social Work, 28*(6), 459–473.

Herzog, J. R., Scott, D., Lewis, M., & Everson, R. B. (2013). Deployment related stress processes in National Guard families: A qualitative analysis. *Humanities and Social Sciences Review, 2*(3), 243–253.

Hiew, C. (1992). Separated by their work: Families with fathers living apart. *Environment and Behavior, 24*(2), 206–225.

Hillenbrand, E. (1976). Father absence in military families. *The Family Coordinator, 25*, 451–458.

Hoge, C., Castro, C., Messer, S., McGurk, D., Cotting, D., & Koffman, R. (2004). Combat duty in Iraq and Afghanistan, mental health problems, and barriers to care. *New England Journal of Medicine, 351*, 13–22.

Jensen, P. S., Grogan, D., Xenakis, S. N., & Bain, M. W. (1989). Father absence: Effects on child and maternal psychopathology. *Journal of the American Academy of Child and Adolescent Psychiatry, 28*, 171–175.

Kelley, M. (1994). The effects of military-induced separation on family factors and child behavior. *American Journal of Orthopsychiatry, 64*(1), 103–111.

Kelley, M., Finkel, L., & Ashby, J. (2003). Geographic mobility, family, and maternal variables as related to the psychosocial adjustment of military children. *Military Medicine, 168*, 1019–1024.

Kelley, M., Hock, E., Smith, K., Jarvis, M., Bonney, J., & Gaffney, M. (2001). Internalizing and externalizing behavior of children with enlisted Navy mothers experiencing military-induced separation. *Journal of the American Academy of Child and Adolescent Psychiatry, 40*(4), 464–471.

Levai, M., & Kaplan, S. (1995). The effect of father absence on the psychiatric hospitalization of Navy children. *Military Medicine, 160*, 104–106.

Mathewson, J. (2011). In support of military women and families: Challenges facing community therapists. In R. B. Everson & C. R. Figley (Eds.), *Families under fire: Systemic therapy with military families* (pp. 215–235). New York: Routledge.

McCubbin, H. I., Thompson, A. I., & McCubbin, M. A. (2001). *Family measures: Stress, coping, and resiliency: Inventories for research and practice*. Honolulu, HI: Kamehameha.

McGoldrick, M., Gerson, R., & Petry, S. (2008). *Genograms: Assessment and intervention* (3rd ed.). New York: Norton.

Motta, R., Joseph, J., Rose, R., Suozzi, J., & Leiderman, L. (1997). Secondary trauma:

Assessing inter-generational transmission of war experiences with a modified Stroop procedure. *Journal of Clinical Psychology, 53*(8), 895–903.

Nash, W. P., & Litz, B. T. (2013). Moral injury: A mechanism for war related psychological trauma in military family members. *Clinical Child and Family Psychology Review, 16*, 365–375.

O'Connor, K. J. (1991). *The play therapy primer: An integration of theories and techniques*. New York: Wiley.

Pierce, P., Vinokur, A., & Buck, C. (1998). Effects of war-induced maternal separation on children's adjustment during the Gulf War and two years later. *Journal of Applied Social Psychology, 28*(14), 1286–1311.

Pittman, J., & Bowen, G. (1994). Adolescents on the move: Adjustment to family relocation. *Youth and Society, 26*(1), 69–91.

Rosenheck, R., & Nathan, P. (1985). Secondary traumatization in children of Vietnam veterans. *Hospital and Community Psychiatry, 36*(5), 538–539.

Ruger, W., Wilson, S. E., & Waldrop, S. L. (2002). Warfare and welfare: Military service, combat, and marital dissolution. *Armed Forces and Society, 29*, 85–107.

Sori, C. F. (Ed.). (2006). *Engaging children in family therapy: Creative approaches to integrating theory and research in clinical practice*. New York: Routledge.

Smith, G. W. (2011) Attachment as a consideration in family play therapy with military families. In R. B. Everson & C. R. Figley (Eds.), *Families under fire: Systemic therapy with military families* (pp. 153–164). New York: Routledge.

Steinberg, A. (1998). Understanding the secondary traumatic stress of children. In C. R. Figley (Ed.), *Burnout in families: The systemic costs of caring* (pp. 29–46). Boca Raton, FL: CRC Press.

Chapter 12

Fostering Change When Safety Is Fleeting

Expressive Therapy Groups for Adolescents with Complex Trauma

CRAIG HAEN

In an adolescent crisis shelter days before Christmas, a ritual took place in a group session: A large gift-wrapped box was passed around the circle, and the group members were asked to tell about the best and worst gifts they'd ever received. Some shared humorous stories of ill-matched presents or touching anecdotes of positive memories. When the box came to 15-year-old Tracey, she hesitated, looked at her peers, and then said in a matter-of-fact tone, "My worst gift was that last year my mother got high and passed out on Christmas. While she was out, her boyfriend raped me twice. I don't have a best gift."

In an article about applying attachment theory to group work, Flores (2010) has noted:

> The strength of a secure base captures one of the important paradoxes of attachment theory: secure attachment liberates. Just as a securely attached child will take more risks exploring a strange room while in the presence of a secure attachment to its mother, a securely attached group member will take more risks in exploring his/her internal world and the relationships with other members in the group if the group environment serves as a secure base. (p. 555)

By describing how groups can function as optimal interpersonal laboratories for securely attached individuals, Flores unwittingly sets the stage for considering a population for whom the paradigm described above represents a paradox. How can group therapy effectively serve young people who are not only *not* securely attached, but who, because of the level of trauma in their lives, have not developed an internalized sense of safety? Can a secure base be established for adolescents who have never known what it is to feel safe, or for whom security is merely fleeting?

This chapter draws on current theory and research to consider how and why group therapy may serve as effective treatment for adolescents with complex trauma. These young people have been underrepresented in the clinical literature, but are overrepresented among the populations in residential treatment, correctional, and hospital settings (Briggs et al., 2012; Green et al., 2010; Ford, Connor, & Hawke, 2009). I present guidelines for effective practice with complexly traumatized adolescents and illustrate how expressive therapy techniques may be used to support these principles.

Although this chapter focuses on expressive therapies techniques, my approach integrates psychodynamic, cognitive-behavioral, systems, interpersonal neurobiology, and trauma-based paradigms. Such integration is in line with practices in the fields of child and adolescent therapy (Drewes, Bratton, & Schaefer, 2011; Gil, Konrath, Shaw, Goldin, & McTaggart Bryan, 2015) that offer adaptable models targeted toward maximizing clinical gains. Integrative approaches are clinically indicated for chronically traumatized young people, among whom there is wide variability in need and symptom profile (Greeson et al., 2014; Lanius, Bluhm, & Frewen, 2013a). This level of complexity often makes existing evidence-based models too narrowly focused to be fully effective, necessitating the incorporation of broader approaches and multimodal techniques (Gaskill & Perry, 2014; Kliethermes & Wamser, 2012; Lanktree & Briere, 2013).

ADOLESCENTS WITH COMPLEX TRAUMA

The peak onset age for most forms of mental illness is 14 years (Lanius, Bluhm, & Frewen, 2013b). Siegel (2013) has hypothesized that the pruning process occurring during adolescent brain development, in which unused circuitry is consolidated, manifests dormant childhood neurobiological vulnerabilities. Research demonstrates that ongoing trauma exposure can lead to long-term alteration of biological stress systems, therefore making it possible to consider trauma "an environmentally induced complex developmental disorder" (De Bellis & Zisk, 2014, p. 187).

The mental health field currently lacks a consensual definition of *complex trauma* or *chronic trauma*. It is variously described in terms of amount of exposure, a child's developmental stage at the time of exposure, and symptom profile (Grasso, Greene, & Ford, 2013; Kliethermes, Schacht, & Drewry, 2014). The diagnostic criteria for posttraumatic stress disorder are insufficient to capture the clinical presentation of youth with complex trauma (Grasso et al., 2013; McDonald, Borntrager, & Rostad, 2014). However, most researchers concur that this disorder is rooted in prolonged exposure to abuse, neglect, violence, and parental misattunement during critical developmental periods (De Bellis & Zisk, 2014). Complex trauma is thought to have its impact on young people through two primary pathways: disorganized attachment and aberrant brain development (Kliethermes et al., 2014; Lanius et al., 2013a). Although symptomatologies vary, adolescents with complex trauma differ from their acutely or singly traumatized peers in the severity and refractory nature of the internal and external manifestations of their illness (Greeson et al., 2014; Tarren-Sweeney, 2013; Wamser-Nanney & Vandenberg, 2013).

These adolescents often have gaps in intellectual, emotional, functional, and self-referential capacities, making the fluctuations between childhood and adulthood that are characteristic of the teen years even more pronounced (Kliethermes & Wamser, 2012). The most salient features of this population are states of extreme arousal coupled with impaired affect regulation (Ford & Cloitre, 2009; Tuber, Boesch, Gorkin, & Terry, 2014). Complexly traumatized adolescents' inability to tolerate and regulate intense feelings often results in their rapidly shifting between poles of hyperarousal and dissociation (Schore, 2013), and between chaotic and rigid behaviors (Mark-Goldstein & Siegel, 2013; Music, 2014).

Due to their impaired abilities to differentiate and make sense of internal states, these adolescents often rely on more primitive processing of external stimuli. As such, they tend to operate with faulty biological alarm systems that signal danger when none is present, or that fail to sound during risky situations (Tuber et al., 2014). Difficulty assessing danger is a particularly important issue for teens, who are already prone to sensation seeking because the brain's incentive processing and cognitive control systems develop at different rates (Chein, Albert, O'Brien, Uckert, & Steinberg, 2010). Adolescents with complex trauma are also vulnerable to developing related mental health and medical disorders because their systems are primed for gross dysregulation and uncontrolled stress (Felitti et al., 1998; Ford, Fallot, & Harris, 2009; Laviola & Marco, 2011).

Other potential challenges that complexly traumatized adolescents face include disturbed self-concept; difficulty navigating interpersonal relationships and social situations; heightened sensitivity to novelty and chaos; impaired executive functioning; inability to use attachment relationships for interactive regulation; difficulty asserting themselves and taking action on their own behalf; ongoing crises from living in chaotic and impoverished environments; and decreased ability to tolerate trauma processing (Frydman & McLellan, 2014; Gaskill & Perry, 2014; Green & Myrick, 2014; Kliethermes & Wamser, 2012; Kliethermes et al., 2014; Lanius et al., 2013b; Music, 2014; Schore, 2013). They often lack an internalized sense of safety, which can lead to cyclical engagement in self-defeating behaviors, in an attempt to shut down the fear that arises from new experiences or from working toward a new level of success (Perry & Szalavitz, 2006). This cycle can stymie mental health professionals, as it can appear that these young people are addicted to their own failures.

As Bendicsen (2013) notes, adolescents who lack an internalized sense of safety are more likely to lapse into primary-process thinking with an absence of metaphorical thought. In these moments, they adopt a myopic view that challenges flexibility, adaptation, and problem solving. Lanius and colleagues (2013a) have suggested that because of repeated experiences of being unable to use their emotions to guide escape, chronically traumatized people develop learned helplessness and a sense that their emotions are useless because they cannot be acted upon. This leads to a compensatory emotional disconnection, or impaired emotional awareness. They may find themselves feeling strong affect without recognizing its presence or being able to locate its source (Music, 2014). As such, these adolescents often reenact trauma-generated themes of shame, distrust, powerlessness, seduction, and threat within the clinical space (Zorzella, Muller, & Classen, 2014).

Many authors have noted that the primary goal in treating youth with complex trauma is expanding their self-regulatory capacities (Green & Myrick, 2014; Lanius et al., 2013b). This aim is a precondition for deriving further benefits from therapy, and is therefore thought to supersede higher-order cognitive and linguistically based skills (Gaskill & Perry, 2014; Ogden & Gomez, 2013). In the words of Music (2014), "We know from both neuroscience and developmental research that we have to feel sufficiently safe and relaxed to be open, curious, to be aware of thoughts and feelings" (p. 12).

GROUP THERAPY

Group therapy is considered ideal treatment for adolescents because it capitalizes on their drive toward social engagement. This modality provides both connection and perspective, as teens find others who not only share their feelings but also may offer alternative ways of understanding those feelings (Malekoff, 2014). Group therapy offers its greatest benefits during work in the here-and-now, which increases immediacy and identification (Kivlighan, 2013). As Herman (1997) has written, "The restoration of social bonds begins with discovering that one is not alone. Nowhere is this experience more immediate, powerful, or convincing than in a group" (p. 215). Research suggests that social support can help provide a buffer for adolescents with complex trauma, countering the isolation characteristic of their past experiences (De Bellis & Zisk, 2014; Ford, Fallot, et al., 2009).

However, despite these benefits, being in a room with others can trigger trauma-related relationship templates and states of arousal, propelling adolescents back to earlier phases of development (Lanktree & Briere, 2013; Marmarosh, Markin, & Spiegel, 2013). This often makes group work an intolerable experience for complexly traumatized young people. As many authors (Mark-Goldstein & Siegel, 2013; Ogden & Gomez, 2013) have posited, each group member has a "window of tolerance," or the amount of arousal he or she can bear while still remaining present. Within this window, cortical functioning remains "online" and the sympathetic and parasympathetic systems stay in relative balance, allowing group members the possibility of integrating their experiences (Jonsson, 2009). For most chronically traumatized adolescents, this window is quite narrow because of their biologically imbedded hypervigilance. Successful group approaches therefore require methods that titrate the intimacy, exposure, and potential contagion of the group experience (Ford, Fallot, et al., 2009).

Arts-based processes may help to resolve the paradox of engaging adolescents in group therapy, despite it being potentially triggering. The multisensory properties of these modalities often serve to dampen arousal enough to quiet the body's alarm system and suppress defenses (Chapman, 2014; Scaer, 2014). In addition, the use of metaphor, which is a core feature of the arts, is thought to engage diverse areas of the brain, contributing to hemispheric integration (Gil, 2014; Mills & Crowley, 2014). Porges (2010) has hypothesized that the arts, particularly music, may support safe interpersonal engagement for patients with dysregulated trauma because they stimulate the social engagement system when verbal intervention is too threatening. Chu (2011) suggests that arts-based approaches may be particularly useful in the beginning stages of trauma treatment to support the processing of experiences for which patients have no words. By giving form to that which is formless, the arts can organize and bring coherence to fragmented trauma memories (Green & Myrick, 2014).

For centuries, societies, groups, and individuals have used the arts as a means of expressing, giving form and coherence to, and integrating traumatic experiences (Bloom, 2010). Adolescence is a developmental stage during which the brain is particularly primed for creativity because of the emergence of abstract and conceptual thinking, increased attraction to reward, and heightened desire for novelty and sensation (Siegel, 2013). The drive toward artistic expression has direct links to childhood play, both of which offer tangible and adaptive benefits to humans (Brown, 2009).

REFRAMING CLINICAL PROCESS WITH THE EXPRESSIVE THERAPIES

"Expressive therapies," also known as "creative arts therapies," integrate the art forms of dance, drama, music, writing, and visual arts into clinical practice. These approaches provide curative embodied experiences, support verbal processing, and allow for alternative pathways of expression. There is currently a dearth of adequate research on the effectiveness of arts- and play-based approaches in groups with adolescents (Bratton, Taylor, & Akay, 2014); nevertheless, Shechtman (2007), perhaps the world's preeminent researcher on child and adolescent group therapy, has advocated for using expressive therapy processes to achieve clinical gains in groups.

Arts-based techniques are either central to or have been incorporated into most established models used with traumatized children and adolescents.

These include the attachment, self-regulation, and competency model (Blaustein & Kinniburgh, 2010); dissociation-focused intervention (Silberg, 2013); eye movement desensitization and reprocessing (Gomez, 2013); integrative treatment of complex trauma (Lanktree & Briere, 2013); the Neurosequential Model of Therapeutics (Gaskill & Perry, 2014); Real Life Heroes (Ford, Blaustein, Habib, & Kagan, 2013); Trauma Affect Regulation: Guide for Education and Therapy (Ford et al., 2013); and trauma-focused cognitive-behavioral therapy (TF-CBT; Cavett & Drewes, 2012; see also Neubauer, Deblinger, & Sieger, Chapter 6, this volume). Many traumatized adolescents will assiduously avoid anything resembling traditional therapy, viewing it as a "one-down" relationship in which they are required to be vulnerable and emote (Gaskill & Perry, 2014). The arts provide a "hook," allowing them to participate on their own terms (Haen & Weil, 2010).

Despite the continued privileging of the verbal, declarative domain in child and adolescent group therapy, and the view of action as defensive or potentially dangerous (Sharp, 2014), neuroscience studies have demonstrated that psychotherapy works on both explicit and implicit levels (Schore, 2011). As van der Kolk (2009) has declared, "The implications of . . . research are clear: Traumatized individuals need to engage in action that is pleasurable and effective, particularly in response to situations where in the past they were helpless and defeated" (p. 463).

Kivlighan (2013) has stated that lasting change in group work is brought about not through the development of insight or skills, but through the provision of these new experiences. The reconsolidation of circuitry taking place during adolescence makes it a time when the brain is particularly plastic and therefore open to modification (Laviola & Marco, 2011; Sercombe & Paus, 2009). For traumatized young people, growth-promoting experiences are either ones that give them a new sense of their voice and their capacities for empathy and distress tolerance, or that counter trauma-based relational schemas related to the dangers of intimacy, the abuse of power, and the silencing of dissent. By facilitating oscillation between experience and conscious reflection, therapists help group members consolidate these experiences (Dies, 2000; Lipton & Fosha, 2011). This movement may also catalyze curiosity among group members about how their minds work (Akhtar, 2011).

The use of expressive therapies can provide an important shift in the clinical space. While the arts are capable of containing the expression of dark material, these methods also tend to generate positive affect and a sense of self-efficacy. Because the arts are essential aspects of human culture, they can be normalizing (Goodman, Chapman, & Gantt, 2009) and empowering as members shift from viewing themselves as "patients" to thinking of themselves as "artists." As Lipton and Fosha (2011) have pointed out, co-regulation hinges partly on a caregiver's ability to amplify positive affect states. Positive emotions are indicative of safety, help to broaden attentional focus and flexibility, and encourage the development of resilience (Barish, 2009; Fosha, Paivio, Gleiser, & Ford, 2009). In recent research, positive experiences are being examined for their potential to contribute to reconsolidation of trauma memories and embedded core beliefs (Ecker, Ticic, & Hulley, 2012).

GUIDELINES FOR INCORPORATING THE EXPRESSIVE THERAPIES INTO GROUPS

A hallmark of arts-based techniques is that they are adaptable and can be used in conjunction with various clinical approaches, or can function as the primary treatment modality. Inherent to the expressive therapies are elements that undergird numerous trauma-based approaches from TF-CBT to exposure therapy, including imaginal exposure, cognitive restructuring, re-storying of traumatic narratives, affect regulation, collaboration, and resilience enhancement (Irwin, 2014; Johnson, Lahad, & Gray, 2009). It is helpful to think of each group session as consisting of three phases: warm-up, action, and closure (Haen, 2005). The warm-up is intended to orient members and help them become a working group by bringing them into similar affective or energetic space. The action phase is the working stage of the session, whereas closure is meant to synthesize the experience and help members to re-regulate themselves and make the transition out of group. Expressive therapies techniques can support each of these phases in work with traumatized adolescents, though it should be noted that this population frequently requires additional time devoted to closure.

The arts exist on a continuum from those whose products are concrete (art, writing) to those whose products are more ephemeral (dance, drama). They also work with varying degrees of embodiment, moving developmentally from kinesthetic to symbolic to lexical modes of representation (Johnson et al., 2009). These differences should be considered in choosing the appropriate art form for a session. During sessions, a therapist should assess a group's needs for expression or containment from moment to moment. Hyperaroused members require interventions that facilitate containment, regulation, and cognition, whereas hypoaroused members benefit from interventions targeting expression, interpersonal connection, and affect.

Within each of the arts modalities are techniques that can be used for expression or containment, and group leaders should be trained in implementing these when using the arts with traumatized people. For example, Gil and Dias (2014) have written about the use of emotional statues and affective scaling from drama therapy in order to promote affect identification, modulation, and expression. For containment, King-West and Hass-Cohen (2008) have noted how pieces of visual art produced by patients can be viewed from a distance, examined from differing perspectives, given titles, and put away in folders or cabinets.

What follows are examples of using expressive therapy techniques to achieve targeted goals with traumatized adolescents. Each section includes a theoretical explanation, suggestions for several arts-based strategies, and clinical vignettes from my work. Most examples emerged naturally as prescriptive interventions to address the needs of a particular group, but have subsequently been used as frameworks for intervening with future groups.

Expanding the Window of Tolerance

Trauma work at its core involves helping people build their capacity to feel emotions and face challenges fully, rather than shrinking from them. This includes assisting adolescents with complex trauma in learning to experience feelings and sensations as "tolerable, helpful, and practically manageable" (Ford & Cloitre, 2009, p. 61), and to differentiate these internal states from harbingers of impending danger. Change is a particularly common trigger for traumatized young people, who cling to predictability and routine. Inherent to expanding the window of tolerance are learning to cope with change as a fundamental part of life, and learning that safety is not the same as comfort—that honesty and interpersonal connection often require some level of risk (Bloom, 2013).

Chapman (2014) theorizes that art facilitates this expansion as it allows for "staying in the right hemisphere long enough for the affect to arise and be tolerated" (p. 113). In more process-oriented (as opposed to product-oriented) art therapy approaches, group members are often invited to draw, paint, or create other visual art in response to a prompt or theme. The emphasis is on following impulses and on tolerating the images and feelings that are generated (Haen & Weil, 2010). Similar approaches exist in dance therapy, in which group members are asked to initiate spontaneous movement in response to music, allowing and trusting their impulses (Wittig, 2010). An entry point for this level of expectation can be warm-ups in which, instead of the classic verbal check-in, the leader can ask group members to express how they are feeling in a simple sound and movement that the group mirrors back to them (Haen, 2015).

Bromberg (2011) has written about the value of providing "safe surprises" that gently push at the outer limits of a patient's window of tolerance. Repeated exposure to such surprises within the relative safety of treatment, he theorizes, helps traumatized people begin to distinguish nontraumatic spontaneity from potential retraumatization. Improvisational methods such as acting and music are particularly adept at creating safe surprises, as they rely on a degree of openness to uncertainty.

In one common acting exercise, two people begin an improvisational scene in the center of the circle. At any point, a member of the audience can call out, "Freeze." The actors pause the scene and hold their bodies still, while the audience member who called out enters the circle and taps one of them out. This member takes the same body position as the group member he or she traded places with, and then utters a new line to which the remaining actor must respond—thus beginning a wholly new scene with new characters. This exercise can continue through many rounds, with members repeatedly freezing the action and starting a new two-person scene. In a musical variation, one member stands in the center of the circle and sings a song of his or her choosing. When this song calls to mind an association for another group member, that member jumps into the circle, taking the place of the original member and singing a new song.

> In an adolescent group in a shelter for victims of domestic violence, the members struggled with the continued uncertainty of their lives—not knowing where they would live next or what would happen to them. They were initially extremely wary of participating in a drama therapy group; however after a few sessions, they became interested in activities that involved intrigue. In one favorite game, a member would leave the room, and the group would come up with an emotion that they would all pretend to have. The member would then reenter the group and interact with them until he or she could accurately "diagnose" the group's feeling. Thirteen-year-old Tia, who had watched her father repeatedly try to kill her mother, was particularly hesitant to be the one to leave the group; she kept saying, "I don't wanna leave and not know what I'm walkin' into." However, when a peer offered to join her, Tia reluctantly took a turn. When she reentered the room, Tia instantly guessed that the group was pretending to be jealous. With a smile, she said, "I'm gonna go out again. Make it harder this time." In later sessions, she would offer to support newer members who were hesitant in the game.

Increasing Cognitive Flexibility

A central executive function, "cognitive flexibility" is broadly thought of as the ability to hold two opposing concepts in mind at once, or to adjust habitual response patterns in light of new information (Malekoff, 2014). Evolutionary research suggests that executive functioning developed in part to negotiate the demands that came with living in groups (Music, 2014). As a survival skill, rigidity helps to divide the world neatly into extremes, so that traumatized people know clearly which people, places, and things to avoid in order to keep themselves safe. Ambiguity and ambivalence are therefore intolerable states.

Adolescents can build cognitive flexibility in groups by playing with paradox and perception, as well as through leaders' encouragement of differences of opinion and complex thinking. Artwork that deals with duality, such as polarity drawings (Chapman, 2014), or activities in which group members have to take other perspectives, such as writing a letter to themselves from someone they struggle to understand, can encourage flexibility. In an exercise derived from psychodrama, a leader might place two chairs in the center of the circle, one behind the other. The leader might then ask members to take turns sitting in the first chair and completing the sentence "People think I am . . ., " and then sitting in the second chair to finish the thought ("But really I am . . ."). This sequence can be used to explore hidden aspects of other people as well.

> In an all-male group with older teens in a residential facility, the members were struggling with self-esteem issues; however, they all remained distant

from their fellow group members and could not be engaged to give positive feedback to one another. The leader devised a game, modeled after a cheesy game show, in which one member was asked to leave the room (pretending to go into the "isolation booth" that is a feature of many game shows). While that member was out of the room, the group, as studio audience, was elicited to come up with three compliments about that member. The absent member was then brought back into the room with much fanfare, was told the three compliments, and had to guess which group member said each one. This process was repeated for each person who wished to be a contestant. Because the emphasis was on guessing, group members with antipathetic relationships would often provide compliments for their peers, saying, "He'll never guess this one is from me." The boys were asked at the end to share the compliment that most surprised them.

Building Identity

Lanktree and Briere (2013) assert that working on identity is an essential clinical goal with complexly traumatized teens because this task, which is central to adolescent development, has frequently been distorted by traumatic exposure. Adolescents often represent who they are through symbols, and their process of identity development can be likened to the trying on of a series of roles (Haen & Weil, 2010). Because symbols transcend cultural barriers, the arts may have particular advantages in working across cultures (Johnson et al., 2009). Asking group members to play songs that resonate with them can allow for safe yet intimate exchanges between members (McFerran, 2010).

Identity can be explored by playing roles that express different aspects of self; by writing poetry or rap lyrics; or by creating visual art, including collages, graffiti, and self-portraits. Art that emphasizes both independence and affiliation helps teens to consider their place within a group.

In one session, group members took individual photos of one another with an instant camera. In the photos, they were asked to represent themselves through one body part—for example, an eye or hand. They were then given markers and invited to write words or draw additional images on the photos. The individual portraits were combined into a collective mobile, which was hung outside the group room.

On a Native American reservation, a group of 16- to 18-year-olds gathered. Under the multiple burdens of historical trauma, as well as of ongoing exposure to domestic violence, suicide, and parental substance abuse, they were sullen, self-conscious, and not at all interested in attempts by two European American therapists to engage them. After some failed attempts to get them to talk, the leaders asked each member to find a spot in the room, to think of an animal that had meaning to him or her, and to take a physical pose that showed that animal. As they did so, they lit up and became animated. They eventually performed monologues in which they portrayed themselves in a year's time, highlighting the dreams they had for themselves and expressing the intergenerational conflicts within their tribe.

Exploring the Future

Flanders (2013) refers to play as an adolescent's "creative way of dreaming, imagining, thinking about a containable, bearable future" (p. 66). For many traumatized young people, however, reality has inhibited the ability to envision anything but a foreshortened future marked by continued victimization or aggression. For these adolescents, the imagination is an untrustworthy place that does not offer respite (Tuber et al., 2014). As a stimulus to safe imagining, the expressive therapies can be used to slowly open up future possibilities (Haen, 2015).

Members can be asked to create sculptures, songs, or movements that represent past, present, and future, with an emphasis on understanding that feelings, people, and circumstances all eventually change, no matter how enduring they seem. The group members can pass around an imaginary crystal ball and share an image they see in it for themselves, other members, or the group as a whole (Haen & Weil, 2010). They also can be invited to write their own future discharge summaries, taking the role of their individual therapists discussing the progress they've made. Homeless teens can be asked to design future homes for themselves and to give the group a "tour."

> In a crisis shelter setting, a group of adolescents who all had similar abuse histories and parents who were either deceased or in prison were asked to imagine themselves in 10 years, looking back on who they were in the present. They were each video-recorded in the role of the future self delivering a message to the present self. They watched these recordings in a subsequent session. Marquis, a 15-year-old who often spoke of prison as his destiny, became tearful as he watched the recording in which his future self shared some of the hard lessons he had learned by being locked up. That week, Marquis called his state worker to initiate discussions about going to a foster home—a possibility he had until then been refusing.

ROLE OF THE THERAPIST

It would be remiss to discuss techniques without outlining the qualities necessary for effective group leadership. Evidence suggests that characteristics of therapists, such as their level of warmth, genuineness, and trustworthiness, account for a greater degree of the variability in treatment outcomes among traumatized patients than do the specific techniques they use (Dalenberg, 2014). In addition, Shechtman and Katz (2007) found in their research that bonding with the therapist had a robust impact on adolescent group effectiveness.

Edgette (2010) has written, "Establishing credibility with adolescent clients is more important for the relationship than establishing rapport" (p. 208). The kind of credibility she is referring to is communicated by stable adult figures who know who they are and are consistent (with reasonable flexibility) in the face of adolescent group members' lack of integration. In particular, adolescents who have been exposed to chronic interpersonal trauma require leaders who model responsible authority; who are playful and humorous, while still maintaining the frame of the group; who encourage differences of thought and opinion; and who can maintain a regulated state in response to limit-testing and hyperaroused acting-out behaviors (Connors, Lertora, & Liggett-Creel, 2011). These qualities are especially important when the power differential is heightened by cultural differences—most often, when a leader represents the majority culture and members are from minority cultures (Harvey, 2011). Rather than using interpretations or silence, the leader can offer his or her ideas as "hypotheses for the group to accept or reject" (Rachman, 1989, p. 37). Rachman (1989) has suggested that in doing so, the therapist allows the group "the psychological room to breathe" (p. 37).

In addition, leaders need to be skillful at tracking both individual members and the group as a whole for signs of "stuckness," dissociation, disengagement, hyperarousal, and confusion. They should know a variety of ways to ground members and reengage them in generative group process (Ford, Fallot, et al., 2009). In these moments of attunement and interactive regulation, the therapist mitigates shame by joining the members—that is, shifting the emphasis away from individual pathology and resistance to a stance of curiosity and shared problem solving (Adams, 2011).

Because traumatized adolescents often engage in the hypertracking of adults (a learned survival skill), it is important for group therapists to be able to make their own internal processes visible to members. They do this through predictability, open co-leader dialogues about decisions in the group, ongoing self-monitoring of internal states and their outward expression, and judicious self-disclosure. This level of transparency helps create safety, as members are likely to misattribute affect they read on a therapist's face as directed at them (Adams, 2011; Silberg, 2013). In addition, therapists should strive to communicate hope by maintaining a firm belief in members' internal wisdom and ability to attain a positive and stable future (Bendicsen, 2013; Kliethermes & Wamser, 2012; Silberg, 2013). As the group develops as a healing entity, the leaders communicate their belief that all the qualities needed for repair already exist among the members (Lipton & Fosha, 2011). Inherent to this message is the group leaders' trust that the members can provide scaffolding for one another and engage in interactive regulation.

CONCLUSION

Although more research is needed to support their effectiveness, expressive therapies represent promising practices for working with adolescents with complex trauma. These modalities may particularly help to engage these young people in group therapy, despite the possibility that groups may stimulate defensive responses. Arts-based processes can be incorporated into a variety of treatment approaches to target expression, self-regulation, expansion of distress tolerance, and development of safe interpersonal connections. By providing positive experiences and empowerment, the expressive therapies may help traumatized young people reclaim a sense of self-efficacy and a connection back to society.

The arts were used for healing long before therapy's existence. Damasio (2010), in considering their evolutionary significance, views them as directly connected to human beings' attempts to give form to trauma. He writes:

> The arts were an inadequate compensation for human suffering, for unattained happiness, for lost innocence, but they were and are compensation nonetheless, an offset to natural calamities and to the evil that men do. They are one of the remarkable gifts of consciousness to humans. (p. 296)

STUDY QUESTIONS

1. Define "complex trauma" and discuss how it differs from other forms of trauma.
2. What benefits might expressive therapies offer that verbal approaches to trauma treatment may not?
3. Pretend you are responding to a program administrator who questions why you are "making art" and "singing songs," rather than working on skill building in your groups. Share how you will justify the work you are doing in concrete terms.
4. Choose one of the challenges listed in the "Adolescents with Complex Trauma" section of this chapter, and brainstorm various ways you might use art, music, movement, role play, storytelling, or creative writing to work on this challenge in treatment.

REFERENCES

Adams, K. (2011). The abject self: Self-states of relentless despair. *International Journal of Group Psychotherapy, 61*(3), 333–364.

Akhtar, M. C. (2011). Remembering, replaying and working through: The transformation of trauma in children's play. In M. C. Akhtar (Ed.), *Play and playfulness: Developmental, cultural, and clinical aspects* (pp. 85–102). Lanham, MD: Aronson.

Barish, K. (2009). *Emotions in child psychotherapy: An integrative framework*. New York: Oxford University Press.

Bendicsen, H. K. (2013). *The transformational self: Attachment and the end of the adolescent phase.* London: Karnac.

Blaustein, M. E., & Kinniburgh, K. M. (2010). *Treating traumatic stress in children and adolescents: How to foster resilience through attachment, self-regulation, and competency.* New York: Guilford Press.

Bloom, S. (2010). Bridging the black hole of trauma: The evolutionary significance of the arts. *Psychotherapy and Politics International, 8*(3), 198–212.

Bloom, S. (2013). The sanctuary model. In J. D. Ford & C. A. Courtois (Eds.), *Treating complex traumatic stress disorders in children and adolescents: Scientific foundations and therapeutic models* (pp. 277–294). New York: Guilford Press.

Bratton, S. C., Taylor, D. D., & Akay, S. (2014). Integrating play and expressive art therapy into small group counseling with preadolescents: A humanistic approach. In E. J. Green & A. A. Drewes (Eds.), *Integrating expressive arts and play therapy with children and adolescents* (pp. 253–282). Hoboken, NJ: Wiley.

Briggs, E. C., Greeson, J. K. P., Layne, C. M., Fairbank, J. A., Knoverek, A. M., & Pynoos, R. S. (2012). Trauma exposure, psychosocial functioning, and treatment needs of youth in residential care: Preliminary findings from the NCTSN core data set. *Journal of Child and Adolescent Trauma, 5*(1), 1–15.

Bromberg, P. (2011). *The shadow of the tsunami and the growth of the relational mind.* New York: Routledge.

Brown, S. (2009). *Play: How it shapes the brain, opens the imagination, and invigorates the soul.* New York: Penguin.

Cavett, A. M., & Drewes, A. A. (2012). Play applications and trauma-specific components. In J. A. Cohen, A. P. Mannarino, & E. Deblinger (Eds.), *Trauma-focused CBT for children and adolescents: Treatment applications* (pp. 124–148). New York: Guilford Press.

Chapman, L. (2014). *Neurobiologically informed trauma therapy with children and adolescents: Understanding mechanisms of change.* New York: Norton.

Chein, J., Albert, D., O'Brien, L., Uckert, K., & Steinberg, L. (2010). Peers increase adolescent risk-taking by enhancing activity in the brain's reward circuitry. *Developmental Science, 14*(2), F1–F10.

Chu, J. (2011). *Rebuilding shattered lives: Treating complex PTSD and dissociative disorders* (2nd ed.). Hoboken, NJ: Wiley.

Connors, K. M., Lertora, J., & Liggett-Creel, K. (2011). Group work with children impacted by sexual abuse. In G. L. Greif & P. H. Ephross (Eds.), *Group work with populations at risk* (3rd ed., pp. 297–315). New York: Oxford University Press.

Dalenberg, C. (2014). On building a science of common factors in trauma therapy. *Journal of Trauma and Dissociation, 15*(4), 373–383.

Damasio, A. (2010). *Self comes to mind: Constructing the conscious brain.* New York: Pantheon.

De Bellis, M. D., & Zisk, A. (2014). The biological effects of childhood trauma. *Child and Adolescent Psychiatric Clinics of North America, 23*, 185–222.

Dies, K. G. (2000). Adolescent development and a model of group psychotherapy: Effective leadership in the new millennium. *Journal of Child and Adolescent Group Therapy, 10*(2), 97–111.

Drewes, A. A., Bratton, S. C., & Schaefer, C. E. (Eds.). (2011). *Integrative play therapy.* Hoboken, NJ: Wiley.

Ecker, B., Ticic, R., & Hulley, L. (2012). *Unlocking the emotional brain: Eliminating symptoms at their roots using memory reconsolidation.* New York: Routledge.

Edgette, J. S. (2010). Avoiding the trap of trying too hard: Appreciating the influence of natural law in adolescent therapy. In M. Kerman (Ed.), *Clinical pearls of wisdom: 21 leading therapists offer their key insights* (pp. 207–218). New York: Norton.

Felitti, V. J., Anda, R. F., Nordenberg, D., Williamson, D. F., Spitz, A. M., Edwards, V., et al. (1998). Relationship of childhood abuse and household dysfunction to many of the leading causes of death in adults: The Adverse Childhood Experiences (ACE) Study. *American Journal of Preventive Medicine, 14*, 245–258.

Flanders, S. (2013). What's so traumatic about adolescence? In E. McGinley & A. Varchevker (Eds.), *Enduring trauma through the life cycle* (pp. 63–81). London: Karnac.

Flores, P. J. (2010). Group psychotherapy and neuro-plasticity: An attachment theory perspective. *International Journal of Group Psychotherapy, 60*(4), 547–570.

Ford, J. D., Blaustein, M. E., Habib, M., & Kagan, R. (2013). Developmental trauma therapy models. In J. D. Ford & C. A. Courtois (Eds.), *Treating complex traumatic stress disorders in children and adolescents: Scientific foundations and therapeutic models* (pp. 261–276). New York: Guilford Press.

Ford, J. D., & Cloitre, M. (2009). Best practices in psychotherapy for children and adolescents. In C. A. Courtois & J. D. Ford (Eds.), *Treating complex traumatic stress disorders: An evidence-based guide* (pp. 59–81). New York: Guilford Press.

Ford, J. D., Connor, D. F., & Hawke, J. (2009). Complex trauma among psychiatrically impaired children: A cross-sectional, chart-review study. *Journal of Clinical Psychiatry, 70*, 1155–1163.

Ford, J. D., Fallot, R. D., & Harris, M. (2009). Group therapy. In C. A. Courtois & J. D. Ford (Eds.), *Treating complex traumatic stress disorders: An evidence-based guide* (pp. 415–440). New York: Guilford Press.

Fosha, D., Paivio, S. C., Gleiser, K., & Ford, J. D. (2009). Experiential and emotion-focused therapy. In C. A. Courtois & J. D. Ford (Eds.), *Treating complex traumatic stress disorders: An evidence-based guide* (pp. 286–311). New York: Guilford Press.

Frydman, J. S., & McLellan, L. (2014). Complex trauma and executive functioning: Envisioning a cognitive-based, trauma-informed approach to drama therapy. In N. Sajnani & D. R. Johnson (Eds.), *Trauma-informed drama therapy: Transforming clinics, classrooms, and communities* (pp. 152–178). Springfield, IL: Charles C Thomas.

Gaskill, R. L., & Perry, B. D. (2014). The neurobiological power of play: Using the Neurosequential Model of Therapeutics to guide play in the healing process. In C. A. Malchiodi & D. A. Crenshaw (Eds.), *Creative arts and play therapy for attachment problems* (pp. 178–194). New York: Guilford Press.

Gil, E. (2014). The creative use of metaphor in play and art therapy with attachment problems. In C. A. Malchiodi & D. A. Crenshaw (Eds.), *Creative arts and play therapy for attachment problems* (pp. 159–177). New York: Guilford Press.

Gil, E., & Dias, T. (2014). The integration of drama therapy and play therapy in attachment work with traumatized children. In C. A. Malchiodi & D. A. Crenshaw (Eds.), *Creative arts and play therapy for attachment problems* (pp. 100–120). New York: Guilford Press.

Gil, E., Konrath, E., Shaw, J., Goldin, M., & McTaggart Bryan, H. (2015). The integrative approach to play therapy. In D. A. Crenshaw & A. L. Stewart (Eds.), *Play therapy: A comprehensive guide to theory and practice* (pp. 99–113). New York: Guilford Press.

Gomez, A. M. (2013). *EMDR therapy and adjunct approaches with children: Complex trauma, attachment, and dissociation*. New York: Springer.

Goodman, R. F., Chapman, L. M., & Gantt, L. (2009). Creative arts therapies for children. In E. B. Foa, T. M. Keane, M. J. Friedman, & J. A. Cohen (Eds.),

Effective treatments for PTSD: Practice guidelines from the International Society for Traumatic Stress Studies (pp. 491–507). New York: Guilford Press.

Grasso, D., Greene, C., & Ford, J. D. (2013). Cumulative trauma in childhood. In J. D. Ford & C. A. Courtois (Eds.), *Treating complex traumatic stress disorders in children and adolescents: Scientific foundations and therapeutic models* (pp. 79–99). New York: Guilford Press.

Green, E. J., & Myrick, A. C. (2014). Treating complex trauma in adolescents: A phase-based, integrative approach for play therapists. *International Journal of Play Therapy, 23*(3), 131–145.

Green, J., McLaughlin, K. A., Berglund, P. A., Gruber, M. J., Sampson, N. A., Zaslavsky, A. M., et al. (2010). Childhood adversities and adult psychiatric disorders in the National Comorbidity Survey Replication: I. Associations with first onset of DSM-IV disorders. *Archives of General Psychiatry, 67*(2), 113–123.

Greeson, J. K. P., Briggs, E. C., Layne, C. M., Belcher, H. M. E., Ostrowski, S. A., Kim, S., et al. (2014). Traumatic childhood experiences in the 21st century: Broadening and building on the ACE studies with data from the National Child Traumatic Stress Network. *Journal of Interpersonal Violence, 29*(3), 536–557.

Haen, C. (2005). Rebuilding security: Group therapy with children affected by September 11. *International Journal of Group Psychotherapy, 55*(3), 391–414.

Haen, C. (2015). Vanquishing monsters: Group drama therapy for treating trauma. In C. A. Malchiodi (Ed.), *Creative interventions with traumatized children* (2nd ed., pp. 235–257). New York: Guilford Press.

Haen, C., & Weil, M. (2010). Group therapy on the edge: Adolescence, creativity, and group work. *Group, 34*(1), 37–52.

Harvey, A. R. (2011). Group work with African American youth in the criminal justice system: A culturally competent model. In G. L. Greif & P. H. Ephross (Eds.), *Group work with populations at risk* (3rd ed., pp. 264–282). New York: Oxford University Press.

Herman, J. L. (1997). *Trauma and recovery* (rev. ed.). New York: Basic Books.

Irwin, E. (2014). Drama therapy. In E. J. Green & A. A. Drewes (Eds.), *Integrating expressive arts and play therapy with children and adolescents* (pp. 67–99). Hoboken, NJ: Wiley.

Johnson, D. R., Lahad, M., & Gray, A. (2009). Creative therapies for adults. In E. B. Foa, T. M. Keane, M. J. Friedman, & J. A. Cohen (Eds.), *Effective treatments for PTSD: Practice guidelines from the International Society for Traumatic Stress Studies* (pp. 479–490). New York: Guilford Press.

Jonsson, P. V. (2009). Complex trauma, impact on development and possible solutions on an adolescent intensive care unit. *Clinical Child Psychology and Psychiatry, 14*(3), 437–454.

King-West, E., & Hass-Cohen, N. (2008). Art therapy, neuroscience and complex PTSD. In N. Hass-Cohen & R. Carr (Eds.), *Art therapy and clinical neuroscience* (pp. 223–253). London: Jessica Kingsley.

Kivlighan, D. M. (2013). Three important clinical processes in individual and group interpersonal psychotherapy sessions. *Psychotherapy, 51*(1), 20–24.

Kliethermes, M., Schacht, M., & Drewry, K. (2014). Complex trauma. *Child and Adolescent Psychiatric Clinics of North America, 23*, 339–361.

Kliethermes, M., & Wamser, R. (2012). Adolescents with complex trauma. In J. A. Cohen, A. P. Mannarino, & E. Deblinger (Eds.), *Trauma-focused CBT for children and adolescents: Treatment applications* (pp. 175–196). New York: Guilford Press.

Lanius, R. A., Bluhm, R., & Frewen, P. A. (2013a). Childhood trauma, brain connectivity, and the self. In J. D. Ford & C. A. Courtois (Eds.), *Treating complex traumatic stress disorders in children and adolescents: Scientific foundations and therapeutic models* (pp. 24–38). New York: Guilford Press.

Lanius, R. A., Bluhm, R., & Frewen, P. A. (2013b). A window into the brain of complex PTSD: Clinical and neurobiological perspectives. In D. J. Siegel & M. Solomon (Eds.), *Healing moments in psychotherapy* (pp. 49–66). New York: Norton.

Lanktree, C. & Briere, J. (2013). Integrative treatment of complex trauma. In J. D. Ford & C. A. Courtois (Eds.), *Treating complex traumatic stress disorders in children and adolescents: Scientific foundations and therapeutic models* (pp. 143–161). New York: Guilford Press.

Laviola, G., & Marco, E. M. (2011). Passing the knife edge in adolescence: Brain pruning and specification of individual lines of development. *Neuroscience and Biobehavioral Reviews, 35*, 1631–1633.

Lipton, B., & Fosha, D. (2011). Attachment as a transformative process in AEDP: Operationalizing the intersection of attachment theory and affective neuroscience. *Journal of Psychotherapy Integration, 21*(3), 253–279.

Malekoff, A. (2014). *Group work with adolescents: Principles and practice* (3rd ed.). New York: Guilford Press.

Mark-Goldstein, B., & Siegel, D. J. (2013). The mindful group: Using mind–body–brain interactions in group therapy to foster resilience and integration. In D. J. Siegel & M. Solomon (Eds.), *Healing moments in psychotherapy* (pp. 217–242). New York: Norton.

Marmarosh, C. L., Markin, R. D., & Spiegel, E. B. (2013). *Attachment in group psychotherapy*. Washington, DC: American Psychological Association.

McDonald, M. K., Borntrager, C. F., & Rostad, W. (2014). Measuring trauma: Considerations for assessing complex and non-PTSD Criterion A childhood trauma. *Journal of Trauma and Dissociation, 15*(2), 184–203.

McFerran, K. (2010). *Adolescents, music, and music therapy: Methods and techniques for clinicians, educators and students*. London: Jessica Kingsley.

Mills, J. C., & Crowley, R. J. (2014). *Therapeutic metaphors for children and the child within* (2nd ed.). New York: Routledge.

Music, G. (2014). Top down and bottom up: Trauma, executive functioning, emotional regulation, the brain and child psychotherapy. *Journal of Child Psychotherapy, 40*(1), 3–19.

Ogden, P., & Gomez, A. (2013). EMDR therapy and sensorimotor psychotherapy with children. In A. Gomez (Ed.), *EMDR therapy and adjunct approaches with children: Complex trauma, attachment, and dissociation* (pp. 247–271). New York: Springer.

Perry, B. D., & Szalavitz, M. (2006). *The boy who was raised as a dog and other stories from a child psychiatrist's notebook: What traumatized children can teach us about loss, love, and healing*. New York: Basic Books.

Porges, S. W. (2010). Music therapy and trauma: Insights from the polyvagal theory. In K. Stewart (Ed.), *Music therapy and trauma: Bridging theory and clinical practice* (pp. 3–15). New York: Satchnote.

Rachman, A. W. (1989). Identity group psychotherapy with adolescents: A reformulation. In F. J. Cramer Azima & L. H. Richmond (Eds.), *Adolescent group psychotherapy* (pp. 21–41). New York: International Universities Press.

Scaer, R. (2014). *The body bears the burden: Trauma, dissociation, and disease* (3rd ed.). New York: Routledge.

Schore, A. N. (2011). The right brain implicit self lies at the core of psychoanalysis. *Psychoanalytic Dialogues, 21*(1), 75–100.

Schore, A. N. (2013). Relational trauma, brain development, and dissociation. In J. D. Ford & C. A. Courtois (Eds.), *Treating complex traumatic stress disorders in children and adolescents: Scientific foundations and therapeutic models* (pp. 3–23). New York: Guilford Press.

Sercombe, H., & Paus, T. (2009). The "teen brain" research: An introduction and implications for practitioners. *Youth and Policy, 103*, 25–37.

Sharp, W. (2014). Sticks and stones may break my bones, but what about words? *International Journal of Group Psychotherapy, 64*(3), 281–296.

Shechtman, Z. (2007). *Group counseling and psychotherapy with children and adolescents: Theory, research, and practice.* New York: Routledge.

Shechtman, Z., & Katz, E. (2007). Therapeutic bonding in group as an explanatory variable of progress in the social competence of students with learning disabilities. *Group Dynamics: Theory, Research, and Practice, 11*(2), 117–128.

Siegel, D. J. (2013). *Brainstorm: The power and purpose of the teenage brain.* New York: Tarcher/Penguin.

Silberg, J. L. (2013). *The child survivor: Healing developmental trauma and dissociation.* New York: Routledge.

Tarren-Sweeney, M. (2013). An investigation of complex attachment- and trauma-related symptomatology among children in foster and kinship care. *Child Psychiatry and Human Development, 44*(6), 727–741.

Tuber, S., Boesch, K., Gorkin, J., & Terry, M. (2014). Chronic early trauma as a childhood syndrome and its relationship to play. In C. A. Malchiodi & D. A. Crenshaw (Eds.), *Creative arts and play therapy for attachment problems* (pp. 215–226). New York: Guilford Press.

van der Kolk, B. A. (2009). Best practices in psychotherapy for children and adolescents. In C. A. Courtois & J. D. Ford (Eds.), *Treating complex traumatic stress disorders: An evidence-based guide* (pp. 455–466). New York: Guilford Press.

Wamser-Nanney, R., & Vandenberg, B. R. (2013). Empirical support for the definition of a complex trauma event in children and adolescents. *Journal of Traumatic Stress, 26*(6), 671–678.

Wittig, J. (2010). The body and nonverbal expression in dance/movement group therapy and verbal group therapy. *Group, 34*(1), 53–66.

Zorzella, K. P. M., Muller, R. T., & Classen, C. C. (2014). Trauma group therapy: The role of attachment and alliance. *International Journal of Group Psychotherapy, 64*(1), 25–47.

Part III

SCHOOL-BASED CRISIS INTERVENTION

Chapter 13

Bullying

Interpersonal Trauma among Children and Adolescents

SUSAN M. SWEARER
HEATHER SCHWARTZ
ALLEN GARCIA

PREVALENCE AND DEFINITION OF BULLYING

In the past few decades, the problem of bullying and interpersonal aggression has gained a great deal of attention in the research and popular literatures. Media attention to these issues has grown exponentially, and understanding the causes and consequences of bullying has become part of worldwide discourse. Bullying, a source of interpersonal trauma, has gained unprecedented attention as a common problem not only for youth, but also for school staff members, families, and communities. Some bullying behaviors may be difficult to detect, and the consequences may be more easily recognized than the actual behaviors. For teachers, discerning the differences among students' "just joking around," students' being "mean," and students' bullying others can be difficult. For researchers, agreeing on a common definition is difficult as well. Given that researchers' definitions of bullying can vary (Smith, Cowie, Olafsson, & Liefooghe, 2002), the reported prevalence rates of bullying behaviors also vary. All these factors make bullying a complex social phenomenon; accordingly, treatment options include individual, group, and systems interventions.

The definition of "bullying" has undergone several iterations, but it is now primarily defined as a relationship marked by a power imbalance in which one or more people act aggressively over time with the intent to harm others (Centers for Disease Control and Prevention, 2014; Olweus, 1999). The main feature that differentiates bullying from other forms of aggression is the power imbalance between a higher-power perpetrator and a lower-power victim. This power imbalance either is perceived by the victim, or is an actual difference (e.g., physical, social) between the bully and victim (Scheithauer, Hayer, Petermann, & Jugert, 2006). Bullying may involve any of the following four methods:

- Physical (e.g., hitting, kicking)
- Verbal (e.g., name calling, saying mean things)
- Relational (e.g., spreading rumors, social exclusion)
- Electronic (e.g., texting, social networking, gaming)

These methods are likely to co-occur (Wang, Iannotti, Luk, & Nansel, 2010). Students involved in bullying tend to fall into one or more roles along the bully-to-victim continuum: "bullies," "victims," "bully-victims," and/or "bystanders" (Haynie et al., 2001). Bullies are those who are involved in the aggressive behaviors. Victims are those who are the targets of aggressive behaviors. Bully-victims are those who both get bullied and bully others. Bystanders are either those who have witnessed bullying situations or those who remain uninvolved or have limited involvement. These roles are not fixed and can change as a child or adolescent encounters new environmental contexts (e.g., new peer groups, new school, new grade level).

Prevalence rates for bullying and victimization vary widely. Some researchers have found that 15–30% of students are directly involved in bullying (Nansel et al., 2001; Seals & Young, 2003; Solberg & Olweus, 2003), while others have found that 10–31% of students report being victimized (Dulmus, Sowers, & Theriot, 2006; Nansel et al., 2001). Researchers have also found that 7–13% of students report bullying others (Boulton & Smith, 1994; Nansel et al., 2001; Peskin, Tortolero, & Markham, 2006), whereas 1–11.5% report both bullying others and being victimized (i.e., bully-victim status; Dulmus et al., 2006; Seals & Young, 2003). Nansel and colleagues (2001) reported that nearly 30% of students in grades 6–10 in the United States were involved in bullying. Given that the reported prevalence of bullying varies so widely in the research literature, it is important for researchers and practitioners to accept a common definition of bullying and for practitioners to understand that definition.

AGE AND GENDER DIFFERENCES IN BULLYING INVOLVEMENT

Of the four methods of bullying, researchers have found that physical bullying increases and peaks during elementary school, and declines in middle and high school; relational bullying tends to follow the opposite trajectory and becomes most prevalent in middle and high school (Cohn & Canter, 2003). In general, researchers have found that as students develop, they become more socially adept and are better able to read social cues, affording more sophisticated methods of bullying. Whereas middle school students may have better social skills than their elementary school counterparts, they often lack emotional maturity and have difficulty resolving complicated interpersonal relationships or social dynamics (Leadbeater, 2010). Therefore, relational bullying becomes more pronounced than physical bullying as children age. Verbal bullying has been shown to remain constant across grade levels.

Although both males and females can engage in any form of bullying, male and female bullies tend to display different forms of aggression toward their victims. Males tend to display more overt, physical bullying behaviors toward others, while females tend to display more covert, relational bullying. Research on aggression has found that similar gender differences exist, and in fact begin to emerge as early as the preschool years, with girls exhibiting lower levels of physical aggression than boys (Loeber & Hay, 1997). Girls, however, display higher levels of verbal and indirect aggression than boys do (Crick & Grotpeter, 1995) and as children grow older, these gender differences in aggressive and bullying behaviors remain consistent (Anderson & Huesmann, 2007). Studies conducted with adolescents have found that boys tend engage in more direct physical and verbal forms of bullying than girls, and that girls engage in more relational forms of bullying than boys (Crick & Grotpeter, 1995). Overall; however, it has been found that boys are involved in bullying at greater rates than girls are (Cook, Williams, Guerra, Kim, & Sadek, 2010).

BULLYING PREVENTION AND INTERVENTION

Bullying is a serious problem among school-age youth that has many adverse effects on the children involved, whether they are bullies, victims, bully-victims, and/or bystanders. Given the prevalence of bullying behaviors among youth of all ages, a vast number of prevention and intervention approaches have been developed; these are targeted at entire schools, whole classrooms, and individual students (Whitted & Dupper, 2005). Furthermore, prevention and policy strategies have also been developed, which focus on (1) systems-level approaches, (2) teacher and/or parent involvement, (3) psychoeducation, (4) student-led initiatives, and (5) specialized interventions intended for students who require more intensive support (Pollack & Swearer, 2011).

Anti-Bullying Campaigns

Although anti-bullying campaigns and organizations are not formal interventions or programs, they are becoming an increased presence in schools. Many of these campaigns have been developed in response to increased public attention to the problems caused by involvement in bullying (i.e., depression, suicidal ideation, anxiety, substance use), particularly suicides related to bullying. These campaigns serve to raise awareness about bullying and its negative impacts, and can be inexpensively implemented across schools and communities. Some examples of anti-bullying campaigns include Stand for the Silent (*www.standforthesilent.org*); the It Gets Better Project (*www.itgetsbetter.org*); the Gay, Lesbian, & Straight Education Network (*www.glsen.org*); Mean Stinks (*www.meanstinks.com*); and Stomp Out Bullying (*www.stompoutbullying.org*). Anti-bullying campaigns have allowed students, specifically victims and bystanders of bullying, to take an active role in speaking out against bullying and participating in efforts to reduce bullying in their schools.

Primary Schoolwide Prevention and Intervention

As the following discussion makes clear, there are numerous intervention options available to address bullying behaviors; however, it is essential to assess the needs of a particular school before choosing a particular approach or approaches, and to ensure that outcomes are continuously monitored to evaluate treatment effectiveness. The best approaches to reduce bullying include schoolwide and communitywide efforts, combined with group and individual interventions.

A multitude of schoolwide bullying prevention and intervention programs exist (Espelage & Swearer, 2011; Zins, Elias, & Maher, 2007). These programs generally involve developing school rules that prohibit bullying; establishing procedures for reporting bullying and for responding to bullying; and psychoeducation for both students and adults. Examples of research-based schoolwide programs for elementary students include the Olweus Bullying Prevention Program (Olweus & Limber, 2002), Bully Busters (Horne, Bartolomucci, & Newman-Carlson, 2003), Steps to Respect (Committee for Children, 2011), the Peaceful Schools Project (Twemlow et al., 2009), and Bully-Proofing Your School (Garrity, Jens, Porter, Sager, & Short-Camilli, 2004).

Secondary and Tertiary Interventions for Bullying and Aggression

Since schoolwide prevention and intervention programs cannot alleviate *all* bullying behaviors, more intensive programs are designed to help the students who are most frequently involved in bullying behaviors as bullies, victims, and/or bystanders. These individualized programs teach replacement skills for social skills and psychological deficits that may be causing these students to bully others or to be at risk for being bullied. For instance, victims may undergo assertiveness training, whereas perpetrators of bullying may be taught nonaggressive problem-solving strategies. Individual therapy approaches, including play therapy, are tertiary bullying interventions.

Play Therapy for Aggressive Children

Although there are few research studies examining the effectiveness of play therapy for bullying behaviors in particular, there is a robust literature on play therapy for aggressive children. Aggression and bullying are related issues that systematically interfere with young people's development in academic, cognitive, behavioral, and social domains. Aggressive children and adolescents are at risk for a host of negative outcomes (Crick & Dodge, 1996), including academic, social, and behavioral difficulties; aggressive behaviors are the leading reason why children are referred for treatment (Kazdin, 1987). Because of these facts, it is important for play therapists to be aware of the recent research on play therapy as an intervention to reduce aggressive and bullying behaviors.

Child-centered play therapy (CCPT) is an approach used by play therapists that encourages children to work through underlying issues (i.e., anger, frustration) and work toward developing a sense of identity and mastery over their environment (Landreth, 2002). In order to facilitate children's healthy development and to create healthy therapeutic relationships, play therapists use genuine interactions, unconditional positive regard and acceptance, and empathetic understanding to create a safe therapeutic space. Once therapists have established trusting relationships with their young clients, they create a condition of self-directed therapy and help their clients work through their aggressive behaviors during the therapeutic process.

Outcomes of CCPT for aggressive children are promising. Young children (ages 4–10) who received short-term, intense CCPT had significant reductions in their externalizing and internalizing problems (Kot, Landreth, & Giordano, 1998). This was one of the first studies that sought to evaluate play therapy for aggressive children. Given that the participants were living in a domestic violence shelter, they likely experienced (observed, encountered, and/or were victimized by) significant aggressive behaviors in their homes. The children in the experimental group had 12 sessions of CCPT across 2–3 weeks. The results indicated significant reductions in externalizing problems (reports of fewer aggressive and delinquent behaviors) rather than internalizing problems (Kot et al., 1998). These findings suggest that CCPT is a promising approach in reducing children's aggressive behaviors.

CCPT has been evaluated in schools as well. In another study, elementary-age students (ages 4–11) who displayed aggressive behaviors in their classrooms were treated with 7–10 weeks of CCPT (Ray, Blanco, Sullivan, & Holliman, 2009). The students included in the study were from diverse and economically disadvantaged backgrounds. Participants in the experimental group received 14 sessions of 30 minutes each in the schools. After treatment, teachers reported significant reductions in aggressive behaviors; however, parents reported moderate effects, with no significant reductions in aggression. During the CCPT intervention, the play therapists included aggressive-themed toys (guns, knives, and handcuffs) in the therapy room. Supporters of using aggressive-themed toys in play therapy have suggested that it facilitates children's aggressive play, leads to adult acceptance, and allows the therapists to understand the children (Trotter & Landreth, 2003). However, others have asserted that play therapists should be cautious in allowing children to use such toys because of outdated research on the topic and insufficient evidence to support the effectiveness of this practice (Schaefer & Mattei, 2005). Although the results indicated no increase in aggressive behaviors, the researchers failed to measure whether or not the clients used the aggressive-themed toys during treatment. Despite these limitations, this study was the first to specifically use CCPT with aggressive-themed toys as an intervention for aggressive students.

Research on the effectiveness of play therapy for aggressive youth has included both group designs and single-case designs. Two case studies of play therapy for aggressive children have recently been conducted. In the first study, two first graders who displayed highly disruptive behaviors in school classrooms received CCPT. Results from teacher reports were more positive for internalizing problems than for externalizing problems: One child's aggressive behavior was reduced, and the other child's behavior remained stable (Cochran, Cochran, Nordling, McAdam, & Miller, 2010). In the second study, Anderson and Gedo (2013) implemented a single-case design in a preschool setting with a 3-year-old boy who engaged in aggressive behavior (hitting, punching, and biting others), was noncompliant, and had difficulties with his mother. The authors hypothesized that his insecure attachment with his mother was the root of his aggressive behaviors. Due to language barriers, his mother was not directly involved in the treatment. Results showed that after 1 year of treatment, the child developed a more secure attachment style, improved his self-coping skills, and decreased his aggressive and externalizing behaviors.

PARENTAL INCLUSION IN PLAY THERAPY FOR AGGRESSION

Although play therapy is an important tool for working with aggressive children, including parents in the process has been hypothesized to be an important extension of such play therapy (Davenport & Bourgeois, 2008). Play therapists can educate parents on practices that will improve their parenting skills. Parents and other primary caregivers are in an excellent position to facilitate the social development of their young children, and play therapists are well situated to teach parents appropriate play and developmental expectations (VanFleet, 2005). Parental training includes educating parents about the increased use of positive parental practices (warm and responsive) and decreased use of negative parental practices (being harsh or intrusive) during children's play. Parent training has also been linked to increased parental engagement in children's play (NICHD Early Child Care Research Network, 2004). Parents who take an active role in their children's play can improve the quality of their play and can reduce the children's aggressive behavior.

In the play therapy literature, CCPT has been the gold standard in work with aggressive children. In order to reduce children's aggression, play therapists have used CCPT to guide their clients through the processes of reducing anger, managing impulsivity, and solving problems effectively. There is support for the use of CCPT as an intervention for children's aggression (Anderson & Gedo, 2013; Kot et al., 1998; Ray et al., 2009); however, the research has produced mixed results in regard to its effectiveness over time (Cochran et al., 2010). In addition to utilizing CCPT as a form of treatment, researchers have supported the use of combined approaches, such as play therapists' providing parents with training in positive parenting practices (Davenport & Bourgeois, 2008) and employing activities that allow children to work through their full range of emotions (Hall, Kaduson, & Schaefer, 2002).

Links between Aggression and Bullying

Aggression has been defined is a negative act with the intent to cause harm (Crick & Dodge, 1996). There are two forms of aggression: proactive and reactive. Proactive aggression is a behavior that is planned with a deliberate purpose of seeking external gains. Reactive aggression is an angered response to a situation that involves provocation. Aggression can appear in two forms, overt (verbal and physical) or indirect (social) (Crick & Dodge, 1996). On the other hand, *bullying* has been defined as repeated occurrences of intentional negative harm, and the person who bullies has a perceived or actual power over the victim (Olweus, 1993). The three key aspects of bullying are intention, repetition, and power imbalance. It can be seen that all bullying is aggressive, but not all aggressive behavior is bullying. Thus bullying is an aggressive behavior with two additional characteristics, repetition and power imbalance.

The outcomes from involvement in bullying may be more deleterious than outcomes from aggression in general (Olweus, 2010). For instance, aggression may be experienced as a one-time incident between two people of the same power, which suggests that both individuals can defend themselves. On the other hand, bullying is characterized as multiple incidents of aggression (repetition), and the victims have difficulty defending themselves (power imbalance). Moreover, researchers have found that the distinction between aggression and bullying may be a result of the instrumentality of behavior, in that not all aggression is connected to negative outcomes and may serve a function of providing access to resources and social opportunity (Hawley, Stump, & Ratliff, 2011). Research has suggested that the use of aggression in school settings is a part of normal child development because aggression has been linked to higher social status and popularity (Hawley et al., 2011).

There are a host of negative outcomes for youth involved in bullying, whether as victims, perpetrators, or bystanders. Some negative consequences include internalizing problems and poor prognoses for future academic, social, and behavioral functioning (Copeland, Wolke, Angold, & Costello, 2013). In addition, students involved in bullying are more likely to experience school and legal consequences (Swearer, Espelage, & Napolitano, 2009). Conversely, some research has reported positive outcomes for students who perpetrate bullying. Some students who bully have achieved higher social status and are seen as more popular (Garandeau, Wilson, & Rodkin, 2010; Hawley, Stump, & Ratliff, 2011).

Cognitive, emotional, and behavioral factors influence children's aggressive and bullying behaviors. The social skills deficit model (Dodge, Pettit, McClaskey, Brown, & Gottman, 1986) has been used to explain why children engage in these behaviors. This model suggests that these youth may have encoding-related problems that lead them to interpret ambiguous or neutral cues as aggressive (Crick & Dodge, 1996). In addition, youth in one study who bullied others, regardless of gender, were likely to have friends who endorsed similar aggressive attitudes and behaviors (Espelage, Holt, & Henkel, 2003). Lack of empathy and lower moral values are additional explanatory factors for bully perpetration (Swearer et al., 2009). Students in one study who perpetrated bullying had lower levels of empathy, and students who were not involved in bullying reported higher levels of empathy (Espelage, Mebane, & Adams, 2004). Relatedly, students who bullied had high levels of moral disengagement, which is a cognitive construct that allows individuals to justify their negative or harmful behaviors (Hymel, Rocke-Henderson, & Bonanno, 2005; Obermann, 2011). These aforementioned cognitive, emotional, and behavioral factors are all areas that can be addressed in treatment for children involved in bullying (Swearer, 2013).

Play Therapy for Involvement in Bullying

Despite the fairly robust literature (described above) on the use of play therapy for aggressive children, there is a dearth of research on the use of play therapy with children involved in bullying. Two important factors may have influenced the lack of research on play therapy and bullying. First, play therapy has traditionally been conducted with younger children, typically in preschool and early elementary school. These younger children may not have the ability to express themselves through verbal communication (Landreth, 2002). Second, although bullying tends to emerge during elementary school, it peaks during middle school (Nansel et al., 2001)—that is, at an age where play therapy is not used by most therapists. Thus, as children increase their engagement in bullying behaviors, they are typically at an age where play therapy is less frequently used. However, counselors who work with adolescents may use various forms of expressive therapies with teenagers, such as art, music, and journaling. They do not usually refer to their methods as "play therapy," even though these same methods are also employed by play therapists with younger children.

Children do engage in bullying and coercive behaviors at earlier ages (preschool and early elementary years) (Hanish, Hill, Gosney, Fabes, & Martin, 2011); however, there has been debate about the appropriateness of the term "bullying" for young children because of the methodological challenges to assessment and measurement of whether young children are actually bullying, teasing, or simply modeling aggressive behaviors (Hanish et al., 2011). Nevertheless, given the promising uses of play therapy for aggressive children, we provide some suggestions for play therapy techniques for children involved in bullying.

BIBLIOTHERAPY

One effective tool for working with young children is the use of children's books on a specific topic—bullying, in this case. A bullying literature project with third-grade students and their teachers found that incorporating books about bullying into the language arts curriculum was an effective way to help these students and teachers to talk about bullying (Swearer et al., 2009). There are many children's books on bullying, and these books can be used by play therapists and kept on a bookshelf in the office or play therapy room (see Table 13.1). Incorporating books into play therapy may be an effective tool for helping children work through bullying issues, whether they are involved as perpetrators, victims, bully-victims, and/or bystanders.

SPECIFIC PLAY THERAPY TECHNIQUES

There are some specific play therapy techniques that can be used in play therapy for aggressive children and children involved in bullying (see Table 13.2). Hall and colleagues (2002) have described 15 child-friendly activities that can be included within play therapy sessions. Two of Hall and colleagues' activities related to aggression are called Balloons of Anger and The Mad Game. Play therapists can use Balloons of Anger to help children learn to appropriately self-manage their negative emotions. A balloon represents a child, and the air inside the balloon represents anger. Play therapists illustrate that when the balloon (child) contains too much air (anger), it can pop, or it can be released slowly. Also, play therapists can use The Mad Game to normalizes the feelings of anger and allow children to express their feelings of anger. As these examples indicate, activities within the play therapy session can be used to help children work through and manage their angry feelings and aggressive behavior.

PROBLEM-SOLVING PLAY THERAPY

In play therapy, bullying can be framed as a problem that needs to be solved, and the POWER acronym can be used to help a young client work through the problem of bullying (Swearer, 2003). The play therapist and the client can draw or paint the POWER acronym, which stands for the following: (1) What is the Problem (i.e., bullying)?; (2) What are Options (e.g., walk away, tell a teacher)?; (3) Which option is best (i.e., walk away)?; (4) Execute the option (i.e., try it); and (5) Rate the option (i.e., did the bullying stop?). This problem-solving technique can be use with children who are bullied, who bully others, and/or who observe bullying. Since a power imbalance is one of the elements in the definition of bullying, using the POWER acronym can be a meaningful technique in play therapy to help children work through their experiences with bullying. Puppets can also be used to demonstrate the POWER acronym during play therapy.

TABLE 13.1. Selected Elementary School Books about Bullying

1. *My Secret Bully*, by Trudy Ludwig
2. *The English Roses*, by Madonna
3. *Don't Be a Bully, Billy: A Cautionary Tale*, by Phil Roxbee Cox
4. *Blue Cheese Breath and Stinky Feet: How to Deal with Bullies*, by Catherine DePino
5. *Bully Trouble*, by Joanna Cole
6. *Umar and the Bully*, by Shabana Mir
7. *The Berenstain Bears and the Bully*, by Stan and Jan Berenstain
8. *Bullies Are a Pain in the Brain*, by Trevor Romain
9. *Amelia's Bully Survival Guide*, by Marissa Moss
10. *The Recess Queen*, by Alexis O'Neill and Laura Huliska-Beith
11. *Cliques, Phonies, and Other Baloney*, by Trevor Romain
12. *How to Handle Bullies, Teasers and Other Meanies: A Book That Takes the Nuisance Out of Name Calling and Other Nonsense*, by Kate Cohen-Posey
13. *Shrinking Violet*, by Cari Best
14. *Enemy Pie*, by Derek Munson
15. *Stand Tall, Molly Lou Melon*, by Patty Lovell
16. *Say Something*, by Peggy Moss
17. *Stick Up for Yourself!: Every Kid's Guide to Personal Power and Positive Self-Esteem*, by Gershen Kaufman, Lev Raphael, and Pamela Espeland
18. *How to Lose All Your Friends*, by Nancy Carlson
19. *Stop Bullying Bobby!: Helping Children Cope with Teasing and Bullying*, by Dana Smith-Mansell
20. *King of the Playground*, by Phyllis Reynolds Naylor
21. *Stop Picking on Me: A First Look at Bullying*, by Pat Thomas
22. *Simon's Hook: A Story about Teases and Put-Downs*, by Karen Gedig Burnett
23. *Don't Laugh at Me*, by Steve Siskin and Allen Shamblin
24. *Nobody Knew What to Do: A Story about Bullying*, by Becky Ray McCain
25. *One*, by Kathryn Otoshi
26. *Bully*, by Patricia Polacco
27. *Mr. Lincoln's Way*, by Patricia Polacco
28. *They Call Me Chicken: A Story of Courage*, by John D. Caporale
29. *Lessons from a Rubber Duck*, by Melissa Saunders
30. *The Bully*, by Thomasina Johnson

Note. From Swearer, Espelage, and Napolitano (2009). Copyright 2009 by The Guilford Press. Adapted by permission.

TABLE 13.2. Play Therapy Techniques for Children Involved in Bullying

Techniques	Description
Cognitive-behavioral play therapy (CBPT; Knell, 1998)	CBPT is based on the principles of cognitive-behavioral therapy, with minor modifications in order to be developmentally sensitive. Therapists use modeling (e.g., with dolls, puppets) to teach children adaptive coping skills that could be used to prevent bullying behaviors, to stop bullying, and/or to respond appropriately to bullying.
Art therapy (Eaton, Doherty, & Widrick, 2007; Nissimov-Nahum, 2008)	Children create a piece of art (i.e., drawing, coloring, painting, and/or clay). The therapist helps children in expressing past trauma and/or problems with bullying. The therapist also works toward helping clients improve self-awareness and self-control.
Sandplay therapy (Richards, Pillay, & Fritz, 2012)	Children create a sandtray scene (i.e., with dry/wet sand, symbols, figures) that represents their world or a personal story. Children express their problems and/or unconscious issues through the sandtray scene they create and through manipulation of the figures.
Including parents (Davenport & Bourgeois, 2008)	The inclusion of parents in the process of play therapy promotes continuity across systems (from therapy to home). Parents are educated to use positive practices during children's play and to facilitate socially appropriate play.
The Solution Drawing (Kaduson & Schaefer, 2003)	Children create a solution to a problem they are encountering. Then, during therapy, children draw an image of that solution. Children are empowered to utilize their drawing as a symbolic tool when faced with the problem in the future.
Draw a Bully (Bully Busters; Newman, Horne, & Bartolomucci, 2000)	Children draw their perceptions of someone who bullies others. This activity helps therapists identify their young clients' beliefs and understand their feelings associated with bullying.
The Mad Game (Hall, Schaefer, & Kaduson, 2002)	Children learn that being angry is an acceptable feeling. Children also have an opportunity to release their negative emotion and learn to process anger so they can express it in a healthy way.
Balloons of Anger (Hall et al., 2002)	Children learn to self-manage their negative emotions. An air-filled balloon is used as a tool to represent a child, his or her negative emotions, and a way to release those emotions.

THE CASE OF MASON, AGE 12

The Target Bullying Intervention Program is an individualized therapeutic intervention that has been used with children and adolescents referred for their bullying behaviors (for more in-depth descriptions, see Swearer, Collins, Radliff, & Wang, 2011; Swearer, Wang, Collins, Strawhun, & Fluke, 2014). Mason, a 12-year-old biracial (African American and European American) male, was referred to the program by his middle school counselor for his physical and verbal bullying behaviors toward other students in his class. Prior to the intervention, he had accumulated 32 office referrals for defiance, disrespect, disrupting the class, inappropriate language, and bullying. Mason reported that he engaged in bullying as a way to stand up to peers, specifically when they talked or made jokes about his family. He felt that the only way to stand up for himself was to "act tough." The school counselor also reported that Mason was easily influenced by others.

The first part of the intervention is a series of self-report questionnaires to help the adults and the client understand some of the related psychological issues that might be influencing the bullying behaviors. Thus Mason completed several measures that assessed for depression, anxiety, self-perception, bullying–victimization, and school climate, as well as an intervention rating profile. Results from these assessments indicated that Mason was not experiencing any depressive symptoms; however, his scores reflected that he might be experiencing a high level of anxiety with respect to making sure he did things that people would like, doing everything exactly right, staying away from things that upset him, and avoiding dangerous situations. It was possible that Mason tried to avoid confrontations; however, when his peers insulted his family, he felt compelled to stand up to those peers. His scores on the self-perception profile were high; however, his scores on scholastic competence and behavioral conduct were relatively lower, perhaps reflecting his expressed desire to do better in school and to deal with problematic peer situations (e.g., people insulting his family) in a more prosocial way. On the survey assessing experiences with bullying and victimization, Mason self-identified as being a victim, a bystander, and a bully. He indicated that he was being bullied one or more times a week in the bathroom, before school, and after school. He noted that older boys, as well as boys in the same grade, often played jokes on him; he further indicated that they sometimes called him names, made fun of him, attacked him, and pushed him. He felt that he was bullied because of his brother, because of his skin color, and because he got angry a lot. Mason also reported seeing others getting bullied one or more times a week, usually during gym class. These other students were often made fun of or attacked for the color of their skin. Finally, he admitted bullying others one or more times a month, primarily in the hallway. He reported that he would sometimes make fun of older boys, as well as boys in the same grade. He noted that he bullied others if they were "wimpy." Finally, on the measure of school climate, Mason indicated a positive perception of his school's climate, and he also stated that he felt the bullying intervention would be helpful.

During the session with Mason, he completed several activities related to the topic of bullying. He participated actively throughout the session, and when given the opportunity to talk about his involvement in bullying others, he was very open and honest in expressing his frustration. Mason completed the self-report measures, participated in a PowerPoint presentation on bullying, and completed a worksheet activity from the Bully Busters curriculum that is designed to equip students with skills to handle future bullying situations. The Knowing My Anger activity was selected because he indicated that he frequently felt angry, but did not know how to cope with his emotions (particularly when people talked negatively about his family) other than physically standing up to them. Through this activity, Mason discussed what made him mad. Mason said that he felt angry whenever his family was talked about or insulted; he felt the need to defend his brother and other family members, and he did that by physically standing up to the peers who insulted them. He would often punch or push the peers. When asked about better ways of handling his anger, Mason said that he had tried asking others, "Please stop it"—but that this had not worked, and it frustrated him that the insults kept happening. When asked whether he had ever told a trusted adult at school, he said that he had once talked about his concerns with a counselor. He said that the counselor helped him through this particular difficult situation, and it made the problem go away. Mason also suggested that he could talk to his family about his problems, and that his parents could handle any significant concerns with the appropriate authority. The therapist and Mason role-played different ways of responding to provoking situations: stopping and walking away; firmly telling the peers to stop; and talking to an adult if he was feeling frustrated. Mason indicated that if he did these things, he would be more likely to avoid getting in trouble.

Throughout the session, Mason openly discussed his engagement in bullying the other students. A major aspect of his bullying discovered during the session was that Mason felt close to his family members and felt that he had to defend them, as described above. During the session, he said he was willing to try to tell an adult at school about the situation before bullying others. He was open and engaged throughout the session, and was able to articulate the effects of his bullying on himself and his peers.

At a follow-up meeting with school personnel, his parents, and Mason, a home–school note that would help everyone keep track of his interactions with his peers was recommended. Mason agreed to begin reporting bullying incidents to trusted school staff members and to his parents, whom he identified as a positive source of support in his life. He indicated that he enjoyed playing board games and basketball with his family, and Mason's parents agreed to increase these positive family engagements. Follow-up office referral data indicated that Mason did not have any additional office referrals after participation in the intervention.

CONCLUSION

Bullying is a significant issue that has many negative effects on children and adolescents and impedes their healthy development. It is clear from the research literature that young people can move among the roles of bully, victim, and bystander, and that many children and adolescents may experience some or all of these roles over time, depending on their school, family, and peer environments. Play therapy is a promising tool for helping children work through the interpersonal trauma caused by bullying and may help prevent future involvement in bullying. It is also vital that bullying prevention and intervention programs address the social ecology in which children reside—namely, families, peer groups, schools, and the broader neighborhoods and communities. It is our responsibility as play therapists to help stop the social scourge of bullying, and to provide appropriate treatments to help individuals involved in bullying live kinder and happier lives.

STUDY QUESTIONS

1. What are the four forms of bullying? How do these forms of bullying change over time and as youth age?
2. What are the three elements in the definition of bullying?
3. What does the POWER acronym stand for?
4. Why is it important for play therapists to work also with parents and other adult caregivers of students and adolescents who are involved in bullying and aggressive behaviors?

REFERENCES

Anderson, C. A., & Huesmann, L. R. (2007). Human aggression: A social-cognitive view. In M. A. Hogg & J. Cooper (Eds.), *The Sage handbook of social psychology* (pp. 259–287). Thousand Oaks, CA: Sage.

Anderson, S. M., & Gedo, P. M. (2013). Relational trauma: Using play therapy to treat a disrupted attachment. *Bulletin of the Menninger Clinic, 77*, 250–268.

Boulton, M. J., & Smith, P. K. (1994). Bully/victim problems in middle school children: Stability, self–perceived competence, peer acceptance. *British Journal of Developmental Psychology, 12*, 315–325.

Centers for Disease Control and Prevention. (2014). Youth violence. Retrieved from *www.cdc.gov/violenceprevention/youthviolence/index.html*

Cochran, J. L., Cochran, N. H., Nordling, W. J., McAdam, A., & Miller, D. T. (2010). Two case studies of child-centered play therapy for children referred with highly disruptive behavior. *International Journal of Play Therapy, 19*, 130–142.

Cohn, A., & Canter, A. (2003). Bullying: Facts for schools and parents. Retrieved from *www.nasponline.org/resources/factsheets/bullying_fs.aspx*

Committee for Children. (2011). Steps to Respect: A bullying prevention program. Retrieved from *http://cfchildren.org/steps-to-respect*.

Cook, C. R., Williams, K. R., Guerra, N. G., Kim, T. E., & Sadek, S. (2010). Predictors of bullying and victimization in childhood and adolescence. *School Psychology Quarterly, 25*, 65–83.

Copeland, W. E., Wolke, D., Angold, A., & Costello, J. (2013). Adult psychiatric outcomes of bullying and being bullied by peers in childhood and adolescence. *Journal of the American Medical Association, 70*, 419–426.

Crick, N. R., & Dodge, K. A. (1996). Social information-processing mechanisms in reactive and proactive aggression. *Child Development, 67*, 993–1002.

Crick, N. R., & Grotpeter, J. K. (1995), Relational aggression, gender, and social-psychological adjustment. *Child Development, 66*, 710–722.

Davenport, B. R., & Bourgeois, N. M. (2008). Play, aggression, the preschool child, and the family: A review of literature to guide empirically informed play therapy with aggressive preschool children. *International Journal of Play Therapy, 17*, 2–23.

Dodge, K. A., Pettit, G. S., McClaskey, C. L., Brown, M. M., & Gottman, J. M. (1986). Social competence in children. *Monographs of the Society for Research in Child Development, 51*(2, Serial No. 213), 1–85.

Dulmus, C., Sowers, K., & Theriot, M. (2006). Prevalence and bullying experiences of victims and victims who become bullies (bully-victims) at rural schools. *Victims and Offenders, 1*, 15–31.

Eaton, L. G., Doherty, K. L., & Widrick, R. M. (2007). A review of research and methods used to establish art therapy as an effective treatment for traumatized children. *The Arts in Psychotherapy, 34*, 256–262.

Espelage, D. L., Holt, M. K., & Henkel, R. R. (2003). Examination of peer-group contextual effects on aggression during early adolescence. *Child Development, 74*(1), 205–220.

Espelage, D. L., Mebane, S. E., & Adams, R. S. (2004). Empathy, caring, and bullying: Toward an understanding of complex associations. In D. L. Espelage & S. M. Swearer (Eds.), *Bullying in American schools: A social-ecological perspective on prevention and intervention* (pp. 37–61). Mahwah, NJ: Erlbaum.

Espelage, D. L., & Swearer, S. M. (Eds.). (2011). *Bullying in North American schools* (2nd ed.). New York: Routledge.

Garandeau, C. F., Wilson, T., & Rodkin, P. C. (2010). The popularity of elementary school bullies in gender and racial context. In S. R. Jimerson, S. M. Swearer, & D. L. Espelage (Eds.), *Handbook of bullying in schools: An international perspective* (pp. 119–136). New York: Routledge.

Garrity, C., Jens, K., Porter, W., Sager, N., & Short-Camilli, C. (2004). *Bully-Proofing Your School: A comprehensive approach*. Longmont, CO: Sopris West.

Hall, T. M., Kaduson, H. G., & Schaefer, C. E. (2002). Fifteen effective play therapy techniques. *Professional Psychology: Research and Practice, 33*, 515–522.

Hanish, L. D., Hill, A., Gosney, S., Fabes, R. A., & Martin, C. L. (2011). Girls, boys, and bullying in preschool: The role of gender in the development of bullying. In D. L. Espelage & S. M. Swearer (Eds.), *Bullying in North American schools* (2nd ed., pp. 132–146). New York: Routledge.

Hawley, P. H., Stump, K. N., & Ratliff, J. (2011). Sidestepping the jingle fallacy: Bullying, aggression, and the importance of knowing the difference. In D. L. Espelage & S. M. Swearer (Eds.), *Bullying in North American schools* (2nd ed., pp. 101–115). New York: Routledge.

Haynie, D. L., Nansel, T., Eitel, P., Crump, A. D., Saylor, K., Yu, K., et al. (2001). Bullies, victims, and bully/victims: Distinct groups of at-risk youth. *Journal of Early Adolescence, 21*, 29–49.

Horne, A. M., Bartolomucci, C. L., & Newman-Carlson, D. (2003). *Bully Busters: A teacher's manual for helping bullies, victims, and bystanders, grades K–5*. Champaign, IL: Research Press.

Hymel, S., Rocke-Henderson, N., & Bonanno, R. (2005). Moral disengagement: A framework for understanding bullying among adolescents. *Journal of Social Sciences, 8*, 1–11.

Kaduson, H. G., & Schaefer, C. E. (Eds.). (2003). *101 favorite play therapy techniques* (Vol. 3). Lanham, MD: Rowman & Littlefield.

Kazdin, A. E. (1987). Treatment of antisocial behavior in children: Current status and future directions. *Psychological Bulletin, 102*, 187–203.

Knell, S. M. (1998). Cognitive-behavioral play therapy. *Journal of Clinical Child Psychology, 27*, 28–33.

Kot, S., Landreth, G. L., & Giordano, M. (1998). Intensive child-centered play therapy with child witnesses of domestic violence. *International Journal of Play Therapy, 7*, 17–36.

Landreth, G. L. (2002). *Play therapy: The art of the relationship* (2nd ed.). New York: Brunner-Routledge.

Leadbeater, B. (2010). Can we see it? Can we stop it?: Lessons learned from university–community research collaborations about relational aggression. *School Psychology Review, 39*, 588–593.

Loeber, R., & Hay, D. (1997). Key issues in the development of aggression and violence from childhood to early adulthood. *Annual Review of Psychology, 48*, 371–410.

Nansel, T., Overpeck, M., Pilla, R., Ruan, W., Simons-Morton, B., & Scheidt, P. (2001). Bullying behaviors among US youth: Prevalence and association with psychosocial adjustment. *Journal of the American Medical Association, 285*, 2094–2100.

Newman, D. A., Horne, A. M., & Bartolomucci, C. L. (2000). *Bully Busters: A teacher's manual for helping bullies, victims, and bystanders*. Champaign, IL: Research Press.

NICHD Early Child Care Research Network. (2004). Affect dysregulation in the mother–child relationship in the toddler years: Antecedents and consequences. *Development and Psychopathology, 16*, 43–68.

Nissimov-Nahum, E. (2008). A model of art therapy in educational settings with children who behave aggressively. *The Arts in Psychotherapy, 35*, 341–348.

Obermann, M. L. (2011). Moral disengagement in self-reported and peer-nominated school bullying. *Aggressive Behavior, 37*, 133–144.

Olweus, D. (1993). *Bullying at school: What we know and what we can do*. Oxford, UK: Blackwell.

Olweus, D. (1999). Sweden. In P. K. Smith, Y. Morita, J. Junger-Tas, D. Olweus, R. Catalano, & P. Slee (Eds.), *The nature of school bullying: A cross-national perspective* (pp. 7–27). London: Routledge.

Olweus, D. (2010). Understanding and researching bullying: Some critical issues. In S. R. Jimerson, S. M. Swearer, & D. L. Espelage (Eds.), *Handbook of bullying in schools: An international perspective* (pp. 9–33). New York: Routledge.

Olweus, D., & Limber, S. P. (2002). *The Bullying Prevention Program: Blueprints for violence prevention*. Boulder, CO: Center for the Study and Prevention of Violence.

Peskin, M. F., Tortolero, S. R., & Markham, C. M. (2006). Bullying and victimization among black and Hispanic adolescents. *Adolescence, 41*, 467–482.

Pollack, W. S., & Swearer, S. M. (2011). Bullying. In G. P. Koocher & A. M. La Greca (Eds.), *The parents' guide to psychological first aid: Helping children and adolescents cope with predictable life crises* (pp. 167–171). New York: Oxford University Press.

Ray, D. C., Blanco, P. J., Sullivan, J. M., & Holliman, R. (2009). An exploratory study of child-centered play therapy with aggressive children. *International Journal of Play Therapy, 18*, 162–175.

Richards, S. D., Pillay, J., & Fritz, E. (2012). The use of sand tray techniques by school counselors to assist children with emotional and behavioural problems. *The Arts in Psychotherapy, 39*, 367–373.

Schaefer, C. E., & Mattei, D. (2005). Catharsis: Effectiveness in children's aggression. *International Journal of Play Therapy, 14*, 103–109.

Scheithauer, H., Hayer, T., Petermann, F., & Jugert, G. (2006). Physical, verbal, and relational forms of bullying among German students: Age trends, gender differences, and correlates. *Aggressive Behavior, 32*, 261–275.

Seals, D., & Young, J. (2003). Bullying and victimization: Prevalence and relationship to gender, grade level, ethnicity, self-esteem, and depression. *Adolescence, 38*, 735–747.

Solberg, M., & Olweus, D. (2003). Prevalence estimation of school bullying with the Olweus Bully/Victim Questionnaire. *Aggressive Behavior, 29*, 239–268.

Smith, P. K., Cowie, H., Olafsson, R. F. & Liefooghe, A. P. D. (2002), Definitions of bullying: A comparison of terms used, and age and gender differences, in a fourteen-country international comparison. *Child Development, 73*, 1119–1133.

Swearer, S. M. (2003). Problem-solving play therapy. In H. G. Kaduson & C. E. Schaefer (Eds.), *101 favorite play therapy techniques* (Vol. 3, pp. 171–174). Lanham, MD: Rowman & Littlefield.

Swearer, S. M. (2013). Treating bullying behaviors among youth. In G. P. Koocher, J. C. Norcross, & B. A. Greene (Eds.), *Psychologists' desk reference* (3rd ed., pp. 391–394). New York: Oxford University Press.

Swearer, S. M., Collins, A., Radliff, K. H., & Wang, C. (2011). Internalizing problems in students involved in bullying and victimization. In D. L. Espelage & S. M. Swearer (Eds.), *Bullying in North American schools* (2nd ed., pp. 45–61). New York: Routledge.

Swearer, S. M., Espelage, D. L., & Napolitano, S. A. (2009). *Bullying prevention and intervention: Realistic strategies for schools*. New York: Guilford Press.

Swearer, S. M., Wang, C., Collins, A., Strawhun, J., & Fluke, S. (2014). Bullying: A school mental health perspective. In M. Weist, N. A. Lever, C. P. Bradshaw, & J. S. Owens (Eds.), *Handbook of school mental health* (2nd ed., pp. 341–354). New York: Springer.

Trotter, K., & Landreth, G. (2003). A place for Bobo in play therapy. *International Journal of Play Therapy, 12*, 117–139.

Twemlow, S. W., Biggs, B. K., Nelson, T. D., Vernberge, E. M., Fonagy, P., & Twemlow, S. (2009). Effects of participation in a martial arts based antibullying program on children's aggression in elementary schools. *Psychology in the Schools, 45*, 947–959.

VanFleet, R. (2005). *Filial therapy: Strengthening parent–child relationships through play* (2nd ed.). Sarasota, FL: Professional Resources Press.

Wang, J., Iannotti, R. J., Luk, J. W., & Nansel, T. R. (2010). Co-occurrence of victimization from five subtypes of bullying: Physical, verbal, social exclusion, spreading rumors, and cyber. *Journal of Pediatric Psychology, 35*, 1103–1112.

Whitted, K. S., & Dupper, D. R. (2005). Best practices for preventing or reducing bullying in schools. *Children and Schools, 27*, 167–175.

Zins, J. E., Elias, M. J., & Maher, C. A. (2007). *Bullying, victimization, and peer harassment: A handbook of prevention and intervention.* New York: Routledge.

Chapter 14

Violence and Traumatic Events in Schools

Crisis Interventions with Students, Parents, and Teachers

JOSHUA MILLER

Shootings and other violent attacks in schools involve the confluence of two areas that terrify and horrify most people. Violent attacks involve death and destruction, but also the realization that the persons committing these attacks intend to hurt other people. Implicit in this is a profound lack of empathy, as well as a process of dehumanization of victims and intended victims. The second area that is difficult to comprehend is the tragedy of children as the targets of such attacks. It is hard enough when children are harmed or killed in "natural" disasters, such as hurricanes or earthquakes, but it is intensely disturbing when children are intentionally victimized. Such incidents generate strong and complex feelings, including fear, rage, guilt, sadness, and anxiety, while also leading to cognitive reactions of disbelief and confusion, precipitating crises of meaning and identity. These reactions do not only occur with families directly affected by the attack, but coalesce collectively. When an event of this type occurs—such as the killing of 20 children at Sandy Hook Elementary School in Newtown, Connecticut, by a lone gunman, Adam Lanza, on December 14, 2012—millions of parents with dependent children around the world face crises of confidence about not only their own ability to protect their offspring, but also the capacity of essential institutions such as schools to keep children safe. In situations of war, intergroup conflict, political repression, and social upheaval, parents, communities, and institutions across the world face this unsettling reality on a daily and prolonged basis: In such situations, adults and children lose a significant amount of control over their ability to maintain their safety and security. An event such as Sandy Hook that has occurred in recent years dissolves the sense of security and social trust that most people in the developed world harbor and expect in social interactions.

According to the Centers for Disease Control and Prevention (CDC; 2014), homicide is the second leading cause of death of youth ages 5–18, and 1–2% of these homicides occur at schools. Overall, the number of homicides of children in schools dropped from 34 in 1992 to 17 in 2009 (CDC, 2014). However, when there are large-scale attacks on children and adolescents in schools, it leads to a collective sense of unease and lack of safety for young people. Several such attacks in the United States have received massive publicity, such as the 1999 attack at Columbine High School in Littleton, Colorado, where 12 teenagers and a teacher were killed (and the two young gunmen then committed suicide). The Sandy Hook Elementary School attack is particularly notable because of the number of children killed (20), their young ages (first graders), the relentless determination of the shooter to kill as many people as possible, and the deaths of six staff members who heroically tried to protect the children—combined with the murder of the attacker's mother and his own self-destruction after his terrible acts of carnage. The scale of this event and the process that followed are difficult to comprehend.

In August 2014, the organization Everytown for Gun Safety listed on its website 74 instances of shootings at schools and colleges *since* the Newtown tragedy. There are also many smaller acts of violence toward children in schools occurring almost continually across the United States; these are often minimally reported in the national media, but nevertheless have chilling consequences for those who attend the school or live in the community. Taken together, all levels of school violence collectively contribute to a sense for parents, teachers, children, and adolescents that schools are no longer safe. Metal detectors, lockdowns, drills for responding to attacks, armed guards, and other signs of vulnerability and attempts at protection are sad daily reminders for many schoolchildren in many communities of how disaster can strike unexpectedly and ubiquitously. When it happens on the scale of the Sandy Hook massacre, it shakes our collective confidence and poses tremendous challenges for those of us responding as therapists and counselors. And yet respond we can and must.

In this chapter, I use the Sandy Hook Elementary School shooting as an example of what mental health workers involved with children and families are confronting and may confront in the future. I consider the dynamics of school shootings and their consequences for children, their parents and siblings, their teachers and other school personnel, and the community at large. I also consider why groups in particular are effective responses to foster healing and recovery. This psychosocial capacity-building approach emphasizes that pain and trauma can intermix with individual and collective strength and resiliency (Miller, 2012). The chapter concludes with specific suggested approaches for social workers and clinicians.

The use of Sandy Hook Elementary School as a case example is both important and complicated. It is valuable to examine such a recent catastrophic event, in order to consider what has helped people to recover and what can be learned by other communities that will, sadly, confront tragic situations in school settings in the future. On the other hand, all such communities, including Newtown, are ambivalent about sharing their tragedies as exemplars with others. Communities do differ in this regard: Oklahoma City is an example of a community that has shared its experiences with other communities as part of its own healing, while other communities are more ambivalent or reticent about receiving such public scrutiny. There are many reasons for this. One is the inevitable conflict within a community about how much to share, what to share, and with whom; members of communities rarely are in unanimous agreement about this. Another reason is that the pain and suffering from such a heartbreaking event are overwhelming, and people and communities seek privacy to avoid having to recall and stir up this pain repeatedly. Many in the community do not want to be defined by the event, which is what often occurs. When Littleton, Colorado is mentioned, for example, most people immediately associate this name with the Columbine shooting (Lysiak, 2013). And lastly, as a colleague working with survivors in Newtown conveyed to me, "We are still in recovery." Such colleagues (and their clients) believe that too much sharing or exposure may be detrimental to the recovery process.

This last point is critical. Although research into mass shootings is important, it should always be secondary to the well-being and the recovery processes of those in the affected communities. We will eventually learn from those who helped and those who were helped. But the immediate needs of those in recovery are more important than constructing randomized controlled trials and other forms of research, as valuable as this research may be for informing best practices.

SCHOOL SHOOTINGS AND THEIR CONSEQUENCES

The Sandy Hook Elementary School Tragedy

On Friday, December 14, 2012, after murdering his mother, 20-year-old Adam Lanza entered Sandy Hook Elementary School; when he was confronted by the school's principal, he fatally shot her and the school psychologist (Owings, 2014). He then roamed the school, entering classrooms that could not be locked from the inside, shooting and ultimately killing 20 first-grade students and 4 other staff members before killing himself approximately 5 minutes after entering the building. Students were hiding under desks and in closets, and many witnessed or heard direct sounds of the attack or the sounds of warnings on loudspeakers. They experienced the arrival of the police 3 minutes after the attack. They were then evacuated from the school 45 minutes after the onset of the violence to the town firehouse, where they were eventually reunited with their distraught parents (Hurley-Hanson & Giannontonio, 2013; Owings, 2014). Teachers led students in songs after leaving the building and reaching safety (Pascopella, 2013).

While all of this was going on, many distressed parents became aware of the attack but did not know the fate of their children. As parents gathered at the firehouse, there were many emotional reunions, but some parents were left without their children. Clergy, grief counselors, and Connecticut Governor Dannel Malloy were present. The police announced the death toll, which led to visible expressions of grief. Finally, Governor Malloy told the remaining parents that their children had not survived (Lysiak, 2013; Owings, 2014). Two days later, at a vigil for families and first responders, President Obama comforted people and read out the names of all 26 victims (Kuhnhenn & Feller, 2012). Many makeshift memorials sprang up in the community, including wooden angels and green and white ribbons (Owings, 2014). There was also an outpouring of public support around the nation, and many cards, teddy bears, and other items were sent to Newtown.

The media spread a great deal of misinformation about the entire situation, including misidentifying the shooter. This was true of social media as well as more mainstream media outlets, such as CNN (Lysiak, 2013). The following week, funerals for all of the victims took place (Lysiak, 2013). Paul Simon and Harry Connick, Jr., performed on behalf of some of the victims (Owings, 2014). Media coverage remained intense, including debates about school safety and mental illness, and a bitter public discourse about gun control. In the longer-term aftermath, three times as many states expanded the right to carry guns as those that restricted gun access (Owings, 2014).

Children eventually returned to school 20 days later at Chalk Hill Middle School in a neighboring county (Lysiak, 2013). The same posters that had been on the walls at Sandy Hook Elementary School were placed in the new location. There was a massive police presence, with bomb-sniffing dogs in the playground. "Comfort dogs," seven golden retrievers, were also brought to the new school (De Santis, 2013). A long process of recovery began.

Circles of Vulnerability

Although most people in the nation were affected by what occurred at Sandy Hook Elementary School, there were varying levels of direct exposure. A tool called "circles of vulnerability" (Rosenfeld, Caye, Ayalon, & Lahad, 2005; see Figure 14.1) helps distinguish these differing levels. Those closest to the event, at the epicenter of these circles, are likely to experience the most severe reactions by virtue of their exposure. When this model is applied to the Sandy Hook event, the center circle might include the children and school personnel who directly experienced and survived the attack, as well as the families of those children and staff who died. Many children who survived the attack lost friends who perished. Extremely close to the center circle are the children, teachers, and staff who were in other parts of the building, as well as law enforcement personnel and other first responders who arrived early on the scene. Parents of children who survived were also deeply affected, especially since many knew some of the children who were killed.

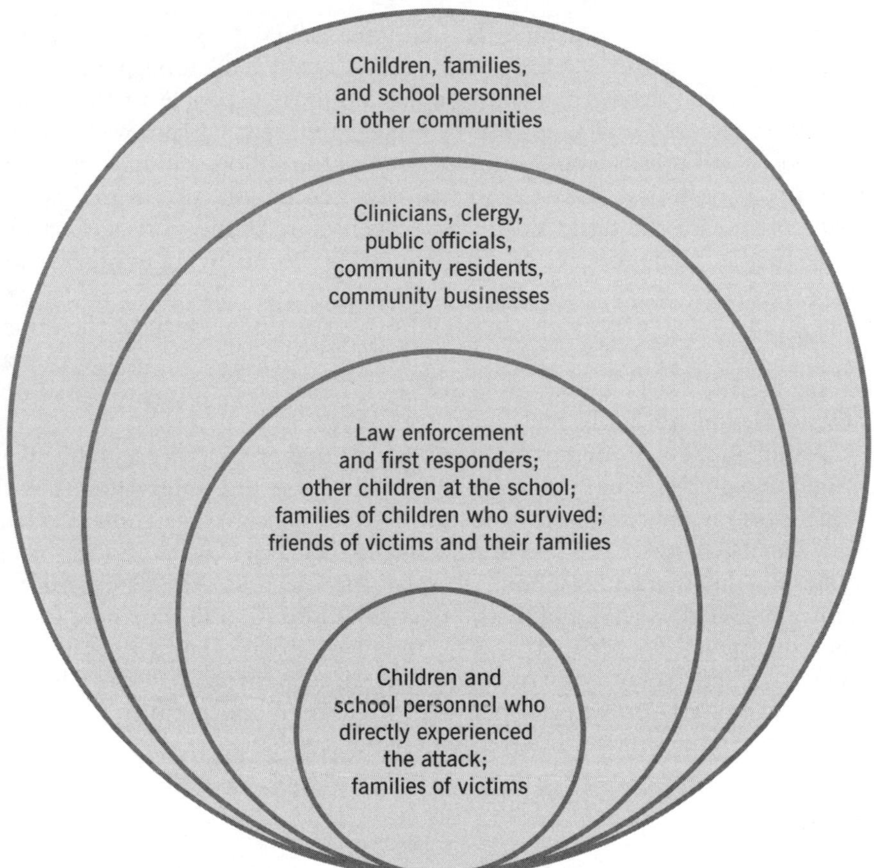

FIGURE 14.1. Circles of vulnerability: Vulnerable groups after school attacks and shootings. From Rosenfeld, Caye, Ayalon, and Lahad (2005). Copyright 2005 by the National Association of Social Workers. Adapted by permission.

Other affected people were those who comforted and counseled others, notably clergy and second-line emergency responders. Despite the training and experiences of both groups, nothing can prepare a professional for a situation such as this. It must also have been emotionally draining for public officials who were trying to respond—including local officials, state bureau chiefs, Governor Malloy, and President Obama. Children at other schools in the community and their families were shaken by what happened. Residents in the community who did not have a direct relationship to the school were similarly stunned. Local businesses were affected by increased and then markedly decreased volumes of business; some have now closed, and their former proprietors have related this to the tragedy (Lysiak, 2013). Counselors and therapists who responded in the aftermath and subsequent months were at risk of "vicarious trauma" (Pearlman & Saakvitne, 1995), "compassion fatigue" (Figley, 1995), "disaster distress" (Miller, 2012), and general burnout.

Further away from the center circle, millions of people in the United States were shocked and saddened by what happened. Parents with school-age children and most school personnel around the nation could identify with those directly affected. Those who had experienced violence in the past or carried other vulnerabilities would have been more prone to triggering and retriggering as a consequence of what happened. People living in other countries were also affected, just as many Americans were struck by large-scale tragedies involving attacks on children in other nations—such as the attack killing 16 children and a teacher in Dunblane, Scotland, in 1996, and Anders Behring Breivik's 2011 killing spree in Utøya, Norway, resulting in the deaths of 69 people (mostly adolescents).

Although these groupings are not complete and are not meant to be taken as rigid categories, I have described them because any interventions with people in the inner circles must necessarily take place in the context of the larger social ecology of the disaster (Miller, 2012). The "social ecology of the disaster" is the interaction among an event, people, and their community as they are shaped by social, political, historical, cultural, and economic forces. This ecology includes personal and community liabilities and vulnerabilities, as well as assets, resources, strengths, and social networks. In this chapter, I focus particularly on ways of helping the children and families within the inner circles in the short-term aftermath of an attack.

Consequences

The consequences of violent attacks are complex, and evaluating their impact often becomes mired in debates over the prevalence of posttraumatic stress disorder (PTSD). How problems are framed has a strong influence on how they are responded to. There are different views of the extent to which reactions are universal and the extent to which they are influenced by culture, social structure, and expectations.

Ramirez and colleagues (2013) found in a review of research of children exposed to extreme violence that 10–80% were reported to develop PTSD symptoms, which is a very wide range. The PTSD was often accompanied by depression, intense fear, and feelings of helplessness. Nader, Pynoos, Fairbanks, and Frederick (1990) studied the reactions of 100 elementary-age children 14 months after a sniper attack on their school in 1984, resulting in one death and in injuries to other children and a staff member. They found that there were still symptoms of PTSD in a significant number of children, particularly avoidance of reminders and fear when thinking of the event. Significantly, there were more lingering, severe symptoms for those children directly exposed to the event than for children who were not directly exposed; the authors concluded that treatment responses should be differentially tailored to children, depending on their degree of exposure. Pfefferbaum and colleagues (2005), in their review of the psychological effects on children of the 1995 Oklahoma City bombing and the September 11, 2001 attacks on the World Trade Center, found similar patterns of more severe and persistent trauma symptoms for those most directly exposed to the violent events. However, they added two other forms of exposure that increased vulnerability: (1) "relationship exposure" (knowing someone who died or was injured); and (2) "media exposure" (prolonged contact with media coverage of the events).

Children's and adolescents' abilities to comprehend school attacks and the ways they express their reactions vary widely, due to many factors—including their developmental levels, their abilities to make sense of what occurred, their family and social supports, and their unique areas of vulnerability and resiliency. Young children, such as the first graders attacked in Newtown, are very reliant on adults (especially parents and teachers) and older children to help them grasp what happened and to offer them a sense of comfort, safety, and security. They rely on predictability and routines, which are at least initially disrupted after a violent attack (Boyden, de Berry, Feeny, & Hart, 2006). Such children are also less able to filter out disturbing and overwhelming images, and rely on adults to help them with this (Pynoos, Steinberg, & Brymer, 2007). This is one reason why it is so important to protect children from overexposure to media coverage of violence. In addition, younger children are prone to blaming themselves for what has happened, and they sometimes employ magical thinking about how some action or misbehavior of theirs might have led to what happened (Rosenfeld et al., 2005, Smith, Dyregrov & Yule, 2002; Webb, 2004). Children who have a prior history of abuse and neglect may even be more vulnerable than others to the negative effects of a violent school attack (Cohen et al., 2006).

Two of the most critical losses for children after a mass shooting at a school are the losses of a sense of safety and of familiar routines (Gordon, Farberow, & Maida, 1999; Jagodic & Kontac, 2002; Miller, 2012; Zubenko, 2002). If young children have lost a teacher, they have lost an adult figure who is one of their caregivers, which can be devastating and contribute to traumatic stress, depression, and anxiety. A violent school attack resulting in the deaths of classmates and teachers creates challenges for children's attachments to others; not only have they lost people to whom they were attached, but the knowledge that someone wanted to harm them shakes the foundation of even the most secure attachments.

Although children are vulnerable and dependent, they are also resilient, even when faced with the terror of school shootings. In a meta-analysis of children's reactions to exposure to disasters and terrorism, Pfefferbaum, Newman, and Nelson (2014) found that the majority of children experienced distress but not psychiatric symptoms, and that the distress subsided over time. Children are adaptable and responsive if a secure holding environment can be reestablished. There are many ways that adults can work with child survivors of school shootings to foster a sense of safety and security, reduce traumatic and depressive symptoms, and facilitate recovery. Such interventions are discussed in the next section.

It is important to note the consequences of events like the Newtown massacre for those charged with caring for children. The shootings at Sandy Hook emphasized to parents around the world that they did not, and do not, have complete control over their children's safety. Parents directly affected also had to grapple with feelings of grief, loss, sadness, anxiety, anger, and despair. For some, there might have been a sense of guilt or even shame over their inability to protect their children. These feelings were likely to ripple out to extended family members, friends, and others in the community.

Teachers and other school personnel also had to contend with the dual challenges of facing their own vulnerability and their personal and professional sense of responsibility for children entrusted to them by parents and the community. Efforts aimed at helping children recover need to consider the importance of also helping parents, teachers, and others in the community to recover.

RESPONDING TO SCHOOL SHOOTINGS

One cluster of responses to events such as school shootings has become familiar to practitioners in the West as "disaster mental health." Some of the characteristics of this approach include an emphasis on trauma (particularly PTSD); the psychological consequences of the attack; and a primary reliance on trained mental health professionals to offer therapy and counseling, often to individuals and families (Miller, 2012). "Psychological first aid" (Bragin, 2014; Miller, 2012) is a central intervention strategy described in greater detail below. Cognitive-behavioral interventions, including exposure and trauma therapy, eye movement desensitization and reprocessing (EMDR), traumatic grief interventions, and psychoeducation, have been demonstrated to be helpful (Pfefferbaum et al., 2014). Some group interventions are also utilized, such as debriefings, group therapy, and support groups.

Psychosocial capacity building (PCB) places an emphasis on enhancement of strength and resiliency, resistance to medicalizing the consequences of the disaster, the use of groups in natural settings, and attention to the significance of culture in shaping both how people react and how they interpret how they react (Miller, 2012). The PCB approach relies less than other approaches do on trained mental health professionals as direct practitioners; it often employs a "training of trainers" model, in which mental health practitioners train local community leaders and paraprofessionals to assist others. This model is particularly useful in situations where there are few trained mental health providers, where seeking counseling and therapy are not normative activities, and/or where sustainability and a sense of community empowerment are high priorities—but it has other advantages, as described below.

In the remainder of this chapter, I suggest a response to situations such as Newtown that integrates disaster mental health and PCB approaches, and that emphasizes the use of various kinds of support groups.

Why Use Groups?

Children are social beings and are used to being in groups at school, in recreational settings, and in organizations such as religious institutions. After violent school shootings, it is critical to help children reestablish routines and reconstruct a sense of safety with what was formerly familiar. In groups, children can explore their reactions with other children, can receive validation and support for what they are experiencing, and can learn from the experiences of others. They can play together, collectively solve problems, and offer a sense of mutual aid and support (Miller, 2012). In groups, unlike in individual treatment, young people can learn from their peers. Groups also offer the potential for creative expression of psychic wounds, overwhelming feelings, and hopes and aspirations (Bryant-Davis, 2005). The opportunity to participate in groups should be offered to not only to children, but to teachers, parents, first responders, and other community members as well.

It is important to consider many variables in setting up groups: membership; whether the group is open or closed; boundaries and confidentiality; facilitation; and an assessment of the maxim "Do no harm" (Miller, 2012). For example, when planning a group's membership, practitioners need to consider the risk of "contagion" of students who did not directly experience school violence by those who did have direct exposure. Both groups of children may benefit from being in a group, but perhaps there are times when they should be in separate groups; groups should not lead to the worsening of any child's symptoms, and the pros and cons of having separate groups need to be assessed according to the unique factors in different situations.

Groups with the following four purposes are particularly helpful after a mass crisis situation such as a school shooting (Miller, 2012):

- Psychotherapy and psychoeducation
- Support
- Recreation
- Task

Some groups are blends of these different sorts of groups. Psychotherapy groups can use psychological first aid (see below) in the immediate aftermath of a disaster, and then move to working with deeper, longer-term reactions to the violence (including trauma and depression), employing cognitive-behavioral treatment approaches (Pfefferbaum et al., 2014) that focus on exposure, desensitization, and traumatic growth. These can be integrated with psychodynamic techniques such as exploring latent fears and concerns, in addition to working to reestablish attachments (Bragin, 2014). Grieving and mourning may occur as well for those who lost a beloved teacher or close classmate. Support groups can involve regular meetings for parents or teachers, offering mutual aid and social support. Recreational groups offer children a chance to reclaim their ability to have fun together as well as engaging creative and pleasurable parts of the brain. Task-oriented groups can involve children and/or adults. For example, older children may meet to plan ways to help younger children directly affected by the violence through offering mentorship or coaching. Parents often come together after a school shooting to establish social action groups and networks that respond to the tragedy. The Newtown Action Alliance (2014) was formed after the Sandy Hook attack to reverse, according to its website, "the escalating gun violence epidemic in this nation through the introduction of smarter, safer gun laws and broader cultural change." This approach exemplifies turning a tragedy into social activism and is also a way of memorializing victims.

Interventions

So how can social workers and other clinicians help children and their families to recover from an attack on a school? Responders have found a range of interventions to be helpful, and some of these interventions have been supported by research. But there are many difficulties with conducting randomized controlled trials under such stressful circumstances, and practitioners must draw upon the accumulated practice wisdom of those who have responded to such situations.

It is important to adapt a social-ecological approach to interventions—an approach that includes children, adolescents, parents, teachers, other school personnel, and community members—and to respect and empower such stakeholders to be partners if not leaders in designing the contours of their own recovery (Bragin, 2014; Miller, 2012). All interventions involve multiple groups of people, and multilevel, multisystemic responses are called for after a major incident of school violence. A community and its many subgroups have been wounded and disrupted, and it takes a communitywide approach to foster lasting healing and recovery. Another important principle is that for youth to recover, their caregivers must also recover and be given the support and tools to help the young people recover. Children are attached to parents, siblings, teachers, and friends, and engaging all of these people in the recovery process is critical for the well-being of exposed youth (Bragin, 2013; Miller, 2012; Pfefferbaum et al., 2014). Children and teens also have attachments to pets and other domestic animals as well as toys, dolls, and other objects, and these relationships can be constructed and reconstructed after a violent attack.

In this section, I consider the following interventions: psychological first aid (PFA); reestablishing safety and routines; rebuilding attachments; encouraging narrative expression; teaching children and adolescents how to calm themselves; providing social support; facilitating grieving and mourning; and reestablishing hope. These are interventions that are suitable for all people exposed to violence, whether they develop symptoms of trauma or not. For those individuals who do develop intractable PTSD, these interventions offer a foundation for response, but additional clinical interventions (e.g., cognitive-behavioral PTSD treatments) may be necessary.

Psychological First Aid

PFA is a helpful way to approach recovery in the early hours, days, and weeks after exposure to severe violence. PFA encapsulates many of the longer-term strategies considered in this section, but does so within a framework of brief crisis intervention. The main emphasis is on immediate coping in the short-term aftermath of a violent encounter. Although the impact of PFA has not been adequately studied, there is a current consensus among disaster responders in the West that it is the most useful protocol for intervening with children, adolescents, and adults who have encountered extreme violence (Pfefferbaum et al., 2014). PFA draws from many theoretical sources and practice methodologies: crisis intervention theory; traditions of mutual aid and support; grief and bereavement work; the value of sharing fears and reactions with others; and the value of telling one's story in an ongoing quest to make sense and meaning of initially unfathomable events (Miller, 2012).

The goals of PFA are to "reduce the initial distress caused by traumatic events and to foster short- and long-term adaptive functioning and coping" (Brymer et al., 2006, p. 5). PFA activities involve reestablishing a sense of safety and security, reinstituting routines, offering comfort and care, fostering social support, and providing short-term crisis intervention. When teachers were sitting with students from Sandy Hook Elementary School and singing familiar songs with them, they were offering a form of PFA. The re-creation of familiar posters at the temporary school and the provision of "comfort dogs" were other ways that PFA was proffered to the same children. Providing crisis counseling, pastoral resources, and locations and opportunities to talk, receive information, and plan for immediate responses to the tragedy are other examples of PFA activities. Coaching parents and teachers about how to respond to children's immediate fears and needs, while also attending to their own direct experiences of trauma, loss, and grief, are still other ways of employing a PFA approach.

Reestablishing Safety and Routines

Hobfoll and colleagues (2007) attempted to establish an evidence-based international consensus about "restoring social and behavioral functioning after situations of disaster and mass casualty" (p. 283) by interviewing an international panel of experts who had responded to such events. Many of their findings support the interventions discussed in this part of the chapter, and first and foremost is the importance of helping children feeling safe again after a school attack. Among the immediate consequences of such attacks are the sense of vulnerability and fragility experienced by young people and their caregivers, as well as the ultimate rupture in attachment when a perpetrator intentionally harms others. The primary foundation block of recovery for youth and caregivers alike is the need to feel safe.

How do we accomplish this? Hobfoll and colleagues (2007) stress the importance of "sustained attachments to loved ones and social groups in combating stress and trauma" (p. 296), which is why working in groups can foster a sense of safety. Bryant-Davis (2005) describes activities that can be done in groups to foster a sense of safety (journaling, singing, movement, drama, arts and crafts, spiritual practices, reconnecting with nature)—all collective ways of creating a sense of solidarity, connectedness, and empowerment. Reassurance is important for children and caregivers after a violent school attack, and participating in these kinds of activities with others is reassuring. Reestablishing routines, offering transitional objects for younger children, having on-site counselors, and offering comfort dogs are all examples of responses that foster a sense of safety. All of these can help children to regain a sense of school as a safe and protected space.

Helping parents to understand how to reassure children and help them to feel safe at home is as important as helping children to feel safe in school. Both parents and children need information and visible indicators that safety precautions are being implemented; in other words, they need the recognition that steps have been taken to prevent future violent occurrences. It is also essential that caregivers filter and protect children from excessive media coverage of the events.

Rebuilding Attachments

The attachment ruptures that come from having been the targets of an attack, as well as from losing friends or classmates, can spill over to other relationships. Reestablishing attachments and building on existing attachments can be achieved through individual therapy, family therapy, and the use of groups in the many ways described above. As Bragin (2014) has discussed, recent attachment-based research has confirmed that both attachment and safety are social and neurobiological processes. Thus strengthening children's ability to "mentalize"—that is, to be able to reflect on what is going on in their minds, as well as the minds of others—is a core ingredient of attachment. Mentalizing occurs in relationships with others. Group activities for children that invite empathy, attunement, sharing, and expression of feelings, as well as the ability to read the feelings of others, are ways of strengthening attachments.

Another aspect of helping children to reattach is to help them express any lingering aggressive feelings, such as their anger and rage about what happened (Bragin, 2014). Without such opportunities for expression, aggression can block the young persons' capacity to trust others, and the results can be isolation and increased vulnerability.

Encouraging Narrative Expression

People of all ages do better after a violent encounter if they can construct a narrative about what occurred that can be shared with others. Telling stories fosters resiliency (Denham, 2008; Landau & Saul, 2004; Miller, 2012). This involves constructing a story that minimally includes the following components: what life was like before the attack; the experience of the attack itself; the residue from the attack, such as fear, anger, anxiety, and despondency; personal, social, and cultural resources and strengths that can be accessed and expanded; and resolutions and hopes for the future. All cultures have collective narratives of strength in the face of adversity, and when personal narratives can draw on these cultural lessons and scripts, they reconnect people with what collectively sustained them before the tragedy.

For young people of all ages, such storytelling can involve a range of expressive media: drawing and art; performances such as singing, enacting dramas, or creating videos; and various forms of writing, such as journaling, poetry, and letters. While all individuals have their own narratives, and it is important that their voices are heard by others, there is even greater power and resonance when narratives are created collectively. This facilitates not only individual expression, but empathy, validation, and taking the perspectives of others (all of which nurture mentalizing). Groups allow narratives to be shared and interwoven with the accounts of other people—peers, teachers, parents, and therapists. Collective storytelling thus creates networks of social support and reinforces the importance of attachment and connection.

Teaching Self-Calming

Hobfoll and colleagues (2007) identified teaching the ability to calm oneself as another foundational method to help people recover from violent attacks. People of all ages can learn simple techniques that help them to calm themselves when anxious or triggered by reminders of violent events. This includes teaching children and adolescents mindfulness exercises, such as focusing on breathing or the EMDR technique of visualizing a safe space. Another EMDR practice—rhythmic bilateral stimulation—also helps children to regain a sense of balance and tranquility. The butterfly method of crossing arms and alternately tapping each shoulder is a form of this. For many children, singing or drumming is soothing. Self-calming techniques can be taught and performed with children in groups, which in turn promotes security and social support.

Providing Social Support

All of the methods discussed in this part of the chapter nurture social support through the use of groups. In addition to formal groups, social support can be provided through friendships, religious affiliations, and recreational activities. Social support can be "horizontal" (i.e., between children of similar ages), but it can also be intergenerational, including older children as well as parents and teachers. A "training of trainers" model is an effective way to generate social support: Clinicians work with older children or teachers and parents to equip them to implement the methods outlined in this section of the chapter. This model is often more effective than direct clinical intervention, as it engages natural helping systems and has the potential for greater sustainability.

Facilitating Grieving and Mourning

It is important to help children grieve—not only for those who literally have been lost, such as other children or teachers who were killed or wounded, but also for the loss of a predictable safe space. As with aggression, failure (or inadequate opportunities) to grieve and mourn can block a child's ability to reestablish and maintain attachments and to regain hope for the future. With school shootings, it is also effective to grieve and mourn collectively, and to create memorials that commemorate the tragedy and the heroism of those who responded and survived. Such memorials can be local, but they can also be created online (e.g., social media) or can take the forms of funds, foundations, and social movements that emerge from the tragedy.

Reestablishing Hope

Even in the wake of such an enormity as the Newtown attack, hope can be instilled. Many survivors of the Columbine High School attacks or the Oklahoma City bombing (where many young people died) not only have regained a sense of hope, but have used what they have learned from their experiences to help others who are suffering. Regaining hope does not come easily or without pain and suffering. But the vast majority of those responding to violence that engulfs youth and families mention sustaining hope as an essential component of the recovery process (Hobfoll et al., 2007). Timing is important—it is difficult to have hope without adequately mourning what has been lost—but for clinicians working with children, adolescents, and communities after violent attacks, one of our roles is to keep the "pilot light" of hope lit for those with whom we work.

CONCLUSION

School attacks and shootings are grievous violations of human dignity and connection. Although such events generate tremendous suffering, this chapter has described ways that social workers and other helping professionals can work multisystemically, integrating mental health techniques with a PCB approach. A tragedy such as Newtown leaves many broken people in its wake, while also straining the fabric of community. Responders carry a precious responsibility: to honor and engage with every wounded individual, while respecting and supporting organizational and community empowerment.

STUDY QUESTIONS

1. All disasters lead to losses and suffering, but what is unique for those who directly experience severe violence, particularly when it occurs in an unexpected setting such as a school?
2. Being a target or witness to violence is challenging for anyone, but what are some of the unique vulnerabilities and sources of resiliency for children and adolescents when they directly experience violence?
3. What are the advantages and drawbacks to using groups in helping young people and their families recover from violent attacks?
4. If you were consulting with school personnel after a violent attack, what questions would you ask and what general suggestions would you make about how to help students, family members, and school employees recover?

REFERENCES

Bragin, M. (2014). Clinical social work with survivors of disaster and terrorism: A social ecological approach. In J. Brandell (Ed.), *Essentials of clinical social work* (2nd ed., pp. 366–401). Thousand Oaks, CA: Sage.

Boyden, J., de Berry, J., Feeny, T., & Hart, J. (2006). Children affected by armed conflict in South Asia: A regional summary. In G. Reyes & A Jacobs (Eds.), *Handbook of international disaster psychology: Vol. 4. Interventions with special needs populations* (pp. 61–76). Westport, CT: Praeger.

Bryant-Davis, T. (2005). *Thriving in the wake of trauma*. Westport, CT: Praeger.

Brymer, M., Jacobs, A., Layne, C., Pynoos, R., Ruzek, J., Steinberg, A., et al. (2006). *Psychological first aid: Field operations guide* (2nd ed.). Los Angeles: National Child Traumatic Stress Network and National Center for PTSD. Retrieved August 27, 2014, from *www.nctsn.org/content/psychological-first-aid.*

Centers for Disease Control and Prevention (CDC). (2014). School associated violent death study. Retrieved June 3, 2014, from *www.cdc.gov/violenceprevention/youthviolence/schoolviolence/savdhtml*

Cohen, J. A., Mannarino, A. P., Gibson, L. E., Cozza, S. J., Brymer, M. J., & Murray, I. (2006). Interventions for children and adolescents following disaster. In E. C. Ritchie, P. J. Watson, & M. J. Friedman (Eds.), *Interventions following mass violence and disaster: Strategies for mental health practice* (pp. 227–256). New York: Guilford Press.

Denham, A. R. (2008). Rethinking historical trauma: Narratives of resilience. *Transcultural Psychiatry, 45*, 391–415.

De Santis, S. (2013, February 6). Lutheran "comfort dogs" welcome students back to Newtown school. *Christian Century*. Retrieved from *www.christiancentury.org/article/2013-01/lutheran-comfort-dogs-welcome-students-back-newtown-school.*

Everytown for Gun Safety. (2014). School shootings in America since Sandy Hook. Retrieved August 7, 2014, from *http://everytown.org/article/schoolshootings/?source=fbno_schoolshootings&utm_source=fb_n_&utm_medium=_o&utm_campaign=schoolshootings.*

Figley, C. R. (1995). Compassion fatigue as secondary traumatic stress disorder: An overview. In C. R. Figley (Ed.), *Compassion fatigue: Coping with secondary traumatic stress disorder in those who treat the traumatized* (pp. 1–20). New York: Brunner/Mazel.

Gordon, N. S., Farberow, N. L., & Maida, C. A. (1999). *Children and disasters.* Philadelphia: Brunner/Mazel.

Hobfoll, S. B., Watson, P., Bell, C. C., Bryant, R. A., Brymer, M. J., Friedman, M. J., et al. (2007). Five essential elements of immediate and mid-term mass trauma intervention: Empirical evidence. *Psychiatry, 70*(4), 283–315.

Hurley-Hanson, A. E., & Giannontonio, C. M. (2013). The Sandy Hook Elementary School shootings. In C. M. Giannontonio & A. E. Hurley-Hanson (Eds.), *Extreme leadership: Leaders, teams and situations outside of the norm* (pp. 224–236). Northampton, MA: Elgar.

Jacodic, G. K., & Kontac, K. (2002). Normalization: A key to children's recovery. In W. N. Zubenko & J. Capozzoli (Eds.), *Children and disasters: A practical guide to healing and recovery* (pp. 159–171). New York: Oxford University Press.

Kunnhenn, J., & Feller, B. (2012, December 16). Obama visits Newtown, Connecticut on Sunday. *Huffington Post.* Retrieved May 30, 2014, from *www.huffingtonpost.com/2012/12/16/obama-newtown-connecticut-sandy-hook-school-shooting_n_2310520.html.*

Landau, J., & Saul, J. (2004). Facilitating family and community resilience in response to major disaster. In F. Walsh & M. McGoldrick (Eds.), *Living beyond loss* (pp. 285–309). New York: Norton.

Lysiak, M. (2013). *Newtown: An American tragedy.* New York: Gallery Books.

Miller, J. (2012). *Psychosocial capacity building in response to disasters.* New York: Columbia University Press.

Nader, K., Pynoos, R., Fairbanks, L., & Frederick, C. (1990). Children's PTSD reactions one year after a sniper attack at their school. *American Journal of Psychiatry, 147*(11), 1526–1530.

Newtown Action Alliance. (2014). About. Retrieved August 12, 2014, from *http://newtownaction.org/about.*

Owings, L. (2014). *The Newtown school shooting.* Minneapolis, MN: ABDO.

Pascopella, A. (2013, June). Sandy Hook Elementary School: Six months later. A conversation with Newtown superintendent Janet Robinson on the tragedy of December 14, 2012, and the continual healing process. *District Administration.* Retrieved from *www.districtadministration.com/article/sandy-hook-elementary-school-six-months-later.*

Pearlman, C. A., & Saakvitne, K. W. (1995). *Trauma and the therapist: Countertransference and vicarious trauma in psychotherapy with incest survivors.* New York: Norton.

Pfefferbaum, B. J., DeVoe, E. R., Stuber, J., Schiff, M., Klein, T. P., & Fairbrother, G. (2005). Psychological impact of terrorism on children and families in the United States. In Y. Danieli, D. Brom, & J. Sills (Eds.), *The trauma of terrorism: Sharing knowledge and shared care* (pp. 305–318). Binghamton, NY: Haworth Press.

Pfefferbaum, B. J., Newman, L., & Nelson, S. D. (2014). Mental health interventions for children exposed to disasters and terrorism. *Journal of Child and Adolescent Psychopharmacology, 24*(1), 24–31.

Pynoos, R. S., Steinberg, A. M., & Brymer, M. J. (2007). Children and disasters: Public mental health approaches. In R. J. Ursano, C. S. Fullerton, L. Weisaeth, &

B. Raphael (Eds.) *Textbook of disaster psychiatry* (pp. 48–68). Cambridge, UK: Cambridge University Press.

Ramirez, M., Harland, K., Frederick, M., Shepherd, R., Wong, M., & Cavanaugh, J. E. (2013). Listen protect connect for traumatized schoolchildren: A pilot study of psychological first aid. *BMC Psychology, 1*(26). Retrieved from *www.biomedcentral.com/2050-7283/1/26*.

Rosenfeld, L. B., Caye, J. S., Ayalon, O., & Lahad, M. (2005). *When their world falls apart: Helping families and children manage the effects of disasters.* Washington, DC: NASW Press.

Smith, P., Dyregrov, A., & Yule, W. (2002). *Children and disaster: Teaching recovery techniques.* Bergen, Norway: Children and War Foundation.

Webb, N. B. (Ed.). (2004). *Mass trauma and violence: Helping families and children cope.* New York: Guilford Press.

Zubenko, W. N. (2002). Developmental issues in stress and crisis. In W. N. Zubenko & J. Capozzoli (Eds.), *Children and disasters: A practical guide to healing and recovery* (pp. 85–100). New York: Oxford University Press.

Chapter 15

Children and Adolescents with Chronic Medical Conditions

Individual and Group Helping in the School

M. CARLEAN GILBERT
RANA HONG

This chapter reviews the multiple problems facing children with serious medical conditions. The focus here is on the challenges of young people with asthma, since this is a disease that affects many youth from preschool through high school. The chapter presents an overview of the illness and its psychosocial impact on a child, family, and school. A case illustrates the impact on a classmate of the tragic death of an asthmatic school-age child, and suggests school-based crisis intervention responses to help those who were most affected by such a death.

ASTHMA AND SCHOOL-AGE CHILDREN

Asthma is one of the most common chronic diseases in childhood, and in 2012 it affected an estimated 7.1 million children under the age of 18 in the United States (Bloom, Jones, & Freeman, 2013). Asthma is a chronic inflammatory condition of the lungs and airways. When a child inhales allergens or irritants into the inflamed lungs, episodes of difficult breathing, wheezing, coughing, and tightening of the chest may be triggered. The subsequent restricted airflow results from the interaction among three factors following exposure to an irritant: (1) airway hyperresponsiveness, which is an exaggerated bronchoconstrictor reaction to the stimuli; (2) bronchoconstriction, which is the contraction of the bronchial smooth muscles and subsequent narrowing of the airways following exposure to an irritant; and (3) airway edema, which is characterized by fluid retention in tissue, increased mucus production, and the formation of mucus plugs that inhibit airflow. Asthma is a serious illness, and in rare instances it can be fatal.

Although the exact causes of childhood asthma are unknown, research findings indicate that both individual vulnerability and environmental conditions are risk factors in the occurrence of asthma (National Heart, Lung, and Blood Institute, 2007). The individual risk factors that contribute to asthma are genetics and an imbalance between Th1-type and Th2-type cytokines, which are proteins that affect cellular activity and inflammation in the immune system. The environmental risk factors that contribute to the development and perhaps severity of asthma are respiratory infections, airborne allergens, and irritants. Common allergens include dust mites, pollens, and molds; cockroaches and their droppings; and dried saliva or dander from the hair and fur of animals and feathers of birds. Smoke from tobacco and wood-burning fireplaces; plants and grasses; unvented stoves; polluted air; scented products; and volatile organic compounds found in materials like paint and new carpet can also increase asthmatic symptoms. Asthma symptoms may be further aggravated by exercise, cold air, or changes in air temperature (Gilbert, 2009).

Two types of pharmaceuticals are commonly used to treat pediatric asthma: short-term and long-term. Physicians generally recommend inhaled corticosteroids (ICSs) such as Alvesco or Flovent, which reduce swelling in the airways and decrease mucus production, for long-term treatment for children. They also may treat children with a combination of ICSs and long-acting beta agonists such as Advair. These prophylactic medications must be used consistently to be effective. When asthma symptoms are exacerbated, oral corticosteroids may be prescribed. The most common side effects of the ICSs are thrush, cough, or hoarseness. Initial concerns that ICSs reduced growth rate (U.S. Food and Drug Administration, 1998) were not substantiated (Agertot & Pederson, 2000).

The prevalence of asthma has been increasing across all ages, both sexes, and all racial groups. For instance, 1 in 12 people (8.3%) had asthma in 2009, compared to 13% in 2012 (Centers for Disease Control and Prevention [CDC], 2014b). Bloom and colleagues (2013) found that in 2012, 15.6% of children between the ages of 5 and 11 years had ever been diagnosed with asthma (according to parental report), and 11% continued to have asthma. Reporting on youth under the age of 18 of various ethnicities, Bloom and colleagues detailed that 21.8% of non-Hispanic black children had ever been diagnosed with asthma, and 16.1% still had asthma; 13.5% of Hispanic children had ever been diagnosed with asthma, and 8.9% still had asthma; the corresponding figures for non-Hispanic white youth were 12.6% and 8%, respectively. Almost 18% (17.9%) of children who had ever been diagnosed with asthma, and 13.3% who still had asthma, lived in families where the family income was below the poverty threshold. In contrast, 12.4% of children who had ever been diagnosed with asthma and 7.9% of children who still had asthma had incomes 200% above the poverty threshold. Although latency-age children were not coded separately, between 2007 and 2009 the asthma death rate for black children ages 0–14 was eight times greater than the death rate of corresponding white children (Gorina, 2012).

Significant differences in asthma care also may exist among racial and ethnic groups. One study of children under age 17 revealed that although their asthma was less severe and they had fewer outpatient visits for asthma, African American youth spent three times as many days in the hospital as Puerto Rican youth (Cohen et al., 2006). One inference is that more frequent clinic visits reduce the occurrence of severe asthma attacks that require hospitalization. Despite growing concerns about health disparities, McManus and Savage's (2012) systematic review identified few culturally sensitive interventions for asthmatic children.

Although childhood asthma is a serious chronic illness with a modest risk of mortality, the frequency of asthma episodes and functional limitations can generally be managed in the outpatient clinic. Numerous evidence-based studies, however, have reported significantly increased risks of asthma severity and/or death for children who are African American, Hispanic, and impoverished. Practitioners working with asthmatic youth must be conscious of these disparities in prevalence rates and utilization of resources when they are completing assessments and planning interventions for children and families who fit these demographics.

IMPACT OF CHILDHOOD ASTHMA ON INDIVIDUAL AND FAMILY FUNCTIONING

Psychosocial Impact of Asthma on School-Age Children

Completing a systematic review of literature published between 1997 and 2012 that focused on the emotional impact of asthma on school-age children, Walker (2012) reported consistent findings that youth with asthma had a higher prevalence of internalizing disorders (such as anxiety and depression) than children without asthma had. This internal distress may be puzzling to children who are unable to label emotions, and it may remain undetected by parents, teachers, and others. Walker's findings appear to be consistent with those of Sawyer and colleagues (2001), whose quality-of-life study of children in third through sixth grades found a significant relationship between the mental health of children with asthma and family functioning, but not between their physical health and family functioning. Single-parent respondents in the Sawyer and colleagues study also reported that their children had poorer physical health, mental health, and social skills than children in two-parent families had.

Asthma is one of the leading reasons for school absenteeism, in comparison to other pediatric medical conditions. Federal government studies found that the respiratory disorder accounted for more than 10.5 million total missed days of school each year (American College of Allergy, Asthma and Immunology, 2012), and that it was the third leading cause of hospitalization among children under the age of 15 (American Lung Association, 2014). Summary data on the general population reported that ill or injured children ages 5–17 from single-mother families, who had a variety of conditions including asthma, were twice (6%) as likely to have been absent 11 or more days of school in a year (Bloom et al., 2013). Another study found that parents who perceived their asthmatic children as vulnerable were significantly more likely to keep them home from school, take them to their primary care physicians, and use preventive medications, regardless of the frequency or intensity of asthma symptoms (Spurrier et al., 2000). Emergency department visits and hospitalizations, however, appeared to be associated with severity of asthma symptoms rather than parental perceptions. Bloom and colleagues (2013) also reported that children in single-mother families were two and a half times more likely (10%) than children in two-parent families to have visited an emergency department within the year. Although these hospitalizations appeared to be based on medical necessity, these findings suggest that clinicians can reduce school absenteeism by encouraging youth's participation in extracurricular activities, monitoring or preventing the overuse of medical resources, correcting parents' distorted images of their children's vulnerability, and identifying resources for single-parent families.

Psychosocial Impact of Asthma on Family Functioning

Clearly, it is very stressful for any family to have a child who is susceptible to having asthma attacks that may seriously impair his or her breathing. Watching one's child gasp for breath can make a parent feel helpless and afraid. Because of this parental vulnerability, it is essential that treatment of the child include important psychosocial information plus support to help the anxious parent(s). Rolland's [ok]family systems–illness model, discussed later in this chapter, presents a detailed overview of typical family challenges in situations of serious illness (Rolland, 1984, 1987, 1994).

Psychosocial Interventions

Clarke and Calam (2012) completed a systematic review of psychosocial interventions intended to improve the physical, social, health, and psychological aspects of asthmatic children's lives. Using the umbrella term "health-related quality of life" (HRQOL), they identified studies of [stet—I think that you change the meaning as there were four studies; as written the studies could have included all four interventions] four interventions that accounted for statistically significant improvement in HRQOL: three asthma education programs, one of which included a problem-solving component, and one art therapy program. Although too few evidence-based studies with adequate effect sizes have demonstrated intervention effectiveness, there are some reports about interventions that may be beneficial to school-age children with asthma. These include the following:

- Stress reduction interventions such as relaxation training and guided imagery (Peck, Bray, & Kehle, 2003)
- Asthma education that includes information about stress, coping, and problem solving, in addition to relaxation training with psychological feedback (Long et al., 2011)
- Biofeedback (Kostes et al., 1991)
- Yoga (Tahan, Gungor, & Bicici, 2014).

Despite evidence that poor family functioning (characterized by family conflict, ineffective parenting styles, and child behavior problems) is associated with poor asthma management and HRQOL of patients (Clarke & Calam, 2012), recent interventions studies designed to improve family functioning of children with asthma are lacking.

THEORETICAL UNDERPINNINGS

Patient Self-Management

Patient self-management programs are designed to improve the health status of persons who suffer from chronic illnesses and to decrease their rates of health care utilization. Self-management is informed by Bandura's (1977) theory of self-efficacy, which contends that a person's beliefs regarding his or her competencies affect the initiation and maintenance of behaviors. In the context of chronic illness, beliefs about medical self-efficacy affect whether individuals attempt to change their health behaviors and whether they accomplish and maintain the changes. Trusting that patients can assume a major role in the management of their illness, clinicians have used Bandura's theory to develop strategies for acquiring disease-related competencies such as problem solving, goal setting, symptom management, and relapse prevention (Bachman, Swenson, Reardon, & Miller, 2006). Several evidence-based studies by Lorig and colleagues (1999, 2001) demonstrated the effectiveness of self-management programs with adults who suffered from coronary disease, lung disease, diabetes, and arthritis.

Shames and colleagues (2004) developed one of the few self-management programs for latency- age children with asthma. In this randomized controlled study, low-income urban children in the intervention group received a three-session curriculum on asthma self-management and a Super Nintendo asthma video game produced under the trademark Bronkie's Asthma Adventure. The video game was developed to increase children's self-efficacy and behavior change by educating and providing feedback on their self-management efforts. The patients also had two clinic visits with board-certified pediatric allergists/immunologists, as well as access to an 18-hour hotline staffed by nurses who had access to the children's individualized treatment plans. Although the intervention group showed a reduction of asthma symptom days in contrast to the control group, findings did not reach statistical significance. Children in the intervention group, however, had statistically significant higher scores in the physical and social activity domains of the Child Health Survey for Asthma. The researchers also found that children in the intervention group had statistically significant more knowledge about asthma self-management at 8 weeks than the children in the control group; at 32 weeks, the knowledge difference between the two pediatric groups was not statistically significant, but the increased knowledge of the intervention parents was. Shames and colleagues acknowledged that the study was limited by the small sample size of 119 children and by unreliable asthma outcome measures.

Family (and Other) Systems

As the literature review above suggests, the management of childhood asthma requires the integration of patient, family, health care, school, and community systems. The family systems–illness model developed by John Rolland (1984, 1987, 1994) has provided a useful framework for the assessment and treatment of children with asthma and their families.

The family systems–illness model provides a normative, preventive approach to the assessment and treatment of patients and families. This social systems approach emphasizes the "goodness of fit" among the psychosocial demands of the illness or disability, the patient, and the family system. Although this model focuses on the family system, which needs to be defined broadly, it recognizes that the child or adolescent and family are imbedded in a larger ecosystem that may include the school, health care system, neighborhood, and community.

Rolland (1984, 1987, 1994) created a psychosocial typology of chronic illness that attends to both the similarities and differences among illnesses and disorders over their clinical courses. He first classified the illnesses and disorders into four types: (1) type of onset, which can be acute (e.g., a sudden clinical presentation) or gradual (e.g., juvenile rheumatoid arthritis); (2) type of course, which can be progressive with continually worsening symptoms (e.g., Type I diabetes), constant with stabilized conditions (e.g., spinal cord injury), and relapsing or episodic with periods of absent or minimal symptoms interspersed with disease flare-ups (e.g., seizure disorders or asthma); (3) type of outcome, which can be nonfatal, causal of a shortened lifespan, or fatal; and (4) type of incapacitation, which can be none, mild, moderate, or severe.

Adding a second dimension, Rolland (1984, 1987, 1994) categorized the time phases of illnesses: crisis, chronic, and terminal. The crisis phase includes the period of symptom development, diagnosis, and initial treatment. During this phase, patients and family members are challenged to attribute meaning to the illness, grieve for the loss of preillness individual and family identity, balance hope with awareness of possible future losses, and demonstrate individual and family system role flexibility. Clinicians are encouraged to monitor organizational shifts in family structure and relationships (e.g., triangles and alliances that may be beneficial or harmful, depending on the time phases). Understanding the clinical course of the illness and requisite tasks is enhanced through the lens of a developmental approach to the individual, family, and illness. The chronic phase covers the time between initial diagnosis and the terminal phase of the illness. This phase of taking "one day at a time" is characterized by progressive, constant, or episodic symptomatology that can be of short or long duration. The terminal phase is characterized by the patient's and family's shift from expectation of a cure to preparation for the inevitable death. Family members are faced with issues of separation, anxiety, grief, and continuation of family life without the deceased member.

The third dimension of Rolland's (1984, 1987, 1994) framework, which is grounded in theories of individual and family developmental life cycles, is family functioning. Although scholars have found it difficult to identify an average age of onset for childhood asthma because of definitional challenges, Wallace, Denk, and Kruse (2004) examined 30,400 records of children hospitalized for asthma and reported that the highest rate of admission was for children ages 1–4. Using Rolland's approach, social workers would view the developmental tasks of preschoolers in terms of their widening social environment and rapidly developing language skills. When they experience asthma, their growing sense of autonomy is threatened by both internal and external limitations. The impact of asthma on a 4-year-old child's psychosocial crisis of autonomy versus shame and doubt, for example, may be expressed in reactions to pain and restrictions on movement caused by medical equipment such as masks and ventilators; struggles for control with medical staff and parents at the "no" stage; separations from major caregivers; and interferences with newly acquired skills of feeding, talking, toileting, and sleeping. As the preschooler approaches age 4, he or she may also develop incorrect ideas about the causes of the asthma, medical terminology, and treatment protocols, while simultaneously being concerned about bodily harm and ashamed of his or her body image.

Rolland's integrative view of the family life cycle also guides assessment and intervention with families. Family members of a 4-year-old child may be young adults who still are adapting to their new roles as spouses or committed partners, parents, in-laws, financial partners, and household managers. Following their child's recovery from a near-death experience like an asthma attack, susceptible parents may develop excessive, long-lasting anxiety about the health of their offspring, even though asthma generally can be managed with medications, reduction of environmental hazards, and patient self-management. The term "vulnerable child," coined by Green and Solnit (1964), is a perception that can develop within the context of this extreme anxiety. Green and Solnit found that a heightened parental view of child vulnerability could lead to overprotective relationships that caused emotional and behavioral problems in the children. Later scholars observed similar interplay between parental perceptions of child vulnerability and mental health problems in pediatric patients with less serious health conditions. Children were found to mirror parents' perceptions of whether they were healthy or helpless victims of their illness (Gilbert, 1995), and vulnerable children had difficulty coping with their illness.

Rolland posited that clinicians cannot fully understand a patient's and family's responses to illness without also understanding the transgenerational history of adaptation to past illnesses and stressors. Because asthma tends to be a familial disorder, understanding the meaning of the illness and of family members' coping styles is an important aspect of assessment. Family myths, taboos, beliefs, and expectations, many of which have cultural origins, are transmitted among the generations (McGoldrick, Giordano, & Garcia-Preto, 2005).

Gestalt Play Therapy

Gestalt play therapy is an important approach to helping young people who either witness or directly experience disturbing events like an asthma attack. An experience such as this can result in serious disruptions in an individual's sensory and thought processing. Developed and first practiced by Violet Oaklander, Gestalt play therapy is a humanistic, existential, and process-oriented approach that includes principles from other theoretical orientations, such as psychoanalysis, Gestalt psychology, and humanistic theories (Oaklander, 2011). A Gestalt play therapist helps a young person improve his or her awareness in the here-and-now; integrate cognitions, senses, emotions and behaviors; and build self-support with various forms and techniques of play (Oaklander, 1992, 1997, 2011).

As already noted, asthma is a serious chronic illness that can, but rarely, results in death. The following case illustrates the impact on classmates of a witnessing a classmate's death from an asthma attack. We illustrate the therapeutic process of Gestalt play therapy with a sixth-grade child who developed an anxiety disorder after watching her friend suddenly die during an asthma attack. The names and identifying characteristics of this case have been altered to protect the anonymity of the child and family.

THE CASE OF JENNIFER, AGE 11

Reason for Referral

Jennifer was referred to me (Rana Hong, a play therapist) by her mother, Laura. Laura reported that Jennifer had been overly anxious and irritable at home for the previous 2 months. About a week prior to the appointment, Jennifer complained of shortness of breath and an accelerated heartbeat while she was doing her assignment after school. Laura recalled that Jennifer began to show difficulty with breathing when she was asked to do her routine chore of cleaning their cat's litter box. The girl frowned, looked upset, and seemed to be out of breath as she refused to clean the litter box. Because of the seriousness of the complaints about difficulty with her breathing, Jennifer was brought to the emergency department (ED) of the local hospital. The doctor on duty at the ED completed a complete evaluation, including cardiopulmonary functioning, and ruled out any physical causes for Jennifer's rapid heartbeat. The physician believed that Jennifer had experienced a panic attack, and she recommended that Jennifer be evaluated further by a child therapist for continued assessment and possible treatment.

Assessment (Session 1)

Initially I completed a biopsychosocial/spiritual assessment with Jennifer and her mother, which confirmed the diagnosis of panic attack suggested by the ED physician. I then conducted an assessment with Jennifer to understand and to explore the roots of her anxiety. Jennifer described her family circumstances as uneventful and free of significant problems. When asked about her school life, however, she brought up the death of a classmate approximately 6 months ago. The classmate, Tom, who sat in the row of desks next to hers, had had a severe asthma attack in the classroom. Jennifer clearly remembered Tom's harsh wheezing, the whistling sounds, and the nonstop coughing as he fought to breathe. Shortly after the paramedics arrived, her classmate stopped coughing and soon died. Although she admitted being "shocked and scared" after witnessing Tom's death. Jennifer stated that she handled her "shock" quite well. When I asked how she handled the "shock," she answered that she tried to calm herself down and to help her friends. That is, Jennifer initially was calmer than the rest of her classmates, so she tried to help other students by listening to them or giving advice whenever her friends appeared to panic or need to talk about the tragedy.

It was apparent that Jennifer began to present anxious behavior after witnessing the tragedy of her classmate's death. In performing her perceived role as a supporter in the shared crisis situation, Jennifer ignored her own feelings, and these later emerged in the form of her recurrent anxious behavior.

After gaining an understanding of Jennifer's current issues, I met with Laura alone to build a therapeutic collaboration for treating Jennifer's issues. Often the role of parents in children's therapy is pivotal, especially when the parent and child have a good relationship. Because of the apparently good relationship between Laura and Jennifer, we planned to have a family check-in time for 15 minutes each week, followed by a 45-minute individual session. During the family check-in time, Laura was advised to present her observations about Jennifer in a supportive manner. In addition, two specific tips were suggested to Laura. First, Laura was not to probe into Jennifer's feelings, but to be active in listening to what Jennifer shared. Also, breathing and relaxation (imagery) exercises were introduced as the tools to enhance

Jennifer's self-nurturing. Laura was guided in how to assist Jennifer with these self-nurturing activities at home.

Gestalt Play Therapy Sessions

Session 2

After we began Session 2 with a 15-minute family check-in session, Jennifer was invited to the play therapy room, where I explained to her that we would play or talk to understand the nature of her worries and to explore some ways to deal with them. Jennifer began this session and the next one by articulately describing her experience of the panic attack and anxious behavior. We explored her first physical response when she felt anxious. She could not identify a physical reaction, so we stood in front of a mirror to observe her different physical responses when she imagined fun experience versus stressful experiences. She learned that when she imagined any stressful experience, she blushed before she noticed the pounding of her heart. She wanted to learn how to handle her anxiety, and we spent a good amount of time in exploring and practicing self-nurturing techniques. These included deep breathing and relaxation exercises that emphasized focusing, and mindfulness methods such as the visualization exercise of creating a safe place.

Sessions 3–5

I became aware that Jennifer and I were developing an "I/Thou" relationship, which is described as a positive attitude in the interactions between therapist and child (Oaklander, 2011, p. 172). I began to explore whether she was making contact with her experience and feelings in association with witnessing the death of her friend at school. When I initially asked her to describe her experience regarding the incident, she did not use feeling-driven words or detailed information. She was unintentionally avoiding acknowledging her contact with the experience, and she was putting more emphasis on reporting others' reactions to it. In Session 5, I decided to help her project her own experience by using a sandtray. The successful use of projection in working with children helps them connect with their own experience. Using Gestalt play therapy concepts, I asked Jennifer to close her eyes and take three deep breaths. I then asked her to think about the incident to see what memories might occur. Then she was invited to find and use the sandtray figures that represented the imagined scene and her current feelings. She selected the following figures: an ambulance, desks, and people.

THERAPIST: Now you can arrange them any way that you would like.

JENNIFER: (*Makes a classroom scene.*) I am done.

THERAPIST: Can you tell me what is happening in here?

JENNIFER: This is about the day that Tom died of the asthma attack.

THERAPIST: I see. I would like to hear more about it. It looks like this is the boy who had the attack. (*Points to a boy figure who is half fallen down, with his hand on his neck.*) Wow, there were many students there at that time. I remembered that you were in the classroom when that happened. Which one are you in here?

JENNIFER: (*Silently points out a girl figure standing right next to the boy figure who has had the attack.*)

THERAPIST: Were you next to him?

JENNIFER: (*Nods.*)

THERAPIST: That seems like a very scary moment for you.

JENNIFER: (*Nods.*)

THERAPIST: Can you give her (*pointing to the figure representing Jennifer*) a voice?

JENNIFER: I can't make a sound because I am so shocked.

THERAPIST: You are right. You couldn't say anything because you were so shocked at that time. But you know what? Since you are with me right now, I think you could make a voice for her. What do you think she could say?

JENNIFER: (*After thinking for a while*) I wanted him to stop coughing.

THERAPIST: You could just say that.

JENNIFER: Why are you coughing next to me? I don't know what to do. Can you please stop?

THERAPIST: You were shocked because you do not know how to stop his coughs. You wanted him to stop coughing.

JENNIFER: (*Sobs.*) I don't know what to feel. I think I was more shocked and scared. I should feel sorry for him, but I was scared of him instead of being worried about him.

THERAPIST: Jennifer, it *is* scary and shocking to witness a severe asthma attack like that. I think your various feelings related to the death of your classmate have been stuck inside of you because you were confused with your feelings. You did not know what to express.

JENNIFER: I was also busy taking care of my friends.

THERAPIST: How did you feel when you took care of your friends? And how do you feel now when you do this?

JENNIFER: It feels good that I can help them out, but I feel more worried about them. I can't sleep sometimes because I am worried about my friends.

THERAPIST: Oh, it seems like taking care of your friends takes lots of your energy out of you and makes you worry.

JENNIFER: Yes. I become more anxious after helping out my friends.

THERAPIST: That is a very good insight. Also, not taking care of your own unpleasant experience with the death of your classmate might be another cause for it.

Using the sandtray helped Jennifer recall her proximity to the crisis situation. It seemed to make it much easier for her to look at her own suffering during Tom's asthma attack. However, her guilty feelings seemed to contribute to her becoming a helper to others, rather than taking care of herself. Due to her unresolved crisis experience, she seemed to absorb her friends' anxiety in her body without any filtering

Sessions 6–8

I gradually shared my understanding of Jennifer's anxiety with her and Laura in the following sessions. In Session 7, Jennifer reported decreased anxiousness after she talked to me about her experience. We continued to work on alternative feelings related to the incident. Jennifer often gave a voice to her self-object, such as "It is OK to feel scared when you see that," or "Who wouldn't be scared of seeing that?" or "I am sorry that happened to you." She also created a "worry box" in which she put all of her worries. She allowed herself 15 minutes per day to use the worry box in the presence of her mother. Laura was the gatekeeper for the worry box, and she closed the box when Jennifer had used it long enough.

Jennifer and I had one more session together 2 weeks later. During the family check-in time, Laura reported that they did not need a worry box any more. She added that Jennifer seemed happier and less stressed lately. Jennifer wanted to do another sandtray in our last session. She wanted to recreate a scene that she had struggled with the preceding week: She put two people across a table from each other, and placed a box next to them. Jennifer explained that she was stressed because her friends talked about their worries repeatedly for a while. Then she decided to give a voice to her figure to talk to the other figure: "Emily, shut up! Stop talking to me about your worries. I am not your worry box. Put your worries in this worry box." We finished the session with laughing and joking by playing out the scene.

The therapy process with Jennifer included both verbal and play-based expressive and projective processes. Her exacerbating symptoms due to an untreated crisis experience were processed through Gestalt play therapy, which helped her integrate her experience. Once Jennifer was able to process the traumatic experience and to "own" aspects of her projection in association with this, she was able to release her negative feelings, to gain coping skills, and even to advocate for her own mental well-being.

DISCUSSION

Despite their youth, latency-age children may sometimes experience the death of a classmate. In 2011, the leading causes of death for children ages 5–9 were unintentional injuries (761), malignant neoplasms (441), congenital anomalies (182), homicide (429), heart disease (92), and chronic lower respiratory diseases including asthma (64). During the same year, unintentional injuries (874), malignant neoplasms (419), suicide (282), congenital anomalies (176), and homicide (154) were the leading causes of death for children ages 10–14. Chronic lower respiratory diseases (72) were the seventh leading cause of death in the older age group (CDC, 2014a). The death of a classmate often starts a "ripple effect" that influences the child's fellow students and their families, teachers, school personnel and administrators, and the community.

Witnessing the death of a fellow student can be experienced as a crisis, which "is a perception of an event or situation as an intolerable difficulty that exceeds the resources and coping mechanisms of the person" (James & Gilliland, 2005, p. 3). The fatality also can be suffered as a trauma, which evokes feelings of terror and helplessness that overwhelm an individual's ability to cope with the experienced event and can result in psychiatric syndromes such as posttraumatic stress disorder (PTSD), depressive disorders, or anxiety disorders (National Child Traumatic Stress Network, 2014). Traumatic reactions are individualized and complex. Factors that affect the duration and severity of such a reaction include the subjective meaning of the event, genetic vulnerability to stress, developmental phase, prior traumatization (including losses), preexisting personality traits (e.g., ineffective use of maladaptive coping strategies, such as denial, passivity, or avoidance), culture, and social support networks. Intrinsic personal characteristics such as healthy self-esteem, self-efficacy, and a range of adaptive coping mechanisms can shield a child from the adverse effects of trauma. External factors such as a dependable primary caregiver, a strong social support system, reliable mentors, a responsive school system, and supportive community environment are also important protective factors. These intrinsic and extrinsic factors, which are specified in Webb's tripartite assessment (see Webb, Chapter 1, this volume), combine to mediate the impact of the crisis or trauma both at the time of the event and during its aftermath.

When a devastating event such as the death of a pupil occurs in a school classroom, all the witnesses experience traumatic anxiety to some degree. Schools should have crisis intervention plans in place to help students, teachers, and staff all express their feelings of horror, anger, and helplessness. Citing Openshaw's (2008) school evaluation tools and sample letters to parents, Anewalt (2010) details four components of a comprehensive school crisis response plan: (1) preparing before a crisis occurs, (2) assessing the impact after an incident happens, (3) responding to the crisis, and (4) collaborating with the community.

In addition to individual treatment for youth whose postcrisis symptoms interfere with daily functioning, students often can benefit from group work. "If trauma isolates, group work connects," writes Andrew Malekoff (2014, p. 286). He has identified principles of group work with youth following a traumatic event. He recommends that sponsoring organizations do the following:

- Provide protection, support, and safety to counteract children's feelings of fear, despair, and hypervigilance.
- Design groups that rebuild disrupted connections to generate mutual support, decrease isolation, and normalize "abnormal" reactions to surreal events.
- Offer opportunities for actions that symbolize victory over feelings of helplessness, grief, vulnerability, shame, and despair. Examples of such actions include writing prose or poetry, playing games such as Ping-Pong Feelings (Malekoff, 2014), creating memory boxes, writing goodbye letters, making a photo album, or writing in a journal (Webb, 2010).
- Be cognizant of the dual challenges of eliciting welcomed remembrances and managing anxiety-provoking reminders of the trauma for the individual and the group.

Debriefing groups may be an especially effective mode of intervention when many school students and personnel have shared the experience of a critical incident or trauma. The time pressures and ratio of crisis staff to sufferers are likely to prohibit professionals from having individual meetings with all persons exposed to a traumatic event. Individual sessions should be reserved for persons who are assessed to be at high risk for psychological disturbance such as PTSD, based on such factors as the subjective meaning assigned to the event, prior traumatization, and diminished social support systems. Openshaw (2008) has described several school-based group programs adapted from Mitchell's (2003) critical incident stress debriefing (CISD) model, which is a strengths-based approach designed to help individuals after their exposure to a shared critical incident. The CISD intervention, which is one component of a comprehensive critical incident stress management (CISM) program (Mitchell, 1983), consists of seven well-defined phases: introduction, fact, thought, reaction, symptoms, teaching, and reentry. The use of debriefing has spawned a contentious debate among crisis response experts. Some researchers have claimed that CISD lacks rigorous research evidence of its effectiveness, may actually do harm, and fails to prevent PTSD (Pack, 2012). Pack (2012) writes that others contend that "Critics who argue that CISD is at best ineffectual or at worst harmful may be throwing the baby out with the bathwater as they fail to understand that debriefing is part of a broader approach to the psychosocial needs of persons affected by trauma to promote resilience" (p. 616).

Morrison (2007) completed one of the very few studies of CISM, including CISD, in school settings. Almost 86% of the participating psychologists and school social workers expressed unconditional positive regard for the structure of CISM and the procedures that they could follow during times of crises. Half of the 28 participants voiced concern that the model needed to be adapted for use with children and adolescents, and 25% of respondents expressed concern that the model failed to address cultural issues. Nevertheless, almost 93% of the practitioners believed that the intervention provided students with a forum in which to express their emotions, connected students to resources, clarified facts and dispelled rumors, and identified pupils who needed counseling.

Although most children return to their previous levels of functioning after a crisis, some youth may develop acute stress disorder, PTSD, an anxiety disorder, or a depressive disorder. Practitioners can use rapid assessment instruments to identify children who may need individual treatment. The Child PTSD Symptom Scale (Foa, Johnson, Feeny, & Treadwell, 2001), for example, can be used to identify children who may be at risk for PTSD. This self-report questionnaire of 20 questions was designed for youth ages 8–18 who have experienced a traumatic event. It assesses for reexperiencing, avoidance, and arousal symptoms, and for functional impairment such as difficulty with school, family members, and friends. Clinicians also may use structured clinical interviews such as the Anxiety Disorders Interview Schedule for Children (Silverman & Nelles, 1988) to guide their assessments.

CONCLUSION

Although asthma cannot be cured, research findings suggest that it often can be controlled by reducing risks through self-management, education, appropriate medical care, and avoidance of environmental triggers.

For children and adolescents who may be indirectly affected by asthma through witnessing peers' asthma attacks at school, it is important for school counselors and social workers to provide some preventive education, such as checklists for their own symptoms and information about when to seek professional help. Those who present with ongoing psychological symptoms can be referred for an integrative approach like Gestalt play therapy, which offers the possibilities of externalizing the experience, improving trauma integration, and building self-support for recovery.

STUDY QUESTIONS

1. How can school personnel effectively deal with the crisis situation of an asthma attack? What steps should be followed in order to assist students and teachers with their anxiety?

2. Given that Laura had a good relationship with Jennifer, she was invited to participate in Jennifer's treatment as a therapeutic collaborator from the beginning of therapy. If you suspected a toxic parent–child relationship, what modifications would you consider in treating Jennifer?

3. If you were a school social worker or counselor at Jennifer's school, what might you do to identify the students who were potentially at risk after the incident of Tom's death?

4. What kinds of visualization and breathing exercises can practitioners use to help them calm themselves down after a crisis?

REFERENCES

Agertot, L., & Pederson, S. (2000). Effect of long-term treatment with inhaled budesonide on adult height in children with asthma. *New England Journal of Medicine, 343*, 1054–1063.

American College of Allergy, Asthma and Immunology. (2012). Asthma facts. Retrieved from *http://acaai.org/news/facts-statistics/asthma*.

American Lung Association. (2014). Asthma and children fact sheet. Retrieved from *www.lung.org/lung-disease/asthma/resources/facts-and-figures/asthma-children-fact-sheet.html*.

Anewalt, P. H. (2010). Violent, traumatic death in schools and community responses. In N. B. Webb (Ed.), *Helping bereaved children* (3rd ed., pp. 190–214). New York: Guilford Press.

Bachman, J., Swenson, S., Reardon, M. E., & Miller, D. (2006). Patient self-management in the primary care treatment of depression. *Administration and Policy in Mental Health and Mental Health Services Research, 33*(1), 76–85.

Bandura, A. (1977). Self-efficacy: Toward a unifying theory of behavioral change. *Psychological Review, 84*(2), 191–215.

Bloom, B., Jones, L. I., & Freeman, G. (2013). Summary health statistics for U.S. children: National Health Interview Survey, 2012. *Vital and Health Statistics, 10*(258). Washington, DC: U.S. Government Printing Office. Retrieved from *www.cdc.gov/nchs/data/series/sr_10/sr10_258.pdf*

Centers for Disease Control and Prevention (CDC). (2014a). 10 leading causes of death by age group, United States—2011. Retrieved from *www.cdc.gov/injury/wisqars/LeadingCauses.html*.

Centers for Disease Control and Prevention (CDC). (2014b). 2012 National Health Interview Survey (NHIS) data. Retrieved from *www.cdc.gov/asthma/nhis/2012/table2-1.htm*.

Clarke, S., & Calam, R. (2012). The effectiveness of psychosocial interventions designed to improve health-related quality of life (HRQOL) amongst asthmatic children and their families: A systematic review. *Quality of Life Research, 21*, 747–764.

Cohen, R. T., Celedon, J. C., Hinckson, V. J., Ramsey, C. D., Wakefield, D. B., Weiss, S. T., et al. (2006). Health-care use among Puerto Rican and African-American children with asthma. *Chest, 130*(2), 463–471.

Foa, E. B., Johnson, K. M., Feeny, N. C., & Treadwell, K. R. H. (2001). The Child

PTSD Symptom Scale: A preliminary examination of its psychometric properties. *Journal of Clinical Child and Adolescent Psychology, 30*(3), 376–384.

Gilbert, M. C. (1995). Differences between "copers" and "non-copers" with pediatric migraine. *Child and Adolescent Social Work Journal, 12*(4), 275–287.

Gilbert, M. C. (2009). Other conditions that may occur in childhood or develop in adolescence. In N. B. Webb (Ed.), *Helping youth and families cope with acute and chronic health conditions: A collaborative strengths-based guide to practice* (pp. 225–240). Hoboken, NJ: Wiley.

Gorina, Y. (2012, May 4). QuickStats: Asthma death rates, by race and age group—United States, 2007–2009. *Morbidity and Mortality Weekly Reports, 61*(17), 315.

Green, M., & Solnit, A. J. (1964). Reactions to the threatened loss of a child: A vulnerable child syndrome. *Pediatrics, 34*, 58–66.

James, R. K., & Gilliland, B. E. (2005). *Crisis intervention strategies* (5th ed.). Belmont, CA: Brooks/Cole.

Kotses, H., Harver, A., Segreto, J., Glaus, K. D., Creer, T. L., & Young, G. (1991). Long-term effects of biofeedback-induced facial relaxation on measures of asthma severity in children. *Biofeedback and Self-Regulation, 16*, 1–21.

Long, K. A., Eving, L. J., Cohen, S., Skoner, D., Gentile, D., Koehsen, J., et al. (2011). Preliminary evidence for the feasibility of a stress management intervention for 7- to 12-year-olds with asthma. *Journal of Asthma, 48*, 162–170.

Lorig, K., Ritter, P., Stewart, A., Sobel, D., Brown, B., Bandura, A., et al. (2001). Chronic disease self-management program: 2-year health status and health care utilization outcomes. *Medical Care, 39*(11), 1217–1223.

Lorig, K., Sobel, D., Stewart, A., Brown, B., Bandura, A., Gonzalez, V., et al. (1999). Evidence suggesting that a chronic disease self-management program can improve health status while reducing hospitalization: A randomized trial. *Medical Care*, 37(1), 5–14.

Malekoff, A. (2014). *Group work with adolescents: Principles and practice* (3rd ed.). New York: Guilford Press.

McGoldrick, M., Giordano, M., & Garcia-Preto, N. (Eds.). (2005). *Ethnicity and family therapy* (3rd ed.). New York: Guilford Press.

McManus, V., & Savage, E. (2012). Cultural perspectives of interventions for managing diabetes and asthma in children and adolescents from ethnic minority groups. *Child: Care, Health, and Development, 36*(5), 612–622.

Mitchell, J. T. (1983). When disaster strikes: The critical incident stress debriefing process. *Journal of Emergency Medical Services, 8*, 36–39.

Mitchell, J. T. (2003). *Crisis intervention and CISM: A research summary.* Ellicott City, MD: International Critical Incident Stress Foundation.

Morrison, J. Q. (2007). Social validity of the critical incident stress management model for school-based crisis intervention. *Psychology in the Schools, 44*(8), 765–777.

National Child Traumatic Stress Network. (2014). What is child traumatic stress? Retrieved from *www.nctsnet.org/sites/default/files/assets/pdfs/what_is_child_traumatic_stress_0.pdf.*

National Heart, Lung, and Blood Institute. (2007). Expert Panel Report 3: Guidelines for the diagnosis and management of asthma (NIH Publication No. 07-4051). Retrieved from *www.nhlbi.nih.gov/files/docs/guidelines/asthgdln.pdf.*

Oaklander, V. (1992). The relationship of gestalt therapy to children. *Gestalt Journal*, 5(1), 64–74.

Oaklander, V. (1997). The therapeutic process with children and adolescents. *Gestalt Review*, 1(4), 292–317.

Oaklander, V. (2011). The Gestalt play therapy. In C. E. Schaefer (Ed.), *Foundations of play therapy* (2nd ed., pp. 171–186). Hoboken, NJ: Wiley.

Openshaw, L. (2008). *Social work in schools: Principles and practice*. New York: Guilford Press.

Pack, M. J. (2012). Critical incident stress management: A review of the literature with implications for social work. *International Social Work, 56*(5), 608–627.

Peck, H. L., Bray, M. A., & Kehle, T. J. (2003). Relaxation and guided imagery: A school-based intervention for children with asthma. *Psychology in the Schools, 40*(6), 657–675.

Rolland, J. S. (1984). Toward a psychosocial typology of chronic and life-threatening illness. *Family Systems Medicine, 2*, 245–263.

Rolland, J. S. (1987). Chronic illness and the life cycle: A conceptual framework. *Family Process, 26*, 203–221.

Rolland, J. S. (1994). *Families, illness, and disability: An integrative treatment model*. New York: Basic Books.

Sawyer, M. G., Spurrier, N., Whaites, L., Kennedy, D., Martin, A. J., & Baghurst, P. (2001). The relationship between asthma severity, family functioning and the health-related quality of life of children with asthma. *Quality of Life Research, 9*, 1105–1115.

Shames, R. S., Sharek, P., Mayer, M., Robinson, T. N., Hoyer, E. G., Gonzalez-Hensley, F., et al. (2004). Effectiveness of a multicomponent self-management program in at-risk, school-aged children with asthma. *Annals of Allergy, Asthma, and Immunology, 92*, 611–618.

Silverman, W. K., & Nelles, W. B. (1988). The Anxiety Disorders Interview Schedule for Children. *Journal of the American Academy of Child and Adolescent Psychiatry, 27*(6), 772–778.

Spurrier, N. J., Sawyer, M. G., Staugas, R., Martin, A. J., Kennedy, D., & Streiner, D. L. (2000). Association between parental perception of children's vulnerability to illness and management of children's asthma. *Pediatric Pulmonology, 29*, 88–93.

Tahan, F., Gungor, H. E., & Bicici, E. (2014). Is yoga training beneficial for exercise-induced bronchoconstriction? *Alternative Therapies, 20*(2), 18–23.

U.S. Food and Drug Administration. (1998, November 9). *Class labeling for intranasal and orally inhaled corticosteroid containing drug products regarding the potential for growth suppression in children* (FDA Talk Paper). Rockville, MD: Author.

Walker, G. M. (2012). Factors related to emotional responses in school-aged children who have asthma. *Issues in Mental Health Nursing, 33*, 406–429.

Wallace, J. C., Denk, C. E., & Kruse, L. K. (2004). Pediatric hospitalizations for asthma: Use of a linked file to separate person-level risk and readmission. *Preventing Chronic Disease: Public Health Research, Policy, and Practice, 1*(2), 1–10. Retrieved from *www.cdc.gov/pcd/issues/2004/apr/03_0009.htm.*

Webb, N. B. (Ed.). (2010). *Helping bereaved children* (3rd ed.). New York: Guilford Press.

Part IV

CRISES IN THE COMMUNITY AND WORLD

Chapter 16

The Mass Traumas of Natural Disasters

Interventions with Children, Adolescents, and Families

JENNIFER BAGGERLY
ERIC J. GREEN

"Is the tornado going to destroy our house and kill us all?" asked a terrified child who was hiding with his mother in the bathroom. This type of life-or-death question could be asked by millions of young people worldwide whose lives will be disrupted by natural disasters. In 2012, a total of 357 natural disasters (e.g., earthquakes, tornadoes, floods, wildfires, and epidemics) across the globe resulted in 9,655 deaths, 124.5 million victims, and $157 billion (in U.S. dollars) in damage (Guha-Sapir, Vos, Below, & Ponserre, 2013). In the United States, Hurricane Sandy alone caused 159 deaths, destroyed 650,000 homes, and resulted in $65.7 billion in damage as it swept across the northeastern states (National Oceanic and Atmospheric Administration, 2013). Scientists predict that, due to the warming of the global environment, approximately 175 million youth annually will be exposed to natural disasters throughout the world over the next decade; this figure represents a 38% increase from the 1990s (Seballos, Tanner, Tarazona, & Gallegos, 2011).

According to standards developed by the American Psychological Association (2015), the Council for Accreditation of Counseling and Related Educational Programs (2009), and the National Association of Social Workers (2003), U.S. mental health professionals must be prepared to mitigate the devastating impact of natural disasters on children and adolescents both nationally and worldwide (Baggerly, 2006). The saying "It takes a village to raise a child" is well known, but it can take a global village to restore children's psyches after a natural disaster. This is an issue of social justice that requires action. Ethically and professionally, mental health professionals have a moral responsibility to advocate for youth in crisis throughout the world and to respond to crises whenever possible. The goal of this chapter is to prepare mental health professionals to intervene with children and adolescents following the crises of natural disasters. Specifically, this chapter addresses (1) the impact of natural disasters on children and adolescents; (2) research on disaster mental health interventions with young people; (3) strategies to prepare for disaster response deployment; and (4) interventions that play therapists can provide for parents, children, and teens after natural disasters.

OVERVIEW OF THE TOPIC: RELEVANT THEORY AND RESEARCH

Although youth have unique individual responses to disasters, research reveals some general responses in the areas of neurophysiology, development, typical symptoms, and clinical symptoms (La Greca, 2008). Trauma resulting from natural disasters can affect children's neurophysiological systems in ways that cause changes in their behavior, cognitive functioning, mental health, and physical development (La Greca, 2008). Natural disasters and their aftermath may create psychological threats that overwhelm youth's typical coping strategies. These threats (both real and perceived) activate the sympathetic–adrenal system, which mobilizes the "fight-or-flight" response of increased breathing and heart rate (Gaskill & Perry, 2012). Ongoing threats or trauma reminders can cause the fight-or-flight mechanism to become stuck in continuous looping, causing hyperarousal, irritability, and sleeplessness; smaller intracranial and cerebral volumes; limited explicit memory; and a diminished sense of identity (Brymer et al., 2006; van der Kolk, 2007). Memories from a disaster may become stored in the brain's right limbic system and produce "flashbacks"—that is, intrusive images, thoughts, smells, and sounds of the terrifying event (Solomon & Heide, 2005). To control hyperarousal and flashbacks, youth may avoid reminders of the traumatic event, such as places, people, or things associated with it (e.g., school classrooms, teachers, or water), which may culminate in various forms of specific phobia.

Natural disasters that disrupt relationships between infants and their primary caregivers can hinder children's brain development—particularly in the prefrontal cortex (i.e., the orbitofrontal cortex and anterior cingulate cortex) and limbic system, and the neural circuits that connect them. Some of these neural circuits are important in psychological, emotional, and physiological development. When these neural structures and pathways are compromised, the future development of empathy and moral judgment can be adversely affected (Solomon & Heide, 2005; van der Kolk, 2007).

Acute Symptoms

Children's and adolescents' typical symptoms after natural disasters may include fear, depression, self-blame, guilt, loss of interest in school and other activities, regressive behavior, sleep and appetite disturbance, night terrors, aggressiveness, poor concentration, and separation anxiety (Brymer et al., 2006). Shioyama and colleagues (2000) studied 9,000 third-, fifth-, and eighth-grade Japanese children affected by the Great Hanshin-Awaji Earthquake. They found that children's symptoms could be factor-analyzed into three broad categories: (1) fear and anxiety, which peaked 4 months after the disaster and decreased as time passed; (2) depression and psychophysical symptoms, which peaked at 6 months and decreased after a year; and (3) prosocial tendencies.

Symptoms may vary from minimum to severe, based on a child's developmental level, personal experiences, and emotional/physical health, as well as the responses of the child's parents to the incident (La Greca et al., 2013; Webb, 2004). Brymer and colleagues (2006) have identified typical symptoms for various age groups. For preschool children, these symptoms include nonverbal fears, expressed in constant crying or whimpering and excessive clinging; nightmares or night terrors; and regressive behaviors such as thumb sucking or bedwetting. For elementary-school-age children, typical symptoms include fear of danger to self and loved ones; increased fighting, hyperactivity, and inattentiveness; withdrawal from friends; school refusal; and reenactment through traumatic play. Typical symptoms of preadolescence and adolescence include physical complaints of headaches or stomachaches; withdrawal; antisocial behavior of stealing or acting out; school problems; risk taking behaviors; and drug and alcohol problems.

The differences between young children's and adolescents' symptoms can be primarily attributed to their cognitive-developmental levels. Since younger children have not developed cognitive permanence, they believe that losses can be undone, and thus they have a difficult time understanding the consequences of natural disasters. In addition, younger children's magical thinking may cause them to believe that their thoughts contributed to or even caused the disaster. Some of their regressive and clinging behavior is an attempt to keep caring adults near them and away from harm (National Institute of Mental Health [NIMH], 2001). Adolescents with preexisting symptoms of rumination and depression may experience exacerbation of these symptoms after a natural disaster, as indicated by research on adolescent survivors of the 2010 flood in Nashville, Tennessee (Felton, Cole, & Martin, 2013).

Chronic Symptoms

Although traumatized youth will typically recover from these symptoms with basic support after a natural disaster, some children experience chronic symptoms. In one of the first prominent studies of children after a natural disaster, Vernberg, La Greca, Silverman, and Prinstein (1996) found that 55% of elementary school children in their study exhibited moderate to severe symptoms 3 months after Hurricane Andrew. More recently, Osofsky, Osofsky, Kronenberg, Brennan, and Hansel (2009) found that 52% of fourth- through sixth-grade children in their study were experiencing severe symptoms warranting a mental health referral within the first year after Hurricane Katrina. Children's chronic symptoms may result in a diagnosis of acute stress disorder (ASD) or posttraumatic stress disorder (PTSD), either of which may be comorbid with anxiety disorders or depressive disorders. Indicators of childhood and adolescent onset of PTSD include the following groups of symptoms that persist longer than 30 days after direct or indirect exposure to a traumatic event: (1) intrusion, such as recurrent and disturbing memories via nightmares or play reenactment; (2) avoidance of thoughts, feelings, or things related to the disaster; (3) negative changes in cognitions and mood, such as self-condemnation and persistent feelings of horror or anger; and (4) changes in arousal and reactivity, such as irritability or difficulty concentrating (American Psychiatric Association, 2013).

Rates of PTSD in children after natural disasters vary, depending on the type of event and the criteria used for a study. For example, 4 months after Typhoon Rusa devastated rural areas in South Korea, 12.3% of elementary school children had either moderate or severe PTSD symptoms, 22.7% had mild symptoms, and 65% had subclinical symptoms (Lee, Ha, Kim, & Kwon, 2004). In contrast, McDermott, Lee, Judd, and Gibbon (2005) found that 22.6% of children in their study had abnormally high emotional symptoms 6 months after exposure to a wildfire disaster. Similarly, approximately 25% of children exposed to an earthquake in Gujarat, India, showed clinical levels of posttraumatic stress symptoms as measured by the UCLA disaster trauma tool (Kumar & Fonagy, 2013). Even higher rates of PTSD were reported by Derivois, Mérisier, Cénat, and Castelot (2014), who found that 42% of children in their study had high levels of PTSD symptoms 16–18 months after the 2010 earthquake in Haiti. In addition, Ayub and colleagues (2012) reported that 64.8% of children in their study had significant PTSD symptoms 18 months after the 2005 Kashmir earthquake in Pakistan. Jaycox and colleagues (2010) found that 60% of children they screened had PTSD symptoms 15 months after Hurricane Katrina.

In their study of children affected by the 2010 Haitian earthquake, Derivois and colleagues (2014) found that girls had significantly higher levels of PTSD symptoms than boys. They also found a significant correlation between PTSD symptoms and social support, indicating that social support can encourage resiliency among youth. McDermott and colleagues (2005) found that younger children and children with higher levels of exposure and threat had a higher prevalence of PTSD than adolescents and youth with lower levels of exposure and threat. Osofsky and colleagues (2009) found that property loss, separation from a caregiver, significant personal loss, and living in a shelter predicted increased symptoms after Hurricane Katrina. Salloum, Carter, Burch, Garfinkel, and Overstreet (2011) found that prior exposure to community violence could amplify the relationship between natural disasters and PTSD.

Adolescents who experience PTSD after a disaster may show severe symptoms, such as increased aggression and lower academic achievement

(Scott, Lapré, Marsee, & Weems, 2014); increased victimization from social ostracism (Terranova, Boxer, & Morris, 2009); and sedentary activity, which is a health risk (Lai, La Greca, & Llabre, 2014). These rates of PTSD and other severe symptoms after natural disasters highlight the need to provide and maintain psychological interventions for teens.

TREATMENT METHOD: DISASTER RESPONSE PLAY THERAPY

After the 2010 Chilean earthquake, children received immediate crisis intervention and school-based group universal prevention via game-like activities (e.g., using a mandala to increase feelings of contentment; drawing pictures of abstract emotions; and role-playing a difficult situation to increase problem-solving skills, self-esteem, self-control, social skills, conflict resolution, and empathy) 3–6 months after the earthquake. Children who received this intervention had significantly less earthquake-related worry and PTSD than the control group (Garfin et al., 2014).

Fifteen months after Hurricane Katrina, 118 children in fourth through eighth grades received 10 group and 1–3 individual sessions of school-based cognitive-behavioral intervention for trauma in schools (CBITS), or 12 individual sessions (with the option of conjoint parent sessions) of clinic-based trauma-focused cognitive-behavioral therapy (TF-CBT) (Jaycox et al., 2010). "Both CBITS and TF-CBT incorporate cognitive-behavioral skills, including psychoeducation, relaxation skills, affective modulation skills, cognitive coping skills, trauma narrative, in vivo mastery of trauma reminders, and enhancing safety" (Jaycox et al., 2010, p. 227). Only 14 of 60 children assigned to the clinic-based TF-CBT group completed treatment, while 57 of 58 children assigned to the school-based CBITS group completed treatment. Results revealed statistically and clinically significant improvement of PTSD for children in both treatment groups, and statistically significant improvement in depression for the group receiving CBITS.

Youth receiving individual and group psychosocial interventions from school-based counselors 2 years after Hurricane Iniki had significant decreases in trauma symptoms, compared to those of control groups (Chemtob, Nakashima, & Hamada, 2002). Youth's adaptive functioning was shown to increase significantly, compared to the functioning of control groups, after teacher-mediated interventions in response to earthquakes in Turkey (Wolmer, Laor, Dedeoglu, Siev, & Yazgan, 2005).

To date, there has been only one play therapy research study with children after a natural disaster. Shen (2002) found that children who received play therapy after the 1999 earthquake in Taiwan showed significant decreases in their anxiety and suicide risk, compared to the control group. However, a meta-analysis by Bratton, Ray, Rhine, and Jones (2005) of 67 play therapy studies shows the effectiveness of play therapy in reducing behavior problems in general. In addition, Schottelkorb, Doumas, and Garcia's (2012) study of refugee children experiencing trauma showed that play therapy reduced their trauma symptoms.

Thus far, cognitive-behavioral therapy has been espoused as the best-validated treatment for children and adolescents who experience traumatic symptoms (Cohen, Deblinger, & Mannarino, 2006). Until research on disaster response play therapy (DRPT) research is conducted, one approach is to integrate play therapy with evidence-informed cognitive-behavioral interventions, such as those used in CBITS and TF-CBT. The principles, preparation, and intervention protocol for DRPT described below are demonstrated in Baggerly's (2007, 2012) videos, as well as in Green's (2014) *The Handbook of Jungian Play Therapy with Children and Adolescents*. We implemented DRPT with children after the deadly tornadoes in Moore, Oklahoma, in June 2013.

Principles and Preparation

As leaders of a DRPT team, we prepared for deployment to Moore by observing several core principles. *The first principle in disaster response is to follow "incident command structures,"* which are paramilitary methods of establishing order in chaos (Federal Emergency Management Agency, 2003). An incident command structure determines who goes where to do a particular job. Mental health professionals should go to a disaster site only if they are deployed to a specific place by an official representative of a government agency or a registered nongovernmental organization (NGO), such as the International Red Cross, Save the Children, EMDR Humanitarian Assistance Programs, or the like. Our University of North Texas at Dallas team was deployed to a specific area in Moore by World Vision, an International NGO that has provided disaster relief for children for over 60 years.

The second principle is to understand the differing objectives for the five phases of a disaster (NIMH, 2002). During the "preincident phase," the objectives are community preparation and improvement of coping strategies. The mental health professional's role includes training, collaboration, informing policy, and setting structure for rapid assistance. During the "impact phase," the objectives are survival and communication. The mental health professional's role emphasizes meeting basic needs of food, shelter, and safety; providing psychological first aid by supporting those who are most distressed; monitoring the environment for stressors; and providing consultation and training for caregivers. During the "rescue phase," the objective is adjustment. The mental health professional's role includes conducting needs assessment, triage, outreach, and information dissemination, as well as fostering resiliency and recovery. During the "recovery phase," the goals are appraisal and planning. The mental health professional's role includes monitoring the recovery environment by listening to those most affected, observing ongoing threats, and monitoring services that are being provided. During the "return-to-life phase," the objective is reintegration. The mental health professional's role is to reduce symptoms and improve functioning via individual, family, and group psychotherapy.

Mental health professionals are most likely to be deployed during the recovery phase. Interventions will need to focus on short-term approaches and referrals to community resources. Our DRPT team members' interventions in Moore focused on psychoeducation about normal symptoms and coping strategies, which are described in detail later. We promoted youth's resilience through play therapy interventions. However, we did *not* provide a long-term psychotherapeutic play therapy structure in sessions because of our conviction that this should be conducted by therapists residing in the Moore area who could provide long-term follow-up.

The third principle of disaster response is to maintain an expectation that young people and their families will have a normal recovery. Rather than seeing all symptoms as pathological, mental health professionals view most youth as simply having normal responses to abnormal experiences.

The fourth principle is to follow the "six C's" of disaster mental health (World Health Organization, 2003). Mental health professionals maintain Calmness through deep breathing and positive self-talk. Common-sense reminders need to be offered to people who are panicking or disoriented. Compassion is expressed through reassuring words and simple acts of kindness. Collaboration is needed with all organizations, professionals, and families. Communication with parents and other professionals about children's needs and therapeutic procedures must be clear. Control of self is maintained by taking breaks as necessary, obtaining emotional support, and developing a "compassion fatigue" resiliency plan (Gentry, Baranowsky, & Dunning, 2002).

The fifth principle for disaster response is to maintain hardiness and flexibility (NIMH, 2002). Disaster response requires physical hardiness for long days in uncomfortable settings. Flexibility is essential in dynamic environmental situations where professionals are often asked to "hurry up and wait," change their locations at a minute's notice, and/or do things that are entirely different from their typical routines. Mental health professionals will also need to be flexible in order to be multiculturally competent. Strategies need to be flexible so that they can be adapted to clients of various ethnicities, races, religions, and cultures.

The sixth principle for disaster response is to utilize developmentally appropriate approaches with children and adolescents. Children are not miniature adults (Landreth, 2012). They must be respected by engaging them in their natural language of play. As Landreth (2012) has said, "toys are children's words and play is their language" (p. 16). Children should be engaged with toys, puppets, art materials, and storybooks (Green, 2014; see also various chapters of the present volume), and should be given plenty of opportunity to play. Our DRPT members provided balls, bubbles, puppets, crayons, and other play materials for children. Also, adolescents do not respond particularly well to coloring books and puppet shows. Developmentally appropriate interventions with adolescents include incorporating expressive art interventions like drawings, paintings, music, board games, video games, social media interaction, journaling, and physical fitness/sport activities (Green, 2014).

The last principle is to gather specific information on the area, the people, and the particular natural disaster that occurred. Awareness of local customs and dress will facilitate rapport between mental health professionals and local residents. Before meeting with children and parents in Moore, our DRPT team members viewed the physical destruction. Concrete slabs covered with debris marked the sites where homes once stood, obliterated by the tornadoes. Yet, in the midst of all this destruction, signs of resiliency could be found. A home with a blue tarp over the roof had a message spray-painted on the garage door: "Hope still lives here."

Interventions and Challenges

Before they begin providing interventions to youth, mental health professionals should consult with parents to assess the disaster's impact on their children and teens and to identify immediate psychosocial needs. Mental health professionals should also address parents' own concerns directly, since their coping ability is a main determinant of how their children will respond (La Greca et al., 2013). If teachers and parents exhibit anxiety about certain issues, youth are likely to mirror that anxiety. Thus practitioners can normalize the symptoms that occur after disaster experiences and can teach parents coping strategies to help mitigate the anxiety they otherwise might project onto their children.

Content of Session	*Rationale/Analysis*
PLAY THERAPIST: Over years of disaster response, we have found that youth and some parents may have nightmares, restlessness, and fear about a disaster happening again. These are usually typical responses. What did you notice in your children and yourself after the tornado?	An attempt to establish empathy with parents concerning the impact of a natural disaster; to normalize typical symptoms after a natural disaster; and to pose a question allowing for the possibilities of differences, honoring a parent's observations, and assessing the parent's perspective.
PARENT: My children talk to others about another tornado coming. Then they all get upset and are afraid to go aside to play. We are running out of things to do inside.	An example of mass sociogenic panic and a resulting need for practical activities.
PLAY THERAPIST: You are worried and tired. The children's fears	Reflection and validation of feelings; normalizing of responses;

are typical after this scary situation. We know some ways to decrease children's anxiety. Would you like to learn? (*Interventions described later are taught.*)

and a suggestion offering hope and giving parents the power of choice.

PARENT: My kids used to ride their bikes down the street, but I told them not to go outside of the yard in case another tornado comes. Now the kids don't even want to walk down the street with me.

An example of how a parent's anxiety is mirrored by children.

PLAY THERAPIST: Sometimes it helps to make up a game to teach your kids the signs of dangerous weather. Before you go for a walk, show them how to calm down their bodies like I just showed you. Each day, walk just a little further than you did the day before.

Practical suggestions of systematic desensitization give parents confidence that they can help children manage their fears.

In addition to addressing parents' or teachers' concerns, mental health professionals should inform them about children's typical and atypical responses to disasters, as well as methods of teaching children coping strategies. We provided parents in Moore with written material available from the National Child Traumatic Stress Network (*www.nctsn.org/trauma-types/natural-disasters/tornadoes#q3*). Another helpful resource is La Greca, Sevin, and Sevin's (2005) workbook *After the Storm: A Guide to Help Children Cope with the Psychological Effects of a Hurricane*. This resource provides basic psychoeducational activities such as a "stress gauge" for parents to assess on a scale of 1–10 how stressed their children are, and a worksheet to plan how to stay healthy. These activities should be assessed for cultural relevance and translated as needed. To make these psychoeducational activities even more developmentally appropriate, mental health professionals should teach parents some basic play therapy techniques, such as puppet play and art activities

Children's interventions in disaster response are most efficiently provided in small- or large-group formats. Felix, Bond, and Shelby (2006; see also Shelby, Bond, Hall, & Hsu, 2004) have recommended integrating play therapy strategies into the *Psychological First Aid Field Operations Guide* (Brymer et al., 2006) protocol for preschool and elementary school children. This protocol focuses on seven objectives, as described below.

Normalizing Symptoms

Mental health professionals should normalize children's responses to disasters, such as bedwetting or aggressiveness, by informing children of typical reactions. This information can be conveyed through symptom charades (i.e., one person acts out a symptom, and others guess what symptom it is), art activities, or puppet shows. A puppet show is described below.

Content of Session	*Rationale/Analysis*
OLD PUPPET: Hello, everyone. My name is Shep the Sheep Dog. I am old and wise.	
YOUNG PUPPET: My name is Sugarloaf the Puppy. I am young and scared.	The play uses a "wise, old" animal and a "young, scared" animal to facilitate the teaching process.
OLD PUPPET: We are here today to learn about the tornado.	Anticipates questions and fears children might have, and projects them onto the young puppet. This validates children's feelings.
YOUNG PUPPET: What is a tornado? Is it a monster?	
OLD PUPPET: No. Do you, children, know what a tornado is? (*Lets children answer; then continues:*) A tornado is a violent, destructive windstorm in the shape of a funnel that can touch the ground.	Assesses children's understanding; then provides factual information in a simple manner.
YOUNG PUPPET: What causes the tornado? Did someone get mad at us and send it? Did a witch make it happen?	Anticipates common cognitive distortions and projects them onto the young puppet.
OLD PUPPET: No? Do you, children, know what causes a tornado? (*Lets children answer; then continues:*) A tornado is caused by very warm and humid air in the lower atmosphere, and cooler air in the upper atmosphere, plus fast wind. The weather reporter on the radio, TV, or computer will tell you when it is coming and when to take shelter.	

YOUNG PUPPET: How can we help ourselves be safe when we know it is coming?	Again, assesses children's understanding; then provides factual information in a simple manner.
OLD PUPPET: Good question. What ways do you know, children? (*Lets children answer; then continues:*) OK. Now we know: (1) Go right away to a nearby underground shelter or to the inside room or hallway away from windows. (2) Sit with knees to your chest and place a jacket or blanket over your head. (3) Stay in place until the bad weather passes your area. Don't go outside until the weather reporter or an adult tells you it is OK.	
YOUNG PUPPET: What happens if the tornado destroys your house?	Assesses children's understanding; then teaches coping strategies and addresses common barriers to coping strategies.
OLD PUPPET: Some people have to move to new places. People are busy cleaning and rebuilding. Many adults and children become sad, worried, scared, confused, or angry.	
YOUNG PUPPET: Is this bad?	Explains expected changes. Validates common emotions.
OLD PUPPET: No, it is normal to feel this way after something scary happens. Many children—even teenagers—will have scary dreams, wet the bed, fight more, or need more attention. Many people cry and don't know why. Many children may want to stay near adults all the time, too. Kids, what other changes might children and teens have? (*Lets children answer.*)	Normalizes common symptoms. Elicits and assesses other symptoms children may experience.

YOUNG PUPPET: I'm glad to hear these are normal things that happen to children and teens after something scary. How long will these things last?	Addresses the concern that symptoms will last forever, and sets expectations of normal recovery while allowing for atypical responses.
OLD PUPPET: For many young people, these changes only last a short time. For some, they last longer. The most important thing is to tell an adult and learn to help yourself and others calm down.	Encourages talking to an adult, and increases sense of hope and power that the children can do something to improve.
YOUNG PUPPET: What can we do to help one another?	
OLD PUPPET: Good question! Kids, what do you do to help others calm down and feel better? (*Lets children answer; then continues:*) Yes, you can (1) pat someone on the back or hold hands, (2) play with each other, (3) sing, (4) dance, (5) breathe deeply and slowly, (6) pray or meditate, (7) read or look at books, (8) say to yourself that you are safe now, (9) think happy thoughts, and (10) talk to an adult.	
YOUNG PUPPET: Will things get better? Will I feel better?	Elicits and confirms positive coping strategies that are culturally and developmentally appropriate.
OLD PUPPET: Yes! We all need to work together to make life better. We will remind ourselves that we are safe now. Tell me what you will do to help yourself and a friend feel better. (*Lets children answer.*)	
YOUNG PUPPET: Let's all try to be happy and dance!	Fosters hope that youth and the community will get better. Reviews coping strategies. Ends on a positive note!

Managing Hyperarousal

Disaster mental health professionals can teach children and teens self-soothing and relaxing techniques to calm their bodies and deactivate their "fight-or-flight" response after a disaster (Brymer et al., 2006). These procedures include (1) taking deep breaths through playful activities such as blowing soap bubbles or balloons; (2) progressive muscle relaxation through tensing and relaxing muscle groups; and (3) focusing on positive images by drawing happy places, engaging in mutual storytelling with a positive ending, or meditating on peaceful places (Felix et al., 2006). A group of children can sing the following words to the tune of "Twinkle, Twinkle, Little Star": "I am safe and I am strong. Take a breath and sing this song. I'm growing stronger every day. I know that I'll be OK. I am safe and I am strong. Take a breath and sing along" (Shelby & Bond, 2005).

Managing Intrusive Reexperiencing

Disaster mental health professionals can teach children and teens methods of managing intrusive thoughts of disaster-related events that are encoded in implicit memory (Brymer et al., 2006). These procedures include (1) "changing the soundtrack" by replacing negative thoughts with a predetermined positive song, story, or saying, such as "I'm safe right now and I know it because I have . . ."; and (2) grounding activities such as rubbing hands on stomach (Felix et al., 2006). Play therapists can also simplify the "5-4-3-2-1" sensory grounding and containment procedure (Baranowsky, Gentry, & Schultz, 2005) by asking children to play a "3-2-1" game. For this game, youth are asked to identify three objects everyone can see, three sounds everyone can hear, and three things everyone can touch; then two things they can see, hear, and touch; followed by one thing they can see, hear, and touch. This activity helps children refocus on the here-and-now and realize that their surroundings are safe.

Increasing Accurate Cognitions

Due to their egocentric and concrete cognitions, some children may misattribute the cause of disaster to their bad dreams or to their own or someone else's bad behavior. Mental health professionals should identify their misattributions and give accurate information. Possible procedures include (1) making a Q-sort of possible reasons for the disaster and asking children to sort them as true or untrue; (2) creating a "blame box" for younger children to put in drawings of who or what they blame, and then drawing the correct reasons together; (3) developing a puppet show in which one puppet asks about misattributions and another puppet gives accurate reasons; and (4) acting out a radio show of people calling in with questions and an expert giving correct information (Felix et al., 2006). When the young puppet in the puppet show described above timidly asked whether the tornado was caused by an angry person or by a witch, the children in Moore loudly responded in unison, "No." Their powerful, united response seemed to alter their collective cognition to an accurate one, which the confident older puppet confirmed.

Increasing Effective Coping

Disaster mental health professionals should help children and adolescents differentiate between effective and ineffective coping strategies, and should help them develop numerous, culturally appropriate adaptive coping strategies (Baggerly & Green, 2013). These procedures may include (1) writing or drawing maladaptive coping strategies on cards, and then telling children to "pass the trash"; (2) playing card games in which children find pairs of adaptive coping strategies and throw out maladaptive strategies; (3) playing coping charades in which children act out positive coping strategies; and (4) organizing developmentally appropriate, cooperative play or games, such as Duck, Duck, Goose and relay races (Felix et al., 2006). For example, our team members guided adolescents in making a "coping bracelet" of five colorful cards on which they drew effective coping strategies (Shelby & Bond, 2005). Green (2014) describes a "coping box," which is a shoebox decorated by an adolescent with various coping strategies written on small squares of construction paper to practice and rehearse with a therapist.

Seeking Social Support

Mental health professionals should teach children and teens appropriate ways of seeking healthy social support and decreasing unhealthy social withdrawal. These procedures (Felix et al., 2006) include (1) role-playing how to ask for social support from four different sources, such as peers, parents, staff members, and teachers; (2) making "support coupons" by writing or drawing requests for help on paper, and giving one of these to a trusted peer or adult when help is needed; and (3) creating a paper doll support chain, in which linked images of dolls are labeled with names of people who provide support.

Fostering Hope

After a disruptive disaster, mental health professionals can be a part of the compassionate humanitarian response that reignites children's hope and positive images for the future (Felix et al., 2006). Procedures to increase hope include (1) role-playing family and community rebuilding efforts; (2) creating stories, poems, or songs that express hope; and (3) identifying community support projects in which children can participate, such as making thank-you cards for police officers or building a rock garden. These interventions foster hope not only in children, but also in adults who witness the therapists working with their children (Baggerly & Green, 2014). A group activity we have used with teenagers is called When the Music Makes Me Smile (Green, 2014). The teens are asked to identify a popular song that they believe represents a part of who they are and conveys some resiliency and inner strength. In a group, we have the teens play the song on YouTube or their iPhones, and we read the lyrics. We then have the teens draw some type of artwork or abstract concept to concretize the feelings associated with the empowering song, derived from the individual expression and metacommunication of strength from the song's lyrics and melodies.

One challenge we faced in Moore with implementing the interventions described above was that we never quite knew how many would attend the sessions. Our team addressed this challenge by being flexible in dividing youth into age-similar groups. One day a group leader might have two children who were 4 or 5 years old, and on the next day the same leader might have six children who were 10 or 11 years old. Another challenge we faced with implementing these interventions was being sensitive to the amount of time each parent or caregiver had available to provide information or receive feedback. Some parents, whose employment had been disrupted by the tornado, were willing to spend as much time as needed to provide information and receive feedback. Other parents were clearly overwhelmed by multiple demands and only had time to sign permission forms. Our team managed this challenge by acknowledging the parents' own needs and providing psychoeducational materials on coping strategies and local resources.

CONCLUSION

As the number of children and adolescents affected by natural disasters continues to increase worldwide, mental health professionals must be prepared as proactive citizens in a global village. Natural disasters can have a clinically significant impact on youth's behavior, cognitive functioning, mental health, and physical development, as well as access to community resources. Most adolescents will experience typical short-term symptoms such as nightmares and avoidance of trauma triggers; younger children may be susceptible because of their more limited coping mechanisms, to full-blown clinical symptoms of PTSD.

Mental health professionals trained in play therapy are uniquely poised with developmentally appropriate knowledge and skills to facilitate children's and adolescents' healing after a natural disaster (Baggerly & Green, 2013; Green, 2014). Play and caring are understood in any language. Mental health professionals are encouraged to follow these guidelines for preparation and intervention, so that they can be global citizens in a global village that helps youth, within the salient context of their families, recover after natural disasters.

STUDY QUESTIONS

1. After a natural disaster, what are the differences between typical and atypical symptoms?
2. How would you design a research study to assess disaster response with children?
3. How will you know whether you, as a mental health professional, are ready to be involved in disaster response? What criteria should you meet before you deploy?
4. What are common concerns and questions that parents may have about their children after a natural disaster? What would you say to parents to respond to these concerns?
5. Describe and demonstrate teaching youth to manage hyperarousal and reexperiencing.

REFERENCES

American Psychiatric Association. (2013). *Diagnostic and statistical manual of mental disorders* (5th ed.). Arlington, VA: Author.

American Psychological Association. (2015). Disaster Response Network. Retrieved from *www.apa.org/practice/programs/drn/index.aspx.*

Ayub, M., Poongan, I., Masood, K., Gul, H., Ali, M., Farrukh, A., et al. (2012). Psychological morbidity in children 18 months after Kashmir earthquake of 2005. *Child Psychiatry and Human Development, 43*(3), 323–336.

Baggerly, J. (2006). Preparing play therapists for disaster response: Principles and procedures. *International Journal of Play Therapy, 15*, 59–82.

Baggerly, J. (2007). *Crisis stabilization for children: Disaster mental health* [Video]. Framingham, MA: Microtraining Associates and Alexander Street Press.

Baggerly, J. (2012). *Trauma informed child centered play therapy* [Video]. Framingham, MA: Microtraining Associates and Alexander Street Press.

Baggerly, J., & Green, E. J. (2013). Playing in peril after a natural disaster: Incorporating play therapy with responsive services. In J. Curry & L. Fazio-Griffith (Eds.), *Integrating play techniques in comprehensive school counseling programs* (pp. 125–139). New York: Information Age.

Baggerly, J., & Green, E. J. (2014). Mending broken attachment in displaced children: Finding "home" through play therapy. In C. Malchiodi & D. Crenshaw (Eds.), *Creative arts and play therapy for attachment problems* (pp. 275–294). New York: Guilford Press.

Baranowsky, A. B., Gentry, J. E., & Schultz, D. F. (2005). *Trauma practice: Tools for stabilization and recovery.* Ashland, OH: Hogrefe & Huber.

Bratton, S. C., Ray, D., Rhine, T., & Jones, L. (2005). The efficacy of play therapy with children: A meta-analytic review of treatment outcomes. *Professional Psychology: Research And Practice, 36*(4), 376–390.

Brymer, M., Jacobs, A., Layne, C., Pynoos, R., Ruzek, J., Steinberg, A., et al. (2006).

Psychological first aid field operations guide (2nd ed.). Los Angeles: National Child Traumatic Stress Network and National Center for PTSD. Available at *www.nctsn.org/content/psychological-first-aid* or *www.ptsd.va.gov/professional/manuals/psych-first-aid.asp*.

Chemtob, C. M., Nakashima, J. P., & Hamada, R. S. (2002). Psychosocial intervention for postdisaster trauma symptoms in elementary school children: A controlled community field study. *Archives of Pediatrics and Adolescent Medicine, 156*(3), 211–216.

Cohen, J. A., Deblinger, E., & Mannarino, A. P. (2006). *Treating trauma and traumatic grief in children and adolescents: A clinician's guide.* New York: Guilford Press.

Council for Accreditation of Counseling and Related Educational Programs. (2009). *2009 standards.* Alexandria, VA: Author.

Derivois, D., Mérisier, G., Cénat, J., & Castelot, V. (2014). Symptoms of posttraumatic stress disorder and social support among children and adolescents after the 2010 Haitian earthquake. *Journal of Loss and Trauma, 19*(3), 202–212.

Federal Emergency Management Agency. (2003). Concept of operations. Retrieved from *www.fema.gov/rrr/conplan/conpln4c.shtm*

Felix, E., Bond, D., & Shelby, J. (2006). Coping with disaster: Psychosocial interventions for children in international disaster relief. In C. Schaefer & H. Kaduson (Eds.), *Contemporary play therapy: Theory, research, and practice* (pp. 307–328). New York: Guilford Press.

Felton, J. W., Cole, D. A., & Martin, N. C. (2013). Effects of rumination on child and adolescent depressive reactions to a natural disaster: The 2010 Nashville flood. *Journal of Abnormal Psychology, 122*(1), 64–73.

Garfin, D., Silver, R., Gil-Rivas, V., Guzmán, J., Murphy, J., Cova, F., et al. (2014). Children's reactions to the 2010 Chilean earthquake: The role of trauma exposure, family context, and school-based mental health programming. *Psychological Trauma: Theory, Research, Practice, and Policy, 6*(5), 563–573.

Gaskill, R. L., & Perry, B. D. (2012). Child sexual abuse, traumatic experiences, and their impact on the developing brain. In P. Goodyear-Brown (Ed.), *Handbook of child sexual abuse* (pp. 30–47). Hoboken, NJ: Wiley.

Gentry, J. E., Baranowsky, A., & Dunning, K. (2002). The accelerated recovery program for compassion fatigue. In C. R. Figley (Ed.), *Treating compassion fatigue* (pp. 123–138). New York: Brunner/Routledge.

Green, E. J. (2014). *The handbook of Jungian play therapy with children and adolescents.* Baltimore: Johns Hopkins University Press.

Guha-Sapir, D., Vos, F., Below, R., & Ponserre, S. (2013). *Annual disaster statistical review 2012: The numbers and trends.* Brussels: Centre for Research on the Epidemiology of Disasters. Retrieved from *www.cred.be/sites/default/files/ADSR_2012.pdf.*

Jaycox, L. H., Cohen, J. A., Mannarino, A. P., Walker, D. W., Langley, A. K., Gegenheimer, K. L., et al. (2010). Children's mental health care following Hurricane Katrina: A field trial of trauma-focused psychotherapies. *Journal of Traumatic Stress, 23*(2), 223–231.

Kumar, M., & Fonagy, P. (2013). Differential effects of exposure to social violence and natural disaster on children's mental health. *Journal of Traumatic Stress, 26*(6), 695–702.

La Greca, A. M. (2008). Interventions for posttraumatic stress in children and adolescents following natural disasters and acts of terrorism. In R. C. Steele, T. D. Elkin, & M. C. Roberts (Eds.), *Handbook of evidence-based therapies for children and adolescents: Bridging science and practice* (pp. 121–141). New York: Springer.

La Greca, A. M., Lai, B. S., Llabre, M. M., Silverman, W. K., Vernberg, E. M., & Prinstein, M. J. (2013). Children's postdisaster trajectories of PTS symptoms: Predicting chronic distress. *Child and Youth Care Forum, 42*(4), 351–369.

La Greca, A. M., Sevin, S. W., & Sevin, E. L. (2005). *After the storm: A guide to help children cope with the psychological effects of a hurricane.* Coral Gables, FL: 7-Dippity.

Lai, B. S., La Greca, A. M., & Llabre, M. M. (2014). Children's sedentary activity after hurricane exposure. *Psychological Trauma: Theory, Research, Practice, and Policy, 6*(3), 280–289.

Landreth, G. L. (2012). *Play therapy: The art of the relationship* (3rd ed.). New York: Routledge.

Lee, I., Ha, Y. S., Kim, Y. A., & Kwon, Y. H. (2004). PTSD symptoms in elementary school children after Typhoon Rusa. *Taehan Kanho Hakhoe Chi, 34*(4), 636–645.

McDermott, B. M., Lee, E. M., Judd, M., & Gibbon, P. (2005). Posttraumatic stress disorder and general psychopathology in children and adolescents following a wildfire disaster. *Canadian Journal of Psychiatry, 50*(3), 137–143.

National Association of Social Workers. (2003). *Disasters. Social work speaks: National Association of Social Workers policy statements, 2003–2006* (6th ed.). Washington, DC: NASW Press.

National Institute of Mental Health (NIMH). (2001). Helping children and adolescents cope with violence and disasters. Retrieved from *www.nimh.nih.gov/publicat/violence.cfm.*

National Institute of Mental Health (NIMH). (2002). *Mental health and mass violence: Evidence-based early psychological intervention for victims/survivors of mass violence. A workshop to reach consensus on best practices* (NIH Publication No. 02-5138). Washington, DC: U.S. Government Printing Office.

National Oceanic and Atmospheric Administration. (2013). Billion-dollar weather/climate disasters. Retrieved from *www.ncdc.noaa.gov/billions/events.*

Osofsky, H. J., Osofsky, J. D., Kronenberg, M., Brennan, A., & Hansel, T. (2009). Posttraumatic stress symptoms in children after Hurricane Katrina: Predicting the need for mental health services. *American Journal of Orthopsychiatry, 79*(2), 212–220.

Salloum, A., Carter, P., Burch, B., Garfinkel, A., & Overstreet, S. (2011). Impact of exposure to community violence, Hurricane Katrina, and Hurricane Gustav on posttraumatic stress and depressive symptoms among school age children. *Anxiety, Stress and Coping: An International Journal, 24*(1), 27–42.

Schottelkorb, A. A., Doumas, D. M., & Garcia, R. (2012). Treatment for childhood refugee trauma: A randomized, controlled trial. *International Journal of Play Therapy, 21*(2), 57–73.

Scott, B. G., Lapré, G. E., Marsee, M. A., & Weems, C. F. (2014). Aggressive behavior and its associations with posttraumatic stress and academic achievement following a natural disaster. *Journal of Clinical Child and Adolescent Psychology, 43*(1), 43–50.

Seballos, F., Tanner, T., Tarazona, M., & Gallegos, J. (2011). Children and disasters:

Understanding impact and enabling agency. Retrieved from *www.unicef.org.uk/Documents/Publications/children-and-disasters.pdf.*

Shelby, J., & Bond, D. (2005, October). *Using play-based interventions in Sri Lanka.* Paper presented at the annual conference of the Association for Play Therapy, Nashville, TN.

Shelby, J., Bond, D., Hall, S., & Hsu, C. (2004). *Operation USA Sri Lanka relief mission treatment manual: Enhancing coping among young tsunami survivors.* Unpublished manuscript.

Shen, Y. J. (2002). Short-term group play therapy with Chinese earthquake victims: Effects on anxiety, depression, and adjustment. *International Journal of Play Therapy, 11*(1), 43–64.

Shioyama, A., Uemoto, M., Shinfuku, N., Ide, H., Seki, W., Mori, S., et al. (2000). The mental health of school children after the Great Hanshin-Awaji Earthquake: II. Longitudinal analysis. *Seishin Shinkeigaku Zasshi [Psychiatria et Neurologia Japonica], 102*(5), 481–497.

Solomon, E. P., & Heide, K. M. (2005). The biology of trauma: Implications for treatment. *Journal of Interpersonal Violence, 20*(1), 51–60.

Terranova, A. M., Boxer, P., & Morris, A. (2009). Changes in children's peer interactions following a natural disaster: How predisaster bullying and victimization rates changed following Hurricane Katrina. *Psychology in the Schools, 46*(4), 333–347.

van der Kolk, B. A. (2007). The developmental impact of childhood trauma. In L. J. Kirmayer, R. Lemelson, & M. Barad (Eds.), *Understanding trauma: Integrating biological, clinical, and cultural perspectives* (pp. 224–241). New York: Cambridge University Press.

Vernberg, E. M., La Greca, A. M., Silverman, W. K., & Prinstein, M. J. (1996). Prediction of posttraumatic stress symptoms in children after Hurricane Andrew. *Journal of Abnormal Psychology, 105*(2), 237–248.

Webb, N. B. (Ed.). (2004). *Mass trauma and violence: Helping families and children cope.* New York: Guilford Press.

Wolmer, L., Laor, N., Dedeoglu, C., Siev, J., & Yazgan, Y. (2005). Teacher-mediated intervention after disaster: A controlled three-year follow-up of children's functioning. *Journal of Child Psychology and Psychiatry, 46*(11), 1161–1168.

World Health Organization. (2003). Mental health in emergencies. Retrieved from *www5. who.int/mental_health.*

Chapter 17

Court Testimony

Animal-Assisted Trauma-Informed Play Therapy to Help Traumatized Child and Adolescent Witnesses

DAVID A. CRENSHAW
LORI STELLA

The use of animals to assist in therapy dates at least back to Sigmund Freud, who included his dog Jo-Fi, a chow, in his sessions with adults. However, the use of facility dogs in trauma-informed play therapy with children who are suffering from complex or developmental trauma is a new approach, and scant if any literature is available about this method. The term "developmental trauma" is used in this chapter because it aptly captures the issues of the children and adolescents we treat. Bessel van der Kolk (2005) first used this term to refer to repeated or chronic exposure to interpersonal trauma, including physical and/or sexual abuse, emotional abuse, witnessing violence, abandonment, or threats to bodily integrity. In addition, since the multiple-trauma exposure occurs in the midst of incomplete development, its impact can include adverse effects on self-esteem, trust, and sense of safety, along with expectations and fears of further victimization.

The use of "facility dogs"—dogs that are graduates of training schools accredited by Assistance Dogs International to accompany vulnerable, often traumatized witnesses while they testify on the stand in court—is a new, promising way of providing comfort to child and adolescent witnesses and reducing the risk of retraumatization. The two of us were involved in a case that made history in the New York State criminal court system: A golden retriever named Rosie accompanied a traumatized adolescent witness on the stand for the first time ever in New York State, thereby enabling her to testify about her extensive sexual abuse by the defendant, who was her father. We have also been active in advocating and lobbying for passage in New York State of a bill named "Rosie's Law," which would make it possible for a wide range and ages of vulnerable witnesses (in addition to children and adolescents) to have the option of a facility dog's comfort while they testify.

BACKGROUND

We knew in the autumn months of 2010 that an adolescent, Jessica (fictitious name)—a resident at the Children's Home of Poughkeepsie (CHP), which serves high-risk foster children and adolescents in a variety of programs—would almost certainly not be able to testify on the stand against her father, since she could barely talk about her repeated and chronic trauma with her therapist (Lori Stella). The two of us (Stella and her supervisor, David A. Crenshaw) discussed nonverbal expressive arts strategies to use with Jessica, since she, like many child trauma survivors, was unable to put into words what happened to her (Crenshaw & Stella, 2011). Fortuitously, Crenshaw attended the annual Association for Play Therapy Conference in October 2010 and learned that highly trained dogs were used in some states to ease the anxiety and potential trauma to child witnesses while the children were testifying (Crenshaw, 2014). Both of us were immediately excited about the possibility that this accommodation, if approved by the court, might be the solution that would empower and enable Jessica to testify. The story of how Rosie enabled Jessica to testify is told later in this chapter. During the time that Rosie was on loan to us for Jessica's use in the courtroom trial, this lovely and loving 11-year-old golden retriever not only opened the door to an innovation in New York State court practices, but also created exciting new possibilities of animal-assisted play therapy for children and adolescents with developmental trauma.

ANIMAL-ASSISTED PLAY THERAPY FOR DEVELOPMENTAL TRAUMA

Developmental trauma dysregulates the lower brain, resulting in increased risk of significant and lasting behavioral, social, emotional, cognitive, and sensory–motor problems (Gaskill & Perry, 2012, 2014; Perry, 2006, 2009; Perry & Dobson, 2013; van der Kolk, 2005, 2006, 2014). The therapeutic task is to calm or soothe the brainstem so that the higher levels of the brain, the emotional (limbic) and cognitive (cortical) centers, become more available to therapeutic interventions. (See Drewes, Chapter,7, this volume, for more discussion of this neurobiologically informed approach to therapy for complex trauma.)

While Rosie was preparing for trial with Jessica, she sat in on therapy sessions not only with Jessica, but with two other children who were also being prepared for court testimony (in a murder trial) and were also in treatment with us. The impact of Rosie's presence in the therapy sessions on all three of the children, as well as on us, was striking. Everyone in the room seemed to feel calmer, even when talking about extremely difficult or painful issues. Rosie's presence was soothing the children's brainstems as well as helping us enable the children to unburden themselves more, which then permitted us to witness and contain this pain. The important implications of this discovery for trauma-informed work with the young people in our multiple programs serving high-risk children and adolescents in foster care led us in August 2011, after the court trials ended, to obtain our own facility dog for CHP—another golden retriever, and a sister of Rosie, named Ivy.

Facility Dogs in the Therapy Room

Ivy, a 9-year-old service-trained dog, was donated to us after the combat veteran she had served for 7 years died quite suddenly. Almost literally overnight, Ivy went from taking care of a veteran to being a facility dog providing emotional support for a group of about 60 children, mostly adolescents. During her first weeks at our program, Ivy was still grieving for the loss of her handler and companion. Ivy's love of children, however, quickly lifted her mood, and the young people in all parts of our program quickly bonded with her. Then in October 2011, we discovered that Ivy was gravely ill with severe and chronic Lyme disease, which had not previously been diagnosed or treated. Ivy nearly died during a period of intensive treatment because the Lyme disease had seriously damaged her kidneys. The veterinarians treating Ivy said that, at most, she would live another 3 months. In fact, Ivy lived another 19 months; we attributed this largely to how much she loved her work with the children and adolescents, which gave her a strong desire to live. A testament to her love of her work came after her retirement on her 11th birthday, February 28, 2013. One week before she died on April 22, 2013—after being so weak the previous 2 days that she could not stand up and had no desire to eat—Ivy rose to her feet, went to where her handler had hung her working vest, and pulled it down from the hook. Ivy insisted on going to work for one last time.

Trauma-Informed Therapy

During her 17 months of working with children and teens with developmental trauma, Ivy, like her sister Rosie, enabled children as young as 3 and teens as old as 19 to create and share their trauma narratives in countless therapy sessions through her calm, gentle presence and love for the young people (Crenshaw, 2012). Trauma narratives are an essential component of empirically supported treatment protocols (Cavett & Drewes, 2012; Cohen, Mannarino, & Deblinger, 2006, 2012), and these stories were often shared by the children or teens while they lay on the floor next to Ivy with their arms around her. Children with ongoing and complex trauma often require more in-depth treatment and more flexible use of the components of empirically supported treatments (Cohen, Mannarino, Kleithermes, & Murray, 2012; Cohen, Mannarino, & Murphy, 2011; Cohen, Mannarino, & Navarro, 2012; Murphy, Cohen, & Mannarino, 2013; Nader, 2011). The key early components of trauma-focused protocols consist of creating safety and strengthening coping. Ivy's consistent and reliable presence in the play therapy sessions did a great deal to increase safety, calm, and trust among the children and adolescents who interacted with her.

Attachment Theory Framework

Attachment theory offers another framework for viewing the benefits of a facility dog in work with severely traumatized children. The children we treat in our foster care programs have suffered repeated interpersonal trauma, including witnessing domestic violence, removal from home, and (in many cases) physical and/or sexual abuse and/or neglect. In a survey of our client population at CHP in 2010 (Crenshaw & Alstadt, 2011), 87% had been exposed to four or more of the adverse childhood experiences included in the Adverse Childhood Experiences (ACE) Study (Felliti et al., 1998). The ACE research has shown that when children are exposed to multiple adverse childhood events, the cumulative impact can include adverse effects not only on the mental health of these individuals, but also on their physical health. Thus CHP serves highly at-risk children who require at least 6–9 months in therapy in order to build a solid bond of trust. That time was reduced significantly when first Rosie, then Ivy, and now Ace (Rosie's grandson and our current facility dog) were included in the therapy sessions because, with few exceptions, the children established trust in the dogs quickly. Since the dogs were already attached to us, the therapists, their presence also reduced the time the children and adolescents needed to trust us.

Case Example 1

Ivy participated in therapy sessions with a preadolescent boy whose trauma had been so chronic and severe that he was unable even to talk about his experience, let alone to begin a trauma narrative, for 2½ years. Due to the overwhelming nature of the interpersonal traumas he had suffered, he experienced periodic crises that led to three psychiatric hospitalizations of several months apiece during that period. Shortly after Ivy was introduced into both individual play sessions and family sessions, however, the boy began to create and share his trauma narrative gradually over a period of 4 months. Because his abuse had been so horrific, the boy could reveal only a little bit at a time. In the first family session when he began to tell his trauma story, Ivy was under the table. This 12-year-old boy crawled under the table, put his arm around Ivy, and began his narrative. In each subsequent session, he positioned himself on the floor—snuggling Ivy, and sometimes laying his head on her—and continued his trauma story until he had disclosed all he could at that time. He shared the trauma events first with Ivy, and then with the therapist and his mother and older sister in the family sessions.

Case Example 2

A 15-year-old girl who, while AWOL from her residential program, was repeatedly raped by a gang of older men, was able to tell her story only in the presence of Ivy. The dog comforted both the girl and her mother throughout the session. Ivy also sat in with the girl when she met a police detective, with the goal of identifying one or more of her attackers from a group of police photographs. Shortly afterward, the overwhelming nature of her trauma led to an episode in which the girl threatened suicide; she was then hospitalized for a 2-month period. On her return to the residential program, she came to my (David A. Crenshaw's) office, saw Ivy, and threw her arms around her, exclaiming, "Ivy, I knew you would be here waiting for me when I came back!" On the day she was discharged from our program, she spent several hours with Ivy, snuggling and taking pictures of her. She told Ivy as she walked out the door, "Ivy, I will never forget you." An adolescent with such an extensive trauma history even before she suffered the horrendous gang rape would generally not be expected to develop a strong attachment to her human therapist, but Ivy enabled this girl to make a meaningful attachment to both the dog and me. In the girl's sessions, she would typically at one point shut down and go into a depressive collapse, dissociate, and become unable to verbalize. When this happened, Ivy would, without prompting, come over and nudge the girl; the adolescent would then pet Ivy and join her on the floor. Ivy's comfort and attention enabled the teen to regroup, to reorient herself to her present surroundings, and then to leave the session feeling able to cope.

More Information about Facility Dogs

Although a body of literature exists on animal-assisted therapy (Chur-Hansen, McArthur, & Winefield, 2014; Dietz, Davis, & Pennings, 2012; Friesen, 2010; Kruger & Serpell, 2006; Lange, Cox, Bernert, & Jenkins, 2007; Lefkowitz, Paharia, Prout, Debiak, & Bleiberg, 2005; Nimer & Lundahl, 2007; Prothman, Bienert, & Ettrich, 2006; Tsai, Friedmann, & Thomas, 2010), and the body of knowledge about and literature on animal-assisted play therapy is growing (Parish-Plass, 2008, 2013; Thompson, 2009; Trotter, Chandler, Goodwin-Bond, & Casey, 2008; VanFleet, 2008; VanFleet & Colţea, 2012; VanFleet & Faa-Thompson, 2010, 2012, 2014, 2015; Weiss, 2009), we could find no publications discussing the use of facility dogs in trauma-informed therapy for youth with developmental trauma.

In fact, the literature reveals considerable confusion about the labels attached to animals utilized in the care, comfort, and mental health treatment of humans, so we provide more information here. The term "facility dogs" in this chapter refers not to therapy dogs that are used by therapists in private practice, or to dogs used for visiting nursing homes, hospitals, or special schools, but rather to *fully trained service dogs that are graduates from training programs* accredited by Assistance Dogs International. When a facility dog finishes its training, instead of being deployed to assist a veteran or a disabled person, the dog is assigned to a program or institution such as CHP, where it provides assistance to a wide range of clients. (Ivy's case was unusual, in that she was originally assigned to a combat veteran, and later in her career came to work as a facility dog at CHP.) The training program for such dogs is 2 years in duration, involving 1,500–2,000 hours during which they learn 80 commands. Our use of facility dogs enables us to involve them in individual play therapy sessions with children, and in verbally expressive therapy with older children, as well as in group play therapy sessions and family sessions. In addition, many children on the campus schedule time to be with and play with our facility dog, which helps them cope when under stress.

In addition, our staff members drop by for brief visits with our facility dog as part of their self-care. A few minutes with our current facility dog, Ace, is extremely helpful to staffers in reducing their level of stress. Ace shares an office with one of us (David A. Crenshaw) and, in his absence, with the other (Lori Stella). The use of a facility dog in court with vulnerable witnesses is discussed in the next section of this chapter, along with Rosie's historic feat in court. Finally, it should be noted that CHP permits several other organizations and individuals to bring therapy dogs once a month to visit children in their cottages. The dogs stay for an hour or two, and the children enjoy these visits. In contrast, facility dogs are working dogs and, as in the case of Ace, may work 3 full days a week or longer.

FACILITY DOGS IN THE COURTROOM

Jessica's Story

Abraham Maslow's (1943) hierarchy of needs includes the fundamental need for safety, including security of one's body, employment, resources, morality, family, and health (Maslow, 1943). It is often the role of a child's parents to provide the foundations of safety. This was not at all the case for Jessica. Jessica did not get to know her parents until she came to the United States at age 10. Her safety was originally established by her grandparents in a Central American country, who raised her from infancy to age 10. Then her mother came to take her away from her grandparents and move her to the United States, and Jessica's initial sense of safety was shaken. Her mother, a stranger, took her on the long journey of undocumented immigration from Central America—a trip through woods and across rivers, many times in the dark with other strangers—to the United States. Jessica's world was turned upside down, and her sense of safety was gone. At one point during the trek, her mother was caught and sent back—leaving Jessica to go on without her, with total strangers, feeling terribly alone.

Upon arriving in the United States, Jessica was introduced to her father. Within weeks, he began sexually abusing her. Jessica's mother arrived in the United States about 1 month after Jessica, but the sexual abuse continued even after the mother's arrival. At some point her mother became aware of the abuse, but turned a blind eye to it. Jessica's abuse continued for 4 years and occurred almost daily, with her father raping her inside the family home or picking her up from school to take her to construction sites. Some people may ask, "Why didn't she tell?" She went to school; she could have told a teacher or counselor. She could have asked for help. What many people outside the child welfare realm do not realize is the depth of the fear that gets instilled in children who are abused. In almost every case, there are forces that silence the victims. In Jessica's case, she was threatened with statements such as these:

> "If you tell, I will kill you."
> "If you tell, you will get separated from your siblings."
> "If you tell, the police will arrest you."
> "If you tell, no one will believe you."

Children who are abused are forced to go to war with their minds. What would be worse, telling and maybe being spared from further abuse? Or telling and being taken far away from their brothers and sisters? And what if they are not believed?

In Jessica's case, her decision to tell came 4 long years after the abuse began. She was picked up by her father from school one day and taken to yet another construction site. This time was different, however: She found the courage and strength to fight back. As he physically tried to pin her down, she kicked, screamed, and hit him. At one point, he grabbed her by the throat and tried to choke her, saying, "I will kill you!" She didn't give up the fight. She fought hard and escaped. She took off running and didn't look back. For the next 2 weeks, no one looked for Jessica—not her mother, nor her father. She was gone. Missing. Finally, the school contacted child protective services (CPS) out of concern because Jessica had not been in school for quite a long time. Once CPS and the police became involved, Jessica was located. She had made it out of state and was staying with a relative. When found by law enforcement and CPS, Jessica told them her story. She wanted to be saved and kept safe; she could no longer be subjected to being brutally raped by her father. CPS and the police believed her and promised her they would keep her safe. Together, both agencies conducted an investigation, and her father was arrested for the crimes he had committed against his daughter.

Due to Jessica's mother's neglect, the girl was unable to return home to her mother. Jessica was placed at CHP, where she would be able to reside in a safe and therapeutic environment. Upon Jessica's first session with me (Lori Stella), she stated that she knew that CHP was a safe place, but she was not sure about anything else. She was quiet and timid, but polite. She was always willing to meet with me, but struggled to engage with me verbally (despite there not being a language barrier, as Jessica spoke English). Jessica spent many sessions in my office unable to express herself, despite our growing relationship. She often would sit in sessions and cry uncontrollably, unable to verbalize what was causing her to cry. Through art, Jessica could express herself somewhat better. Many of her paintings and drawings were bright and vibrant. However, there was always a man watching the other characters in the pictures—a man who was not colored in and did not have a face. This man appeared in many of her drawings, but she was never able to identify who he was; she always described him as a person who was not like the rest of the group.

Jessica and Rosie

Despite the fact that the Sixth Amendment to the U.S. Constitution gave her father the right to face Jessica in court, both of us strongly believed that Jessica also had rights. "A child witness may testify by alternative methods where by clear and convincing evidence, adequate showing has been made of the child's vulnerability to severe mental and emotional harm" (Dellinger, 2009, p. 178). Although there are alternatives to a child's testifying in court face to face against the defendant, such as testimony via closed-circuit television, this method is often not utilized because the verdict is subject to appeal based on the rights of the accused to confront the accuser, as was affirmed by the U.S. Supreme Court (*Crawford v. Washington*, 2004). The jury viewing the witness in person is often effective in prosecutors' efforts to put offenders away. According to the assistant district attorney who prosecuted Jessica's case, "In my 20 years of prosecuting, we have never used closed-circuit television."

As the trial approached and the use of closed-circuit television did not appear to be an option, we both began to have significant concerns that Jessica would struggle to testify against her father. Although Jessica had been at CHP for almost 1 year, she still had not been able to talk at all about what her father did to her, or even acknowledge him at all. I (Lori Stella) took Jessica to her first trial preparation meeting with the assistant district attorney. Despite the attorney's compassionate and empathetic approach with Jessica, Jessica significantly struggled to answer the prosecutor's questions. She cried throughout the hour-long preparation and appeared as though she was being traumatized all over again. This was no fault of the prosecutor, as this was her job. However, for Jessica, who had not been able to discuss her trauma effectively even with me, this was just too much. Strong concerns arose as to whether Jessica would be able to testify against her father at all, and, furthermore, whether her emotional well-being would be endangered if she was put on the stand. Judicial processes are frightening to children, especially in cases where youth are being asked questions by strangers involving sexual content, exacerbating the children's trauma (Makin, 1999). Jessica's sense of safety and security had already been torn away from her when her father repeatedly raped her.

While I (Stella) worked with Jessica in therapy to provide her with emotional support and psychoeducation on the judicial processes, Crenshaw attended the aforementioned conference in which someone spoke about the use of courthouse dogs in other states. After the conference, the two of us discussed the possibility of researching the use of courthouse dogs and determining whether this comfort tool would be effective for Jessica during her testimony. Courthouse dogs provide a comfortable atmosphere for witnesses, by assisting them in testifying in an effective and clear manner (Sandoval, 2010). When we began to review all of the documented benefits from the use of courthouse dogs, it became clear that having such a dog available would be a strong protective factor for Jessica on the stand. Crenshaw approached the district attorney's office and asked whether or not the use of a courthouse dog would be a possibility. The district attorney's office was quite open to the idea, even though the staff quickly learned that there was no precedent for it in the history of the New York State court system (whose records date back to 1691).

While the district attorney's office worked to get the necessary approval from the judge, the two of us (along with others staff members of CHP, who later became informally known as "Rosie's team") worked to locate a dog that would be reliable and appropriate to use in the courthouse. Dale Picard, owner of Educated Canines for Assisting Disabilities in Torrington, Connecticut, generously offered the use of his dog, Rosie, a retired trained facility dog. The very first session between Jessica and Rosie created the path to Jessica's healing. Although Jessica had built quite a strong therapeutic relationship with me (Stella), she still was unable to express her emotions regarding the trial, her parents, or any conflict in general. With Rosie present, even in the first session, this all changed. Jessica, I, and Rosie went for a walk around the CHP grounds and settled in at a picnic table overlooking the woods. Rosie jumped right up next to Jessica and sat there with her on the picnic bench. As Rosie sat with Jessica, Jessica petted the dog and talked with me about an argument she had gotten into with her roommate. For Jessica, this was enormous progress, as she had never opened up about any conflict or feelings during prior sessions. Rosie had successfully assisted not only in opening the door for me to lend an ear to Jessica's expression of feelings, but in creating an opportunity for a stronger, more trusting relationship between Jessica and myself. Dogs are unusually intuitive and are able to sense humans' emotions and dissipate feelings of distrust and fear (Dellinger, 2009). For several weeks, Jessica and I utilized Rosie in our therapy sessions. With Rosie's presence, Jessica opened up much more about her feelings regarding the trial and about her fears. The confidence and empowerment that emerged with Rosie present were astonishing.

In addition to the therapy sessions in which Rosie participated, Rosie began to accompany Jessica to the district attorney's office for her trial preparation meetings with the assistant district attorney who would be prosecuting the case. The level of stress that Jessica had experienced during the first preparation meeting was greatly decreased with Rosie present. Jessica's engagement with the prosecutor was much more precise and clear, and Jessica was able to remember and verbalize more specific details of the crimes that were committed against her. Witnesses having access to a properly trained dog during the proceedings experience a calming environment that encourages them to be more forthcoming in giving testimony (Dellinger, 2009). Jessica no longer appeared to be frozen by the fear of having to disclose embarrassing and private details of her life to a stranger.

As Jessica worked with Rosie in therapy and prepared for the trial, the prosecution made an application for a hearing to be held in order to gain the judge's permission to utilize Rosie during Jessica's testimony. I (Lori Stella) was called to testify as to the benefits of having Rosie accompany Jessica to the witness stand. I provided ample evidence regarding the revictimization Jessica would be subjected to if she was required to testify against her father face to face without support. According to criminal procedure law in New York, there are many issues to be considered in order to provide accommodations to vulnerable witnesses, including factors that would cause the witness to sustain serious mental or emotional harm by being required to testify within the presence of the defendant. Consideration is also given to whether during the alleged offense the defendant held authority over the witness, and whether the offenses are considered heinous (New York State criminal procedure law can be accessed at *http://ypdcrime.com*). In Jessica's case, all of these factors surely needed to be considered. I provided additional information as to how Rosie would provide Jessica comfort while testifying, in order to assist in maintaining Jessica's emotional well-being while allowing the defendant his Sixth Amendment rights. "Studies have confirmed that animate touch (holding a dog's leash or petting the dog while testifying), often leads to a psychological sense of well-being, decreased anxiety, lowered heart rate, increased speech and memory functions, and heightened mental alertness" (Sandoval, 2010, p. 17). Furthermore, providing Jessica the opportunity for Rosie to accompany her to the stand would not only benefit Jessica, but also assist both the prosecution and the defense in obtaining effective testimony. The judge agreed with my testimony at the pretrial hearing and decided to allow Rosie to accompany Jessica to court.

In the summer of 2011, on a warm sunny day, Jessica and Rosie made their way to the courthouse for Jessica's testimony. Rosie was placed carefully on the stand by her handler, while I accompanied Jessica into the courtroom. This was the first time in over a year that Jessica was faced with the man who had habitually sexually abused her. Jessica took the stand with Rosie at her feet. For over an hour, Jessica testified and was able to provide clear answers to both the prosecution and the defense. Furthermore, Jessica was provided with direct comfort by Rosie throughout her testimony—something that closed-circuit television would not have been able to provide her. Testifying with Rosie at her feet not only allowed Jessica to maintain her emotional health intact, but also provided her with an empowering experience, which created a path for healing. The trial lasted 1 week, and within 1 day, Jessica's father was subsequently found guilty and sentenced to 25 years to life in prison. For this, Jessica is grateful—and, though it has now been several years since the trial, she gives credit to Rosie. To this day, she states that she could never have testified without the comfort that Rosie provided her on the witness stand.

Advocating for Vulnerable Witnesses

In preparing for the trial with Rosie, we discovered that although there are procedures within U.S. court systems to provide child witnesses with alternatives to testifying in open court, this often does not happen; therefore, many such cases cannot be prosecuted, especially since the *Crawford* decision by the U.S. Supreme Court in 2004. Exploring policies and procedures within other countries makes it astonishingly clear how differently child witnesses are treated in the justice system. For instance, in some member states of the European Union, "all minors under the age of 18 fall within the category of vulnerable witness" (Crime Victim Compensation and Support Authority, 2010, p. 53). In other countries, not only the witness's age but also his or her mental and cognitive abilities are taken into consideration. In Jessica's case, I (Stella) was able to provide expert testimony regarding Jessica's posttraumatic stress disorder and the exacerbation of symptoms that could potentially occur without appropriate accommodations in court. However, in other countries, proving the child's risk of retraumatization is not necessary. For example, the presence of child victims under the age of 18 in court occurs only in exceptional cases in Lithuania (Crime Victim Compensation and Support Authority, 2010). In Sweden, a child age 15 or younger is not required to be present in court, since the child's statements may be recorded, and thus his or her physical presence within the court is not necessary (Crime Victim Compensation and Support Authority, 2010). Malaysia allows a supportive person to accompany a child while the child is giving testimony (Vasudevan, Ibrahim, & Kamini, 2007). If a child's statements are required in court, there are several alternative methods for doing so. For example, in Ireland, a child's parent or guardian may make a victim statement on his or her behalf if the child is under the age of 14 (Crime Victim Compensation and Support Authority, 2010).

In addition to the strong possibility that a child victim's presence in court will be intimidating and possibly detrimental to the witness, the questioning of the young witness raises concerns for that child's well-being. In Germany, "the examination of witnesses under the age of 18 shall be conducted solely by the presiding judge and although other parties are entitled to ask questions, it is the judge that forwards the questions to the child in a way that is most appropriate" (Crime Victim Compensation and Support Authority, 2010, p. 96). Such accommodations should be strongly considered for adoption in the United States. Many U.S. defense attorneys take advantage of having a child witness and do not conduct themselves with compassion or empathy. In Jessica's case, the defense attorney disclosed very personal information while she was on the stand—information that he had been instructed before the trial not to bring up. Unfortunately, some attorneys try to confuse a child witness by asking questions in a tone that may bewilder the witness; they then imply that the child is not being truthful (Cunningham & Hurley, 2007).

TRAUMA-SENSITIVE COURTS

Mental health professionals rarely have the opportunity to be involved in a history-making court case, as we did. Our intent was to find a way to enable a severely traumatized adolescent girl to tell her story in court in a complete way without undue risk of retraumatization. We were guided in the process by the pioneers of the Courthouse Dogs movement: Ellen O'Neill-Stephens, a former prosecutor in Seattle who founded the program, and Celeste Walsen, a veterinarian, who is its executive director (see *www.courthousedogs.com* for a wealth of information about the training and use of courthouse dogs). We followed closely the appeals process in New York State because the verdict of the trial court was appealed by the defense on the grounds that the dog elicited sympathy from the jury for the witness, and therefore deprived the defendant of a fair trial. However, in July 2013, the appellate court rejected unanimously the defense's argument and upheld the conviction of the defendant. The appellate court not only affirmed the trial court judge's decision to make a highly trained dog available to the witness to reduce the risk of retraumatization, but expressed the view that this accommodation should be considered a best practice. The defense then appealed to the Court of Appeals, the highest court in New York State. In April 2014, the Court of Appeals announced its decision not to review the appellate court's decision, thus affirming this decision.

Ironically, the strength of the appellate court's decision has made the progress of the proposed Rosie's Law through the New York legislature difficult because of the mindset "If it's not broken, don't fix it." Given how clear and affirming the trial and appellate court decisions have been, the reluctance of legislators, prosecutors, and judges to seek legislation in a difficult matter that pertains to children is understandable. The two of us, however have advocated for Rosie's Law (see *www.nysenate.gov/press-release/senator-gipson-and-assemblyman-skartados-rosie-s-law-would-help-children-and-disabled-*) because its passage would give legislative approval for extending this accommodation to other vulnerable witnesses—such as adults testifying to domestic violence, older adults testifying to elder abuse, or adult witnesses suffering intellectual or emotional challenges that would make it difficult for them to communicate effectively on the stand. The legislation at this writing is pending approval in the Senate and Assembly of New York State.

Our involvement in the court system and legislative process as advocates for one vulnerable young witness has led to our advocacy for a more trauma-sensitive court system for *all* child (and vulnerable adult) witnesses. Judith Herman (2003) has poignantly expressed her concern about the experience of child witnesses in the U.S. court system: "Indeed, if one set out intentionally to design a system for provoking symptoms of posttraumatic stress disorder, it might look very much like a court of law" (p. 159). There are enormous differences and conflicts between the ways that mental health professionals elicit trauma narratives in a therapeutic manner and the requirements of the legal system. As Herman explains, "Victims need an opportunity to tell their stories in their own way, in a setting of their choice; the court requires them to respond to a set of yes–no questions that break down any personal attempt to construct a coherent and meaningful narrative" (p. 160).

Perhaps the most troubling and potentially harmful aspect of courtroom testimony for the child is the face-to-face confrontation with the defendant. Herman (2003) states, "Victims often need to control or limit their exposure to specific reminders of the trauma; the court requires them to relive the experience by directly confronting the perpetrator" (p. 160). Child sexual abuse, to which the child is often the only witness, is by far the most likely cause of a child's testifying in court (Goodman, 2005). Is it any wonder, given the intimidating conditions of a courtroom trial that surveys of adults who acknowledge that they were sexually abused as children reveal that only 10% ever disclosed their sexual abuse during childhood (Lyon, 2014)? Abused children are particularly at risk when testifying because the legal process itself is an ongoing trauma reminder (Saxe, Ellis, & Kaplow, 2009).

Many children, too terrified and intimidated to give direct testimony in court, are deprived of any sense of justice, let alone compassion. Lyon and Dente (2012) report that many criminal convictions around the country have been overturned because children's out-of-court statements were admitted after they failed to testify. "These cases include allegations of sexual abuse, physical abuse, and domestic violence, the types of cases in which child witnesses are often called to testify" (p. 1183). The U.S. Supreme Court's *Crawford* decision in 2004 has made it difficult to prosecute cases in which the child witness initially reported the crime to the authorities but later was too afraid, intimidated, or traumatized to testify (Lyon & Dente, 2012).

The legal system has unwittingly and unintentionally contributed to the silencing of child and adolescent victims because of the high-stress conditions that courtroom trial conditions impose on young witnesses, many of whom are already traumatized by their exposure to abuse or violence. Under the best of circumstances, youth typically disclose these events with significant reluctance and great emotional distress to a trusted family member or a clinical therapist with whom they have developed sufficient trust to risk such exposure. Events like sexual abuse or witnessing violent crimes, particularly when such events involve a family member, are inextricably linked to stigma and a painful sense of shame—factors that often effectively silence victims, particularly children and adolescents.

Emotionally disturbing questions during testimony can trigger acute trauma reactions. One of the most common responses in children is dissociation, which is a common coping response when an experience is terrifying to the point of overwhelming a person's psychological resources. When young people are exposed to potential threats or stressors, their brains initiate a cascade of events known as the "stress response system." The brain releases numerous transmitters, hormones such as cortisol, and peptides throughout the body, all directed at coping with the stressful situation (Crenshaw, 2013; Thoman, 2014). These internal threat-induced responses interfere with cognitive and language processing at the exact times when youth are called upon to give precise and clear answers to questions during court testimony. In addition, the stress factors tend to increase under cross-examination because the defense attorney in the adversarial position may ask questions in a hostile or angry tone, employ questions using developmentally inappropriate language, or ask the same questions in many different ways to create confusion and establish inconsistencies in a child's testimony.

CONCLUSION

The two of us were gratified to be part of a history-making court case that has established a strong legal basis for using courthouse dogs in New York and has influenced this movement throughout the country. When Jessica and Rosie went to trial in 2011, there were 10 states that allowed the use of courthouse dogs; at this writing, there are now 26. When we started, we only had Jessica as the focus of our concern and caring. We now recognize that child and adolescent witnesses in courts throughout the United States are often deprived of their chance for justice, due to the intimidating nature of the legal process superimposed on the trauma they have already suffered. Our effort at this point, in honor of the courage and heroic feat of Jessica and Rosie, is to join with other crime victim advocates in efforts to achieve the goal of making U.S. Courtrooms more sensitive to the needs of all traumatized victims.

STUDY QUESTIONS

1. What cultural barriers are important to consider in working with a vulnerable child witness whose culture, religious background, or cultural beliefs are different from your own? What may be some challenges the therapist and vulnerable child witness may face in sessions, due to cultural differences and language barriers?
2. How do you think Jessica benefited from utilizing art in her therapy sessions? What other creative arts strategies could be utilized with nonverbal, vulnerable child witnesses?

3. Do you think Jessica faced challenges after the completion of the trial? If so, what might some of those challenges have been?

4. In what ways did Rosie help Jessica to find her voice? How did Rosie's presence contribute to Jessica's ability to communicate effectively on the stand during her testimony?

5. What changes should be made within the U.S. court system to make the courts more trauma-sensitive in the treatment of child witnesses? What are some of the barriers to creating such changes?

REFERENCES

Cavett, A. M., & Drewes, A. A. (2012). Play applications and trauma-specific components. In J. A. Cohen, A. P. Mannarino, & E. Deblinger (Eds.), *Trauma-focused CBT for children and adolescents: Treatment applications* (pp. 124–148). New York: Guilford Press.

Chur-Hansen, A., McArthur, M., & Winefield, H. (2014). Animal-assisted interventions in children's hospitals: A critical review of the literature. *Anthrozoös, 27*(1), 5–18.

Cohen, J. A., Mannarino, A. P., & Deblinger, E. (2006). *Treating trauma and traumatic grief in children and adolescents.* New York: Guilford Press.

Cohen, J. A., Mannarino, A. P., & Deblinger, E. (Eds.). (2012). *Trauma-focused CBT for children and adolescents: Treatment applications.* New York: Guilford Press.

Cohen, J. A., Mannarino, A. P., Kleithermes, M., & Murray, L. A. (2012). Trauma-focused CBT for youth with complex trauma. *Child Abuse and Neglect, 36,* 528–541.

Cohen, J. A., Mannarino, A. P., & Murray, L. A. (2011). Trauma-focused CBT for youth who experience ongoing traumas. *Child Abuse and Neglect, 35,* 637–646.

Cohen, J. A., Mannarino, A. P., & Navarro, D. (2012). Residential treatment. In J. A. Cohen, A. P. Mannarino, & E. Deblinger (Eds.), *Trauma-focused CBT for children and adolescents: Treatment applications* (pp. 73–102). New York: Guilford Press.

Crawford v. Washington, 541 U.S. 36 (2004).

Crenshaw, D. A. (2012, June). Secrets told to Ivy: Animal-assisted play therapy in a children's residential facility. *Play Therapy,* pp. 6–9.

Crenshaw, D. A. (2013). Trauma-sensitive courts. Retrieved from *http://courthousedogs.com/legal_trauma_sensitive.html.*

Crenshaw, D. A. (2014, December). Advocacy for vulnerable child witnesses. *Play Therapy,* pp. 20–23.

Crenshaw, D. A., & Alstadt, C. (2011). *A study of the adverse childhood events (ACES) in the last 100 admissions to the Children's Home of Poughkeepsie.* Unpublished study.

Crenshaw, D. A., & Stella, L. (2011, December). The play therapist as an advocate for children in the court system. *Play Therapy,* pp. 6–9.

Crime Victim Compensation and Support Authority. (2010). *Child victims in the Union—Rights and empowerment.* Umea, Sweden: Author. Retrieved September

24, 2011, from *www.unicef.org/ceecis/Child_victims_in_the_Union_CURE.pdf.*

Cunningham, A., & Hurley, P. (2007). A full and candid account: Using special accommodations and testimonial aids to facilitate the testimony of children. Retrieved September 24, 2011, from *www.lfcc.on.ca/full_and_candid_account.html.*

Dellinger, M. (2009). Using dogs for emotional support of testifying victims of crime. *Animal Law Review, 15*(2), 171–192.

Dietz, T. J., Davis, D., & Pennings, J. (2012). Evaluating animal-assisted therapy in group treatment for child sexual abuse. *Journal of Child Sexual Abuse, 21*, 665–683.

Felitti, V. J., Anda, R. F., Nordenberg, D., Williamson, D. F., Spitz, A. M., Edwards, V., et al. (1998). Relationship of childhood abuse and household dysfunction to many of the leading causes of death in adults: The Adverse Childhood Experiences (ACE) Study. *American Journal of Preventive Medicine, 14*(4), 245–258.

Friesen, L. (2010). Exploring animal-assisted programs with children in school and therapeutic contexts. *Early Childhood Education Journal, 37*, 261–267.

Gaskill, R., & Perry, B. D. (2012). Child sexual abuse, traumatic experiences, and their impact on the developing brain. In P. Goodyear-Brown (Ed.), *Handbook of child sexual abuse: Identification, assessment, and treatment* (pp. 30–47). Hoboken, NJ: Wiley.

Gaskill, R., & Perry, B. D. (2014). The neurobiological power of play: Using the Neurosequential Model of Therapeutics to guide play in the healing process. In C. A. Malchiodi & D. A. Crenshaw (Eds.), *Creative arts and play therapy for attachment problems* (pp. 178–194). New York: Guilford Press.

Goodman, G. S. (2005). Wailing babies in her wake. *American Psychologist, 60*(8), 872–881.

Herman, J. L. (2003). The mental health of crime victims: Impact of legal intervention. *Journal of Traumatic Stress, 16*(2), 159–166.

Kruger, K. A., & Serpell, J. A. (2006). Animal-assisted interventions in mental health: Definitions and theoretical foundations. In A. H. Fine (Ed.), *Handbook on animal-assisted therapy: Theoretical foundations and guidelines for practice* (pp. 21–38). Amsterdam: Elsevier Academic Press.

Lange, A. M., Cox, J. A., Bernert, D. J., & Jenkins, C. D. (2007). Is counseling going to the dogs?: An exploratory study related to the inclusion of an animal in group counseling with adolescents. *Journal of Creativity in Mental Health, 2*(2), 17–31.

Lefkowitz, C., Paharia, I., Prout, M., Debiak, D., & Bleiberg, J. (2005). Animal assisted prolonged exposure: A treatment for survivors of sexual assault suffering posttraumatic stress disorder. *Society and Animals, 13*, 275–295.

Lyon, T. D. (2014). Interviewing children. *Annual Review of Law and Social Science, 10*, 73–89.

Lyon, T. D., & Dente, J. A. (2012). Child witnesses and the confrontation clause. *Journal of Criminal Law and Criminology, 102*(4), 1181–1232.

Makin, K. (1999, October 16). Top courts stands up for child witnesses: Judges say using hearsay evidence can be better than making a child testify. *The Globe and Mail* [Toronto], p. A1.

Maslow, A. (1943). A theory of human motivation. *Psychological Review, 50*(4), 370–396.

Murphy, L. K., Cohen, J. A., & Mannarino, A. P. (2013). Trauma-focused cognitive behavioral therapy for youth who experience continuous trauma exposure. *Peace and Conflict: Journal of Peace Psychology, 19*(2), 180–195.

Nader, K. (2011). Trauma in children and adolescents: Issues related to age and complex traumatic reactions. *Journal of Child and Adolescent Trauma, 4*, 161–180.

Nimer, J., & Lundahl, B. (2007). Animal-assisted therapy: A meta-analysis. *Anthrozoös, 20*, 225–238.

Parish-Plass, N. (2008). Animal-assisted therapy with children suffering from insecure attachment due to abuse and neglect: A method to lower the risk of intergenerational transmission of abuse? *Clinical Child Psychology and Psychiatry, 13*(1), 7–30.

Parish-Plass, N. (2013). *Animal-assisted psychotherapy: Theory, issues, and practice.* West Lafayette, IN: Purdue University Press.

Perry, B. D. (2006). Applying principles of neurodevelopment to clinical work with maltreated and traumatized children. In N. B. Webb (Ed.), *Working with traumatized youth in child welfare* (pp. 27–52). New York: Guilford Press.

Perry, B. D. (2009). Examining child maltreatment through a neurodevelopmental lens: Clinical application of the Neurosequential Model of Therapeutics. *Journal of Loss and Trauma, 14*, 240–255.

Perry, B. D., & Dobson, C. L. (2013). Application of the Neurosequential Model of Therapeutics (NMT) in maltreated children. In J. D. Ford & C. A. Courtois (Eds.), *Treating complex traumatic stress disorders in children and adolescents* (pp. 249–260). New York: Guilford Press.

Prothman, A., Bienert, M., & Ettrich, C. (2006). Dogs in child psychotherapy: Effects on state of mind. *Anthrozoös, 19*, 265–277.

Sandoval, G. (2010). Court facility dogs: Easing the apprehensive witness. *The Colorado Lawyer, 39*(17), 17–23.

Saxe, G., Ellis, H., & Kaplow, J. B. (2009). *Collaborative treatment of traumatized children and teens: The trauma systems therapy approach.* New York: Guilford Press.

Thoman, D. H. (2014). Testifying minors: Pre-trial strategies to reduce anxiety in child witnesses. *Nevada Law Journal, 14*, 236–267.

Thompson, M. J. (2009). Animal-assisted play therapy: Canines as co-therapists. In G. R. Walz, J. C. Bleuer, & R. K. Yep (Eds.), *Compelling counseling interventions: VISTAS 2009* (pp. 199–209). Alexandria, VA: American Counseling Association.

Trotter, K. S., Chandler, C. K., Goodwin-Bond, D., & Casey, J. (2008). A comparative study of group equine assisted counseling with at-risk children and adolescents. *Journal of Creativity in Mental Health, 3*(3), 254–284.

Tsai, C.-C., Friedmann, E., & Thomas, S. A. (2010). The effect of animal-assisted therapy on stress responses in hospitalized children. *Anthrozoös, 23*(2), 245–258.

van der Kolk, B. (2005). Developmental trauma disorder: Toward a rational diagnosis for children with complex trauma histories. *Psychiatric Annals, 35*(5), 401–408.

van der Kolk, B. (2006). Clinical implications of neuroscience research in PTSD. *Annals of the New York Academy of Sciences, 107*, 277–293.

van der Kolk, B. (2014). *The body keeps the score: Brain, mind, and body in the healing of trauma.* New York: Viking Press.

VanFleet, R. (2008). *Play therapy with kids and canines: Benefits for children's developmental and psychosocial health.* Sarasota, FL: Professional Resource Press.

VanFleet, R., & Colţea, C. G. (2012). Helping children with ASD through canine-assisted play therapy. In L. Gallo-Lopez & L. C. Rubin (Eds.), *Play-based interventions for children and adolescents with autism spectrum disorders* (pp. 39–72). New York: Routledge.

VanFleet, R., & Faa-Thompson, T. (2010). The case for using animal assisted play therapy. *British Journal of Play Therapy, 6*, 4–18.

VanFleet, R., & Faa-Thompson, T. (2012). The power of play, multiplied. *Play Therapy Magazine of the British Association of Play Therapists, 70*, 7–10.

VanFleet, R., & Faa-Thompson, T. (2014). Including animals in play therapy with young children and families. In M. R. Jalongo (Ed.), *Teaching compassion: Humane education in early childhood* (pp. 89–107). New York: Springer.

VanFleet, R., & Faa-Thompson, T. (2015). Animal-assisted play therapy. In D. A. Crenshaw & A. L. Stewart (Eds.), *Play therapy: A comprehensive guide to theory and practice* (pp. 201–214). New York: Guilford Press.

Vasudevan, V., Ibrahim, A., & Kamini, R. S. (2007, June 26). Children to give evidence without being seen in court. *New Straits Times* [Kuala Lumpur, Malaysia], p. 14.

Weiss, D. (2009). Equine assisted therapy and Theraplay. In E. Munns (Ed.), *Applications of family and group Theraplay* (pp. 225–233). Lanham, MD: Jason Aronson.

Chapter 18

Crisis Intervention Therapy with Children, Adolescents, and Family Members after Shootings in the Community

NANCY BOYD WEBB
VALERIE L. DRIPCHAK

Since the terrorist attacks of September 11, 2001, Americans have witnessed—and the mass media have reported—numerous episodes of violent shootings that killed and wounded innocent bystanders, ranging in age from preschoolers to the elderly. These tragic events have occurred at various times of day in various community settings, such as schools, a movie theater, university campuses, a naval base, and an outdoor political rally in front of a supermarket. For surviving victims, witnesses, and families of the victims and bystanders, the tragedies have resulted in a loss of a sense of safety and predictability in their worlds. This increased sense of vulnerability has made children and adolescents aware that adults cannot always protect them or their loved ones. Some survivors have begun to "watch their backs," because they now consider the world a very dangerous and unpredictable place.

The total number of deaths by firearms in the United States in 2013 was approximately 32,000 (*unconservatives.about.com*). This compares with about 1,609 people who lost a spouse or partner in the 9/11 World Trade Center attacks, and 3,051 children who lost a parent ("The Awful Numbers," 2002). Unpredictable shootings victimize young children, teens, their friends, parents, family members, and teachers. Because this problem is so widespread and growing, it is essential that mental health specialists, schools, and community programs serving young people prepare for the prospect of future tragic deaths, with plans for crisis intervention and bereavement counseling for the traumatized survivors, family members, and friends of the shooting victims.

This chapter first reviews the phenomenon of traumatic bereavement as it affects young children and adolescents, and then provides examples that demonstrate possible responses among schoolchildren of different ages to deaths caused by traumatic shootings. Because mass shootings affect *all* members of a community, it may be difficult for adult family members who are grieving to focus adequately on helping the young survivors. Therefore, a therapist may include a parent in conjoint crisis intervention play therapy with an affected child to encourage a mutual grieving and recovery process. Other forms of crisis intervention play therapy include individual counseling and support groups for traumatically bereaved relatives and friends of the victims.

TRAUMATIC BEREAVEMENT IN CHILDREN AND ADOLESCENTS

In this chapter, "traumatic bereavement" refers to grief and other reactions to an event (e.g., a shooting) in which one or more deaths or life-threatening injuries occurred. The combination of grief and trauma presents a challenge for therapists because the survivors' traumatic memories interfere with the process of remembering the person(s) who died (Gil, 2010; Nader, 1997; Webb, 2010). The term "childhood traumatic grief" has been used by Mannarino and Cohen (2011) to refer to a situation in which posttraumatic reactions hinder a young person's progression through the mourning process. Traumatic grief differs from ordinary bereavement because preoccupation with the details of the trauma dominates and blocks the normal grieving process (Cohen, Mannarino, & Greenberg, 2002; Pynoos, 1992). As a result, a therapist must address components of the trauma before the individual can tolerate and process his or her grief (Nader, 1996, 1997; Webb, 2010). Some specific treatment techniques intended to help a child or adolescent deal with traumatic memories, so that he or she can move on to grief processing, include the following:

- Stress management exercises, such as relaxation, guided imagery, safe-place drawings, and age-appropriate deep breathing exercises (e.g., asking the youth to pretend to blow up a balloon or blow bubbles).
- Psychoeducation about typical reactions to trauma (e.g., "It's OK to be scared and to have bad dreams; you'll feel better after a while").
- The creation of a story about the traumatic death (the "trauma narrative"). This is done gradually, at the individual's developmental and tolerance levels, over several sessions. Sometimes a young person draws a picture of the trauma; at other times, he or she may use dolls, puppets, or other toys to recreate it.
- Correction of inaccurate cognitions (such as guilt about what caused the death, and/or how it might have been prevented).
- Creation of a pretrauma (intact) memory image of the deceased. This may be accomplished by looking at old photographs that stimulate positive memories.

All of these approaches require great sensitivity on the part of the therapist, in order to avoid flooding the youth with anxiety related to the trauma and with feelings of grief about the loss. The timing and pacing of the work will vary, depending on developmental factors and on the youth's ego strengths and coping resources (Crenshaw, 2006). The therapist must move carefully between activities that generate anxiety and those that help to contain it. After the child or teen has begun to attain some distance from the trauma, and to put it clearly in the past, he or she may feel able to begin the mourning process.

Posttraumatic Play

Children often express their symptoms of trauma through their play. Whereas typical play tends to be free-flowing and to change over time, the term "posttraumatic play" has been used by Malchiodi (2008) and others (e.g., Gil, 2006; Shelby & Felix, 2005) to describe the play of children that is ritualistic, constricted, repetitious, and without resolution in enacting a traumatic event. In this type of play, children are not in control of their fantasies, and they often remain trapped with internal conflicts in their play (Dripchak, 2007).

As mentioned in Chapter 3, Terr (1989, p. 15) notes that "traumatized youngsters appear to indulge in play at much older ages than do nontraumatized youngsters." This is probably because they do not want to remember and talk about their frightening experiences. Therefore, the opportunity to play or engage in creative activities such as art facilitates the *symbolic* expression of experiences that are too horrible to verbalize.

Developmental Considerations

Attachment and Loss

Biologically driven attachment responses are universal, and they exist for the purpose of providing protection and security. The hallmark of attachment is proximity-seeking behavior, which a toddler achieves by staying close to the important people in his or her life. The typical preschool child has multiple attachments, with the mother generally serving as the primary attachment figure, while the father and other regular caregivers may function as secondary attachment figures (Davies, 2011). As the child gradually develops the ability to form a mental representation of significant people ("object constancy"), he or she begins to be able to regulate anxiety without immediate help from a parent (Davies, 2011). However, this progress is sporadic and subject to reversal under stressful conditions: The young child who is upset or frightened quickly reverts to wanting to be close to a parent for comfort and security. When an attachment figure disappears suddenly from the child's life because of death, the youngster may experience intense feelings of distress, confusion, anger, and separation anxiety.

The impact of any unpredictable traumatic death, such as occurs in motor vehicle accidents, war, natural disasters, or shootings, depends on the young person's and family's circumstances before the death, the child's age, the circumstances of the traumatic event, and the nature of the community response. Webb refers to the assessment of these factors as the "tripartite assessment" and has described it in Chapter 1 of this volume.

The Preschooler's Understanding of Death and World Events

Children's understanding of death parallels their cognitive development (Webb, 2010). As reviewed in detail previously, the concepts of the permanence, irreversibility, and universality of death develop gradually over time. A preschool child believes in magic and typically has an exaggerated view of his or her own power. Piaget (cited in Davies, 2011) describes this stage as characterized by the child's inability to discriminate between thoughts and deeds. This combination of egocentric and magical thinking makes most preschool children unable to fully comprehend the reality and finality of death. In addition, they cannot understand causality and have a very literal and sometimes distorted view of how and why a particular death has occurred. When a preschooler comes to realize that no amount of magic or ritual will bring a dead person back, he or she may become very confused and angry.

Cultural, religious, and family beliefs influence how a family responds to any death and whether or not the children are included in various ceremonies. For example, therapists working with bereaved Christian families need to be alert for preschool children's possible misconceptions regarding their families' beliefs and teachings about heaven and God. It is very difficult for a preschool child to comprehend the distinction between the body and the spirit; when he or she hears a minister or priest say, for instance, "God wanted your father and took him to heaven," the child may begin to resent God and/or to wonder whether and when it might be possible to travel to heaven to pay a visit to the dead parent!

The Elementary-School-Age Child's Understanding of Death and World Events

Children of elementary school age gradually understand that death is irreversible and that it will happen to everybody "sometime." However, children of this age believe that death happens primarily to the elderly and weak, and that young people their age usually do not die. When children reach 9 or 10 years of age, they may develop a more realistic understanding of death, although they still may have difficulty dealing with it. In summary (see Ch. 1 of Webb, 2010, for a fuller review), some typical responses of school-age children (6–12 years old) to death include the following:

- They may be unable to deal with death.
- They may use denial to cope with the loss, and may act as if the death did not occur.

- They may hide their feelings in an effort not to seem childish, and may do their grieving in private (this is especially true for boys).
- They may feel guilty and/or different from peers because of the death.
- They may express anger or irritability rather than sadness.
- They may overcompensate for feelings of grief by becoming overly helpful and taking care of others (this is especially true for girls).
- They may develop somatic symptoms or hypochondria.
- Anxiety may occur, due to increased fear of death.

This list can be used as a guide for therapists attempting to help elementary-school-age children after a traumatic event such as a shooting.

The Adolescent's Understanding of Death and World Events

After age 9 or 10, when the youngster's thinking becomes increasingly logical, children acquire a more realistic perception of the finality and irreversibility of death. Bereaved adolescents may respond as follows:

- They may feel helpless, frightened, or numb.
- They may behave in a manner younger than their years (regression).
- They may feel conflicted between the desire to behave in an adult manner and the wish to be taken care of as children.
- They may experience guilt about typical teen behaviors, which were a normal part of the individuating process, in which they were engaging at the time of the death.
- They may use anger to defend against feelings of helplessness.
- They may respond in a self-centered or callous way.

Deaths Resulting from Deliberate Actions

The traumatic deaths of 9/11 involved not only the tragedy of mass destruction and multiple deaths, but the additional complicating fact that these were caused deliberately with the intent to bring about the maximum of psychological, economic, and physical distress to the citizens of the United States. Since that time, numerous shootings have received extensive attention in the mass media, and the reports of each shooting have stated detailed information about the perpetrator's identity, the nature of the weapon(s) used, and the perpetrator's preparation to carry out the shooting. Parents and teachers often struggle to decide what and how much to tell the children about the perpetrators. Guidelines posted on the Internet following the 9/11 tragedy recommended that parents relay limited information to their children about the event and the perpetrators, while also trying to reestablish the children's usual routine as much as possible (Brymer et al., 2006). When a youth's parent is among the victims, it will be extremely difficult for the surviving mother or father to muster the emotional resources to carry out these guidelines, and the parent and family will benefit from support and counseling from friends and professional therapists.

Mediating Factors Following Shooting Deaths

The Critical Role of a Surviving Parent

Numerous articles and chapters in the professional literature emphasize the importance of surviving parents' being able to deal with their own traumatic grief in order to be able to support their children (Osofsky, 2004; Rossman, Bingham, & Emde, 1997). According to Van Horn and Lieberman (2004, p. 118), "The caregiver's capacity to cope with a child's response after a trauma has been found to be the strongest predictor of child outcome, with increased levels of maternal support predicting lower levels of symptomatology and higher levels of adjustment in children." The same principle applies to the need of grieving adolescents for support. Therapists must focus on helping these parents so that they can then more effectively attend to their children.

Influence of Extended Family and Community Supports

The comfort and support of extended family members can be critical for a family that suffers a death in a shooting. Families always tend to come together at times of bereavement, but situations of *public* bereavement add a further layer of grief on top of their personal loss. Often the tragic event affects many people, as in the case of the Gabrielle Giffords shooting in Arizona in 2011, following which there was an outpouring of grief and helping efforts in the community and from the nation (Giffords & Kelly, 2011). Such displays of mass mourning and support may be quite meaningful to adults, but probably are irrelevant to young people who are focused on their personal loss of a father, mother, friend, or grandparent. The threat of unknown danger presents an additional source of stress for children and teens bereaved by traumatic shootings because as children age, their ability to comprehend danger increases (Fletcher, 1996). When children are told that the "bad guys killed your father [or mother] and a lot of other people," the world can then seem a very dangerous place.

TREATMENT ALTERNATIVES FOR TRAUMATIC GRIEF

Numerous examples in this book describe different play therapy approaches that focus on the individual child, or the parent and child (Echterling & Stewart, 2008), and on adolescents in group formats. It is not possible to discuss all treatment alternatives here, but we have created two case examples to illustrate two different clinical interventions. One is trauma-focused cognitive-behavioral therapy (TF-CBT), and the other is parent–child conjoint therapy. The examples are based on our extensive clinical experiences with trauma victims of all ages. The cases are typical of interventions that are appropriate for use with traumatized children following shooting incidents that they witnessed or they learned about later. Space limitations do not permit inclusion of an example of a group with traumatically bereaved adolescents, but Haen (Chapter 12, this volume) discusses the use of expressive therapy in groups for adolescents with complex trauma.

Evidence-Based and/or Evidence-Informed Treatment Options

Despite the changes made in the *Diagnostic and Statistical Manual of Mental Disorders*, fifth edition (American Psychiatric Association, 2013) to the diagnosis of posttraumatic stress disorder (PTSD) in children, the helping professions continue to remain divided on the use of treatment practices. However, there is growing agreement that when children are left untreated, they may experience serious problems later. Therefore, doing nothing is not an option.

Glicken (2009) suggests that in the current practice of psychotherapy with children, professionals often rely on "clinical wisdom," with little evidence that what is being done actually works. This type of practice is based on intuition, subjectivity, and years of experience, which some therapists still believe allow them to make their own decisions. However, members of the helping professions are increasingly seeking treatment approaches based on evidence-based practice (EBP). The Council for Training in Evidence-Based Practice (2008) defines EBP as "making decisions about how to promote healthful behaviors by integrating the best available research evidence with practitioner expertise and other resources, and with the characteristics, state, needs, values and the preferences of those who will be affected" (p. 3). For the time being, a starting point for research in EBP can be anecdotal reports and single-case designs.

Many studies of the effectiveness of different therapies in reducing child trauma symptoms favor the use of cognitive-behavioral therapy (CBT) over other methods. Possibly because the goals of CBT are so specific, they lend themselves more easily to measurement. Nevertheless, Webb (2006) has argued earlier that the fact that other child treatment approaches, such as play therapy, have not been studied in comparable controlled outcome research does not mean that these treatment methods may not also help traumatized children.

Chapter 3 reviews some of the most current research on EBP in child trauma treatment (Bratton, Ray, Rhine, & Jones, 2005; Cohen, Mannarino, & Deblinger, 2006), but these studies are still quite limited in number, and some child therapists prefer to use the terminology "evidence-*informed* practice" to include approaches that look promising in terms of practitioners' and clients' satisfaction with the outcomes.

CBT and TF-CBT

Researchers on CBT methods have reported high levels of success in the treatment of traumatized children and adolescents. The early work in what is now called TF-CBT focused on young victims of sexual abuse (Cohen & Mannarino, 1993, 1996). It merged play therapy methods such as the use of dolls, puppets, and art with cognitive techniques such as thought stopping, cognitive reframing, positive imagery, and parent training in a short-term (12-session) model, which was found to bring about significant symptom improvement. Neubauer, Deblinger, and Sieger (Chapter 6, this volume) describe the use of the TF-CBT approach with an adolescent victim of sexual abuse and witness of domestic violence.

Cohen and colleagues (2001) have developed a TF-CBT model to treat traumatic grief in children. The main components of this model are summarized by the acronym PRACTICE: Psychoeducation and parenting; Relaxation; Affective expression and modulation; Cognitive coping; Trauma narrative development and processing; *In vivo* exposure; Conjoint parent–child sessions; and Enhancing safety and future development. The research findings indicate that children and caregivers who received TF-CBT showed significantly greater improvements with respect to PTSD than children who received child-centered play therapy, and these improvements were sustained over a 1-year follow-up (Deblinger et al., 2012; Neubauer et al., Chapter 6, this volume).

Some of the key elements in TF-CBT involve the use of cognitive techniques, such as relaxation methods, increasing the individual's sense of safety, increasing his or her ability to discuss the traumatic death without extreme distress, and correcting any misconceptions about the trauma. The following case illustrates this method with a child witness to a shooting in which he lost his father. The case is blended from several others, with all identifying information changed.

The Case of Joe, Age 8

BACKGROUND

Joe, an 8-year-old boy, lived with his parents, Ann and Staff Sergeant Walter Syms, and his younger sister, Ashley (age 2). Sergeant Syms had been stationed at an Army base in the Pacific Northwest with his family for the 2 years prior to the traumatic event.

TRAUMATIC EVENT

The incident occurred on a Saturday morning when Joe was visiting the base commissary with his dad. While they were selecting a few items for a picnic that the family planned to take later in the day, a soldier came into the commissary with a loaded gun. Joe heard him mumble some words, but he couldn't make out what the man was saying. The man's voice was drowned out by the sounds of a gun firing a series of bullets. In what seemed like an instant, Joe felt someone push him to the floor and then felt his father lying on top of him. Then there was silence, but Joe felt as if he could not move. Minutes later, some soldiers rushed into the commissary and told everyone to remain where they were and be quiet. Joe tried to whisper to his father; but his father did not respond, so Joe thought that he had to be silent as well.

After what seemed like a long time, Joe was helped to his feet, and he saw people lying on the floor covered with blood. Joe then saw his father on the ground, surrounded by people who were trying to take care of him. Joe was taken outside, and he saw his mother standing by one of the ambulances. She rushed to him, gave him a hug, and carried him to the ambulance; they then went to the hospital. On the way, Joe asked if his father was going to be at the hospital too, but his mom did not answer him. He later learned that his father had died when the gunman shot him. Three other people also were killed by the gunman, who subsequently killed himself. Ann took her two children and returned to her family's home out of state to make funeral arrangements.

SYMPTOM PRESENTATION

Ann decided to stay with her family at least until the end of the school year, so 2 weeks after the funeral, she enrolled Joe in a new school. As time went on, she noticed that Joe was undergoing some changes. He was having nightmares about "monsters" taking away his mother and sister. He began to refuse to go to school and would cry continually whenever his mother left the house. Joe also became hypervigilant and strongly reacted to any loud noise by running out of the room with his hands cupped over his ears, screaming. During this time, Ann was trying to deal with her own grief and trauma after the death of her husband, so she decided to seek professional help for Joe.

INTAKE TELEPHONE CONTACT

Throughout the initial intake call, Ann described the issues surrounding the death of her husband, and Joe's reactions to his being present when the shooting occurred. Ann found it reassuring to learn that Joe's responses were not unusual, and she was further validated by the therapist's reassurance that she was doing "all the right things to help Joe," including contacting the agency for help. The therapist reviewed the symptoms of childhood PTSD with Ann, as well as how TF-CBT would be used to help alleviate these issues. Joe and his mother were given an appointment.

INITIAL SESSION: PSYCHOEDUCATION

During the first session, Joe and his mother were seen together. They discussed the reasons for being there, and learned what the process would be. This introduction helped the therapist to begin establishing rapport with Joe and Ann. After validating Joe's feelings, the therapist taught Joe a relaxation exercise of blowing bubbles in a slow and methodical fashion. Future appointments were set.

PARENTING SESSIONS WITH THE MOTHER, ANN

Several sessions were spent with Ann in reviewing parenting skills. During these sessions, the therapist and Ann discussed times when it might be best to ignore certain of Joe's behaviors, and when to address them. There also was a discussion of how to manage Joe's nightmares. The plan was to leave the door of Joe's bedroom slightly ajar, so that when Ann heard her son crying at night, she could go to his room and comfort him.

Ann was also informed about other behaviors that might occur—for example, selective attention, irritability, or peer relationship issues. Although Ann had not noticed any of these responses from Joe, this discussion provided her with some information about possible future occurrences.

RELAXATION TECHNIQUES WITH JOE

Joe liked blowing bubbles, and this activity helped him to relax. However, Joe continued to dwell on some scary thoughts that he said his "mind would go to." The therapist introduced the concept of "thought stopping," which involves stopping intrusive thoughts and replacing them with pleasant ones. This technique was practiced in sessions, as well as at home and then in school.

AFFECTIVE EXPRESSION AND REGULATION TECHNIQUES WITH JOE

Early in the therapeutic process, the therapist and Joe worked together to identify as many of his feelings as possible. Each of these feelings was rated on an "emotion thermometer" (see Figure 18.1) for intensity of affect, as well as in terms of "what I like to feel" and "what I don't like to feel."

Storytelling helped Joe express different emotions in a variety of situations. Ann also was taught this strategy, and she used it with Joe at home. This exercise permitted Joe to develop a higher level of comfort with expressing his feelings. However, the circumstances surrounding his father's death were not brought up at this point in the therapy.

COGNITIVE COPING AND PROCESSING WITH JOE

The differences between thoughts and feelings were emphasized with examples from Joe's own life. One example Joe gave was when his mother reprimanded him after he took one of his sister's toys away from her. Joe was able to identify his thought as being "I should be able to play with her toys because I let her play with some of mine." He further recognized that he felt "mad" about this. The next step in the process was to have Joe learn how to come up

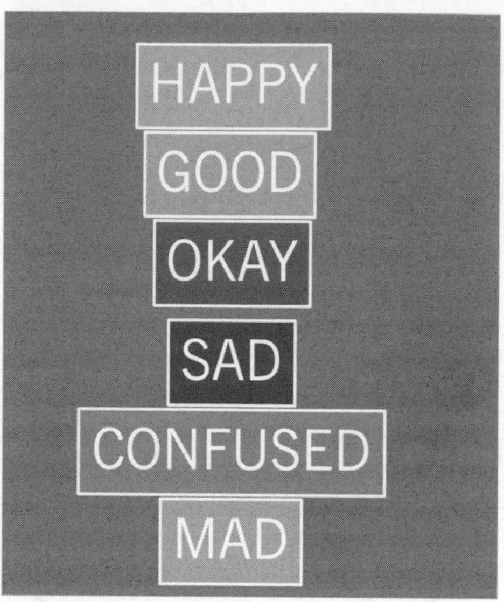

FIGURE 18.1. Emotion thermometer blocks.

with a different thought, in order to generate a more positive feeling. Joe came up with the idea that "I probably could have played with Ashley's toy, if I'd asked." He said that he would then feel "good."

After Joe was able to differentiate between thoughts and feelings, he was shown a picture of a triangle with the words "thoughts," "feelings," and "behaviors" printed at its angles (see Figure 18.2). The therapist discussed with Joe the relationships among these concepts; and they practiced with "real-life" examples of how to change thoughts, in order to generate different feelings and behaviors.

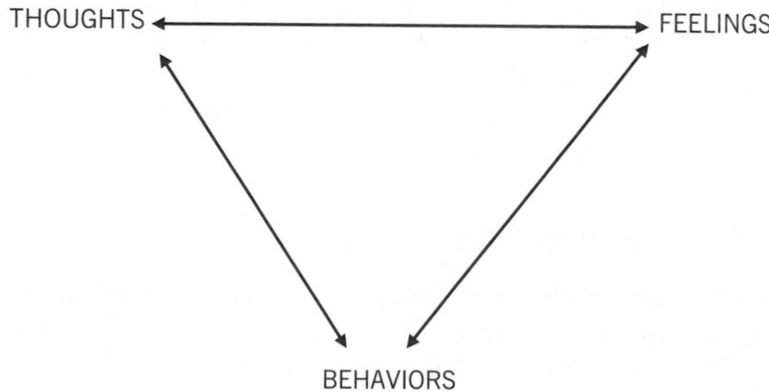

FIGURE 18.2. The cognitive triangle. From Dorsey and Deblinger (2012, p. 60). Copyright 2012 by The Guilford Press. Adapted by permission.

TRAUMA NARRATIVE DEVELOPMENT AND PROCESSING

All the early therapy sessions led up to creating a "trauma narrative," which is the central focus in TF-CBT. The goal in doing this is to help the traumatized individual gradually become able to tolerate the memory of the trauma. Over the course of several sessions, Joe created a book about his father. This began by presenting some basic information, such as his dad's name, activities they had enjoyed doing together (fishing, playing, and watching baseball games), the names of his mother and sister, and the nature of his dad's work in the Army. After writing this information in his book, Joe drew a picture of him and his dad fishing together.

In the next step, Joe was encouraged to talk about shopping for a family picnic. He described the store and the types of food that they would eat on a picnic. Joe then drew a picture of a family having a picnic.

The next step involved Joe's telling what happened before, during, and after the shooting, along with his thoughts and feelings at each stage. At particular intervals, the "emotion thermometer" was used to rate the intensity of his feelings and help him modulate his responses.

The therapist encouraged the narrative by asking Joe what was the worst part of this experience, and Joe drew a picture of "bodies that had blood around them." He added that he did not see any blood on his father, and drew a picture of his father in his uniform. As Joe shared his story during successive sessions, he provided more details; the therapist helped him "turn over" his thoughts to regulate his feelings.

IN VIVO MASTERY

Joe continued to have difficulties with being separated from his mom. Therefore, as he was finishing his book about his father, the therapist and Joe decided to create a plan for him to go to school and have other periods of separation from his mom. Ann also needed to be comfortable with the plan, which provided for gradual steps for separation between Joe and his mother. School was used as the initial focus, and Joe was given permission to use a telephone at specific intervals of the school day to call his mother. When Ann needed to be away from Joe, she in turn would contact him.

CONJOINT PARENT–CHILD SESSIONS

Each session with Joe was discussed with Ann, and there were times when Ann was included in the sessions with Joe. In this way, Ann was able to learn about the treatment methods and duplicate some of the approaches used in the sessions at home. This participation gave Ann a greater degree of involvement in her son's recovery process. The conjoint sessions also allowed Joe to share his trauma narrative with his mother and to experience a sense of pride about its creation. This helped to bring about more mother–son communication around the events of the trauma.

ENHANCING SAFETY AND FUTURE DEVELOPMENT

Another part of the TF-CBT model involves teaching skills to children to ensure their safety. In Joe's case, this evolved into reassurances that he had done the best thing possible during the shooting by lying still and listening to the rescue workers when they arrived on the scene.

FACILITATING JOE'S MOURNING PROCESS

Once Joe was able to complete his trauma narrative, it became possible for him to express his feelings of sadness and anger connected to the death of his father. He admitted to feeling guilty because his dad had chosen to lie on Joe's back and protect him. Instead, he wished he had run out of the store, so his dad would not have thought that he had to shield him. Sometimes at night he cried because he felt that his dad had died for him. He also cried because he missed his dad so much, and he missed his friends and his old school as well.

These feelings were normalized by the therapist, who said that good fathers and mothers always did everything possible to protect their children. The therapist explained to Joe that he had done exactly what his father wanted him to do. Ann was included during some of these sessions, and Joe and Ann took turns reading out loud from a book, *The Invisible String* (Karst & Stevenson, 2013). They took breaks from reading when Joe wanted to ask questions. The metaphor of the invisible string was used to suggest to Joe that he was "connected" to his dad in a very special way.

In continuing with the mourning process with Joe, the therapist helped Joe make a list of all the activities that he missed about his dad. Each activity was shared through a story that Joe told. In subsequent sessions, Joe and the therapist made another list of things that Joe would miss in the future without his dad. As "homework," Joe and his mother put together a shoebox of memories of Walter for Joe to keep in his room. Joe brought in the shoebox during one of the sessions and discussed each item (and memory) that was contained in the box, including a letter to his dad that he wrote during one of the sessions. During some of these appointments, Joe and Ann would become tearful and cry. These expressions of emotions were met with support in normalizing the process of grief. Eventually, Ann and Joe planned a special memorial celebration of Walter's life, which was held in a park with some friends and relatives.

COMMENTS

The use of TF-CBT requires specialized training. It is important not to move too quickly through the process. When it is done well, the outcomes for a child like Joe and his mother may have long-term successes.

Conjoint Parent–Child Therapy

Therapy with a parent and child together is referred to as "conjoint therapy." The focus of such therapy is on the parent–child relationship and how to improve it. There are several circumstances in which this approach may be considered. Webb (2010) suggests that it is useful when the child cannot tolerate any separation from the parent, as in the case of Joe. It also is used when a behavior modification program has been implemented, so that both parent and child can monitor progress. Another use is to improve the parent–child relationship and to help parent and child work through a shared issue, such as traumatic grief. This was the case in the example of Mary and her mother, below. This case is blended from several others, with all identifying information changed.

The Case of Mary, Age 5, and Her Mother, Jane

PRESENTING PROBLEM: REFERRAL INFORMATION

The referral was made by Mary's kindergarten teacher, who stated that Mary's behavior had changed drastically since her father's death 2 months ago at a political rally, where a lone gunman had shot 10 people dead and wounded 5 others. Mary was no longer interacting with the other children in her classroom, and often spent time just staring out the window. At home, Mary had become very clingy toward her mother, Jane. She followed Jane from room to room, and did not want to sleep alone in her bedroom at night. She was waking at night with bad dreams, and in the morning Jane had difficulty getting her ready for school. Since her husband's death, Jane herself had given up some of her usual activities (such as wanting to talk with her friends), and she had trouble even performing routine food shopping. She admitted that she cried a lot.

FAMILY BACKGROUND

Mary's father, John, was 37 years old when he died. He was a reporter for the local newspaper. Jane was 39 and not employed. Mary, age 5, was in kindergarten, and she liked her school.

John's parents and married brothers lived on the West Coast and did not have much contact with John and his family. Jane's parents lived close by, as did Jane's unmarried sister. There was frequent contact between Jane's family and her relatives. Mary was extremely close to her aunt, Susan, who spent a great deal of time with her during family get-togethers.

FIRST SESSION WITH JANE

After I (Nancy Boyd Webb, the therapist in this case) obtained information about her family and about Mary, as reported above, Jane began to cry and admitted that she resented being a mother when she herself felt so depleted. She said that her husband had always been kind and attentive to her feelings, and that now she felt alone. At times she wondered how she could carry on, but she admitted that her parents and sister provided great support, and that she owed it to her wonderful husband to take good care of his only child, Mary. I asked Jane if she would consider a bereavement group for herself; she said that she had gone to one session of a group, but couldn't stand to hear about everyone else's problems and didn't go back. Jane said that she was very concerned about Mary, and she hoped that I could help her, adding that she herself felt like a "basket case."

Assessment and Treatment Plan

Because it was apparent that both Mary and her mother were suffering from traumatic bereavement, conjoint parent–child therapy was the treatment of choice in this case.

Mary's clinging behavior toward her mother suggested that she was afraid that she would lose her also, and this made it difficult for her to concentrate in school. On the other hand, Jane felt so depleted and so overwhelmed with her own feelings that she seemed unable to give her daughter the reassurance and comfort the girl needed. She had become somewhat depressed and emotionally distant since her husband's sudden and tragic death.

I hoped that the conjoint sessions would permit this girl to express her fears, and that the time alone with her mother would prove beneficial for both. Clearly, the mother's grief also needed to be expressed; I hoped that in time she would consider individual therapy for herself.

GOALS OF TREATMENT

The primary goal of treatment was to improve the parent–child relationship. This would be addressed by helping the mother take pleasure in her daughter's very appealing qualities, and by helping the two to find mutually satisfying activities in which to engage together.

A secondary goal of treatment was to identify the signs of traumatic grief in either the mother or the daughter, and to permit the expression of such grief either verbally or in play. Mary, as a preschool child, might not comprehend accurately the circumstances of her father's death, and her understanding probably needed to be clarified with facts. The girl's feelings about her loss, including some inevitable anger, could be permitted in play, but not in interpersonal actions directed at her mother.

BRIEF VIGNETTE OF A SESSION

There was some tension between Mary and her mother, as reflected in the girl's repeated attempts to cuddle up to her mother, and Jane's tendency to pull away from her child. Mary obviously wanted reassurance and comfort from her mother, but Jane was not particularly responsive to her daughter's needs. Jane appeared to be quite "strung out,"and her emotional capacity seemed to have reached its limits. She seemed to want Mary to be more mature than the child was capable of being.

At first I directed the conjoint sessions by asking Jane to get down on the floor and play with Mary. Mary was thrilled and set up a block play situation with a lot of people, which might have been her version of the scene in which her father died. She said, "The people are standing around and waiting." Jane immediately changed the play to one in which the people were watching a parade. Mary startled all of us when she announced, "Something bad is going to happen." I commented on how scary it is when bad things happen when people are just trying to have fun. Jane moved away, and Mary moved close to her. I suggested that they give each other a hug, and Mary immediately responded. I noticed tears in Jane's eyes, and I said that sometimes mothers get sad when bad things happen, but hugging can help a lot.

OVERVIEW/SUMMARY OF TREATMENT

There were eight conjoint mother–child sessions and one session with the mother alone. During almost every session, Mary would set up a scene with a lot of people and a stage in front. She then would destroy the scene and say that all the people were getting killed. Sometimes she picked an adult male and said, "He is the reporter, and he's going to get killed." My role as therapist was to try to make Jane aware of her child's feelings and to help her to verbalize them. The mother learned to follow my lead and often repeated what I said, such as "That's so sad when good people die."

In a session alone with Jane, she admitted that she got furious with Mary because Mary kept waking at night and wanting to come into her bed. She missed her husband so much at night when she was alone in her bed that she couldn't stand having her daughter try to sleep in his place. She confessed that she did not find much joy in her child; rather, she felt a sense of heavy responsibility and obligation. She knew that Mary wanted more from her than she could give. I agreed that Mary seemed to want and need a lot of reassurance from her, and I normalized this in terms of her probable fear that she (Jane) might die and disappear from her life also. I suggested that Jane could help her daughter by setting aside some time alone for her, and that, as a result, the girl might become less demanding. For example, she could tell Mary that coming for therapy was "her special time with Mom."

In the following two sessions with Mary, Jane brought photos of her husband and Mary together. Mary was more calm than usual during these sessions. She put her head on her mother's lap and smiled. It seemed to help her when her mother made it possible to remember and talk about "the good times." There was a definite change in Mary's play during this period, from the earlier repeated death reenactments to calmer, less pressured play. Jane, although still feeling overwhelmed, became more able to focus on her daughter and to participate with her in her play. I felt that Mary had experienced some cathartic relief in playing and replaying the death scenes; equally important was that the parent–child relationship seemed warmer and more mutually satisfying.

COMMENTS

This case illustrates the value of conjoint parent–child treatment in a situation of traumatic grief in which the surviving parent was unable to meet the needs of her preschool child. Because of the critical importance of a mother's ability to help her child during the bereavement process, conjoint crisis intervention play therapy proved to be the treatment of choice in this situation; it resulted in a reduction of the girl's problematic behaviors and a greatly improved mother–daughter relationship. This child's play therapy demonstrates how a preschooler will repeatedly "play out" his or her confusions in an attempt to comprehend a traumatic event.

The mother–child relationship was clearly in a crisis state at the beginning of treatment, and it is possible that without therapy, the girl and her mother would have grown farther apart and the girl might have become more symptomatic. The mother's own need for therapy was evident, and I hoped that a positive experience with her child would make Jane more open to obtaining her own treatment.

CONCLUSION

Different play therapists will select particular helping interventions with traumatized children and adolescents on the basis of many factors, such as a client's age, the nature of the traumatic event, the child's or adolescent's symptoms, and the therapist's own training and experience in using different modalities of treatment. A play therapist who is trained as an art therapist will obviously use that helping method more often than will a different therapist who prefers to use sandtray work with children and adolescents. To our knowledge, few if any studies have been done to evaluate the effectiveness of one method over another, and most clinicians agree that the most important element in successful treatment is the therapeutic relationship, not the method or theoretical views of the therapist.

The cases illustrate two effective forms of crisis intervention play therapy: TF-CBT and conjoint parent–child treatment. Both proved to be effective in situations of traumatic grief that resulted in a surviving parent's inability to meet the needs of a child adequately. In both examples, the mother–child relationship was clearly in a crisis state at the beginning of treatment.

Both cases demonstrate how children use play to express their confusions in an attempt to comprehend a traumatic event and reduce their anxiety. The use of CBT methods provides a child and parent with specific activities for dealing with their stress. The parent–child approach relies on helping a parent emotionally and cognitively to comfort a grieving child. Appropriate treatment by either method serves to enhance children's natural resiliency.

STUDY QUESTIONS

1. Discuss factors other than Jane's grief that may have had an impact on her relationship with Mary. Consider the girl's temperament and gender in your response.
2. Compare and contrast the use of conjoint parent–child therapy with the use of TF-CBT in situations of traumatic bereavement.
3. Consider the issue of secondary traumatization as it may have affected the therapist in these cases. How can the therapist guard against becoming preoccupied with a case involving a traumatic event that has been widely publicized?
4. Discuss the developmental factors that apply to girls or boys whose fathers die when they are preschoolers or in elementary school. What predictions can you make about Mary's or Joe's future ability to cope without a father?

REFERENCES

American Psychiatric Association. (2013). *Diagnostic and statistical manual of mental disorders* (5th ed.). Arlington, VA: Author.

The awful numbers: Death, destruction, charity, salvation, war, money, real estate, spouses, babies, and other September 11 statistics. (2002, September 11). *New York*. Retrieved from *nymag.com/news/articles/wtc/1year/numbers.htm*

Bratton, S. C., Ray, D., Rhine, T., & Jones, L. (2005). The efficacy of play therapy with children: A meta-analytic review of treatment outcomes. *Professional Psychology: Research and* Practice, 36, 376–390.

Brymer, M., Jacobs, A., Layne, C., Pynoos, R., Ruzek, J., Steinberg, A., et al. (2006). *Psychological first aid: Field operations guide* (2nd ed.). Los Angeles: National Child Traumatic Stress Network and National Center for PTSD.

Cohen, J. A., Greenberg, T., Padlo, S., Shipley, C., Mannarino, A. P., & Deblinger, E. (2001). *Cognitive-behavioral therapy for childhood traumatic grief.* Unpublished manuscript, Drexel University College of Medicine.

Cohen, J. A., & Mannarino, A. P. (1993). A treatment model for sexually abused preschoolers. *Journal of Interpersonal Violence, 8*, 115–131.

Cohen, J. A., & Mannarino, A. P. (1996). A treatment outcome study for sexually abused preschool children: Initial findings. *Journal of the American Academy of Child and Adolescent Psychiatry, 35*, 42–50.

Cohen, J. A., Mannarino, A. P., & Deblinger, E. (2006). *Treating trauma and traumatic grief in children and adolescents.* New York: Guilford Press.

Cohen, J. A., Mannarino, A. P., & Greenberg, T. (2002). Childhood traumatic grief: Concepts and controversies. *Trauma, Violence, and Abuse, 3*, 307–327.

Council for Training in Evidence-Based Practice. (2008). *Definition and competencies for evidence-based behavioral practice*. Kirkland, WA: Northwest University.

Crenshaw, D. (2006). Neuroscience and trauma treatment: Implications for creative arts therapists. In L. Carey (Ed.), *Expressive and creative arts methods for trauma survivors* (pp. 21–38). London: Jessica Kingsley.

Davies, D. (2011). *Child development: A practitioner's guide* (3rd ed.). New York: Guilford Press.

Deblinger, E., Cohen, J. A., & Mannarino, A. P. (2012). Introduction. In J. A. Cohen, A. P. Mannarino, & E. Deblinger (Eds.), *Trauma-focused CBT for children and adolescents* (pp. 1–26). New York: Guilford Press.

Dorsey, S., & Deblinger, E. (2012). Children in foster care. In J. A. Cohen, A. P. Mannarino, & E. Deblinger (Eds.), *Trauma-focused CBT for children and adolescents* (pp. 49–72). New York: Guilford Press.

Dripchak, V. L. (2007). Posttraumatic play: Towards acceptance and resolution. *Clinical Social Work Journal, 35*, 125–134.

Echterling, L. G., & Stewart, A. (2008). Creative crisis intervention techniques with children and families. In C. A. Malchiodi (Ed.), *Creative interventions with traumatized children* (pp. 189–210). New York: Guilford Press.

Fletcher, K. E. (1996). Childhood posttraumatic stress disorder. In E. J. Mash & R. A. Barkley (Eds.), *Child psychopathology* (pp. 242–276). New York: Guilford Press.

Giffords, G., & Kelly, M. (2011). *Gabby: A story of courage and hope*. New York: Scribner.

Gil, E. (2006). *Helping abused and traumatized children: Integrating directive and nondirective approaches*. New York: Guilford Press.

Gil, E. (Ed.). (2010). *Working with children to heal interpersonal trauma: The power of play*. New York: Guilford Press.

Glicken, M. D. (2009). *Evidence-based practice with emotionally troubled children and adolescents*. San Diego, CA: Elsevier Academic Press.

Karst, P., & Stevenson, G. (2013). *The invisible string*. Camarillo, CA: De Vorss.

Malchiodi, C. A. (Ed.). (2008). *Creative interventions with traumatized children*. New York: Guilford Press.

Mannarino, A. P., & Cohen, J. A. (2011). Traumatic loss in children and adolescents. *Journal of Child and Adolescent Trauma, 4*, 22–33.

Nader, K. O. (1996). Children's exposure to traumatic experiences. In C. A. Corr & D. M. Corr (Eds.), *Handbook of childhood death and bereavement* (pp. 201–220). New York: Springer.

Nader, K. O. (1997). Childhood traumatic loss: The interaction of trauma and grief. In C. R. Figley, B. E. Bride, & N. Mazza (Eds.), *Death and trauma: The traumatology of grieving* (pp. 17–41). Washington, DC: Taylor & Francis.

Osofsky, J. D. (2004). Different ways of understanding young children and trauma. In J. D. Osofsky (Ed.), *Young children and trauma: Intervention and treatment* (pp. 3–9). New York: Guilford Press.

Pynoos, R. S. (1992). Grief and trauma in children and adolescents. *Bereavement Care, 11*, 2–10.

Rossman, B. B. R., Bingham, R. D., & Emde, R. N. (1997). Symptomatology and adaptive functioning for children exposed to normative stressors, dog attack, and parental violence. *Journal of the American Academy of Child and Adolescent Psychiatry, 36*, 1089–1097.

Shelby, J. S., & Felix, E. D. (2005). Posttraumatic play therapy: The need for an integrated model of directive and nondirective approaches. In L. A. Reddy, T. M. Files-Hall, & C. E. Schaefer (Eds.), *Empirically based play interventions for children* (pp. 79–103). Washington, DC: American Psychological Association.

Terr, L. C. (1989). Treating psychic trauma in children: A preliminary discussion. *Journal of Traumatic Stress, 2*, 3–20.

Van Horn, P., & Lieberman, A. F. (2004). Early intervention with infants, toddlers, and preschoolers. In B. T. Litz (Ed.), *Early intervention for trauma and traumatic loss* (pp.112–146). New York: Guilford Press.

Webb, N. B. (Ed.). (2006). *Working with traumatized youth in child welfare*. New York: Guilford Press.

Webb, N. B. (Ed.). (2010). *Helping bereaved children: A handbook for practitioners* (3rd ed.). New York: Guilford Press.

Chapter 19

Multiple Traumas of Undocumented Immigrants

Crisis Reenactment Play Therapy

ROWENA FONG
ILZE EARNER

The population of undocumented and illegal immigrants in the United States is growing, despite the U.S. government's strong and persistent efforts to increase border security and tighten legislative policies. In 2010, the total foreign-born population in the United States was reported to be nearly 40 million, with 17,476,000 naturalized citizens and 22,480,000 noncitizens (U.S. Census Bureau, 2012). But, in contrast, in June 2014 the U.S. Customs and Border Protection Agency reported more than 52,000 unaccompanied children crossing the border with Mexico; most of these children and youth were actually coming from Central America, specifically Honduras, El Salvador, and Guatemala. President Barack Obama met with Texas Governor Rick Perry in Dallas to discuss the state's tense border crisis with Mexico (Cohen, 2014).The attempts to crack down on this undocumented population are affecting children, youth, and family members who are struggling to survive. Gleeson (2013) reports the confusing and conflicting inclusion and exclusion experiences of undocumented young adults who are trying to find jobs or receive financial assistance in schools; too often, the results have been life-threatening suicide attempts because of the great disappointments and high levels of stress related to the barriers these young people encounter.

Citizenship status has now become a major contributing factor to the mental health problems experienced by both immigrants and refugees. As Delgado, Jones, and Rohani (2005) stated a decade ago, "It is important to reemphasize that the difference between a refugee and an immigrant or undocumented person may have more to do with the political situations of the United States than any other factor" (p. 18). The current U.S. political situation is not uniformly favorable—indeed, is often hostile—toward undocumented persons, and the hostility is contributing to major mental health stressors for this population. Lee and Matejowski (2012) report that noncitizens were 40% less likely to use mental health services than U.S. citizens, for reasons such as lack of insurance coverage. Fear of parental deportation, poverty, discrimination, and unreported domestic violence were other kinds of stressors faced by many undocumented immigrant children and youth; such stressors, according to Henderson and Bailey (2013), increased the risk for developing psychopathology.

The situations of these undocumented families vary, but most of them have endured multiple traumas, which can subsequently result in the mental health conditions of "complex trauma" (Kliethermes, Schacht, & Drewry, 2014) and/or, for children, "developmental trauma" (van der Kolk, 2005). Many undocumented families are leaving countries where poverty and often violent living conditions have forced them to choose immigration so they can feed their children or make decent wages. Other families have decided to leave countries where political and/or religious strife has created a hazardous, war-torn environment. In either case, these families are desperate to leave their countries of origin and hope someday to become legal, permanent U.S. residents; they either may be smuggled into the United States or may have legitimate documents when they leave their homelands. However, even those who initially entered through legal means may later be designated illegal and no longer have valid documentation to stay in the United States. Still other people, such as students, tourists, or businesspersons, may initially come to the United States with legal documents for temporary residence, but overstay the length of their authorized visits (for various reasons), thus losing their legal status and privileges. Their skill levels and needs will be very different from those of persons who are illiterate and without employment experience or skills. Because many different types of situations cause undocumented persons to come to the United States, it is very important for social workers, counselors, and therapists to know the circumstances and conditions in which such children and families come for help.

The literature on immigrants and refugees (Delgado et al., 2005; Dettlaff & Fong, 2012; Foner, 2001; Fong, 2004; Garcia, 2012; Potocky-Tripodi, 2002; Sládková, in press) is beginning to include works that focus solely on undocumented individuals and families (Ellis & Chen, 2013; Gilchrist, 2013; Gleeson & Gonzales, 2012; Gonzales, Suárez-Orozco, & Dedios-Sanguineti, 2013; Henderson & Bailey, 2013; Jerome-D'Emelia & Suplee, 2012). As an addition to this literature, this chapter begins by describing the multiple traumas experienced by undocumented families at different stages of migration; manifestations of trauma in undocumented children and teens; and crisis reenactment play therapy with this population. A case of a 12-year-old girl in an undocumented family is then presented.

TRAUMAS OF UNDOCUMENTED FAMILIES AT DIFFERENT MIGRATION STAGES

Undocumented individuals and families endure multiple traumas, which take a lot of time and patience to work through in therapy. The traumas may be related to what they endured in their homelands, what they experienced in their journeys to America, and/or what they are subjected to when they make adjustments to living in the United States (Balgopal, 2000; Fong, 2004; Webb, 2007). Zuniga (2004, pp. 186–187) describes the five stages of migration originally outlined by Sluzki (1979); although these five stages do not pertain specifically to *illegal* migration, they provide a framework that can help professionals determine the nature and extent of traumas endured by undocumented individuals and families.

Stage 1 is the "preparatory stage"—a time when a person or family makes the decision to leave the homeland. For some people, this decision is carefully thought out and planned, with consideration of all family members' needs. For most families, however, time pressure does not allow careful and detailed planning, so not knowing the details of what lies ahead and feeling a loss of control generate many worries and fears. For undocumented families, this preparatory stage can be particularly stressful because of their unauthorized status and the haste and uncertainty that may accompany the decision-making process.

Stage 2 is the "act of migration." A wide variety of circumstances may surround the actual journey. Zuniga (2004) describes the situation of many undocumented families: "For those who enter without documents, the horrors of exploitation, assault, and rape can be realities, replete with traumatic memories that impact their future ability to adapt and cope" (pp. 186–187). Bevin (1999) presents the case of a 9-year-old boy who witnessed his mother's rape by the "coyote" (guide) who had led the family across the border into the United States. For families leaving their countries of origin, there is much grief for the people, places, and things that are left behind. There may be physical and emotional hardships, as well as social conflicts with other undocumented immigrants. If families can come directly to the United States, they will not experience waiting periods in holding places such as refugee camps; such waiting can add further stressors to the accruing traumas.

Stage 3, the "period of overcompensation," involves some kind of honeymoon period after entry into the new country. For undocumented persons, the sense of newness is mixed with anxious discomfort at not knowing enough about the new country, and being unable to find out more because of fear of exposure and eventual deportation. This stage quickly leads toward *Stage 4*, which is a "period of crisis and decompensation"—a time when the members of an undocumented family come to realize how much their illegal status prevents them from receiving help and resources. Unmet expectations, unrealized hopes, and numerous frustrations plague all family members.

Stage 5, called "transgenerational impact," is a time when immigrant families work through the integration of old and new values, allowing the younger generation to function better in society. This stage may not apply to undocumented persons because, whether they are young or old, persons without legal papers cannot fully function in the new country. For example, transgenerational issues may manifest themselves primarily in terms of legal versus illegal status upon the birth of a child. When undocumented parents have a child born in the United States, the child becomes a U.S. citizen, whereas the older siblings may (like their parents) have illegal status because of their lack of proper documentation upon entry into the United States. Despite his or her legal status, the child who is a citizen still endures many tensions and fears similar to those that the undocumented family members have to endure. Sometimes feelings of resentment build up because the undocumented children/teens cannot engage in educational or social activities, due to the limitations placed upon them by their illegal status. In situations like these, the multiple frustrations and traumas never cease, despite years of acculturation into the United States. Undocumented children and youth have the ongoing tension of physically existing in an environment where they are labeled "illegal." They also have to deal with the psychological torment of existing in a society where they are not allowed to be fully visible or viable participants in everyday community life.

MANIFESTATIONS OF TRAUMA IN UNDOCUMENTED CHILDREN

Cynthia Monahon (1993) defines "trauma" as follows: "Trauma occurs when a sudden, extraordinary, external event overwhelms an individual's capacity to cope and master the feelings aroused by the event" (p. 1). We use the term in Monahon's sense in this chapter, although her characterization of a traumatic event as "a sudden, extraordinary, external event [that] overwhelms an individual's capacity to cope" is somewhat broader than the American Psychiatric Association's (2013) current criterion of being exposed to threatened or actual major injury, sexual violence, or death. Undocumented children/adolescents do not experience a single traumatic event (in this broader sense), but *multiple* events; this fact makes it very challenging for professionals to discern and link any one antecedent event that produces new or reinforces old traumas. The terms "complex trauma" (Grasso, Greene, & Ford, 2013) and "developmental trauma disorder" (van der Kolk, 2005) more accurately describe the experiences and reactions of undocumented immigrants to the unending series of losses, frightening events, and ongoing ordeals they must endure.

Counselors must be aware of the reality of this immigration ordeal. Delgado and colleagues (2005) warn:

> Even if the social worker's role in working with the newcomer youth does not require or allow for any discussion of such trauma, it is critical to be aware of the degree of likelihood of traumas having occurred. Further, if the youth themselves arrived at such a young age that they have no memory of the trauma, it is important to recognize that they may be parented by

> those who do, and indeed the trauma may be an integral part of the "family story." (p. 49)

Young children are very aware of their parents' anxieties, and this awareness in itself can lead to feelings of being unsafe (Timberlake & Cutler, 2001; Webb, 2007) see also various chapters in the present volume). Increased difficulties occur when the child and parent have been separated during the early years, and human attachment and trauma issues may be present. James (1997) emphasizes the need to review the traumatic experience slowly and carefully, in order for the child or youth to understand both the experience and the feelings related to the traumatic aspects of those experiences.

Undocumented children and adolescents experiencing trauma can have varying reactions. Their signs of trauma may include panic attacks, separation anxiety, other fears and anxieties, physiological reactions, denial, behavioral regressions, and loss of pleasure. Some youth may withdraw from or restrict their peer interactions (Bevin, 1999). Others may have sleep-related difficulties. It is not uncommon for undocumented young people to experience frightening dreams and nightmares related to their intense fears of being exposed and deported. Complaints of headaches and other aches and pains may represent the somatization of unspoken mental health disturbances (Carlson, 1997; deVries, 1996). Personality changes may also occur, as once happy and outgoing children and adolescents become sullen and withdrawn youngsters struggling to cope with the major stressors they are facing (Canino & Spurlock, 1994; Lynch & Hanson, 1998). Immigrant youth, whether they are undocumented or U.S. citizens, who have been traumatized by suffering physical or sexual abuse and/or neglect may also sometimes manifest extreme behaviors of hoarding (Iwaniec, 2006). Total or partial avoidance to deal with the trauma, or the need to talk about and retell their traumas, may initially consume undocumented youth until they feel they have regained some control over their lives and situations (Suárez-Orozco & Suárez-Orozco, 2001).

CRISIS REENACTMENT PLAY THERAPY

Talking about trauma is not always comfortable or safe for individuals, especially undocumented children and adolescents. Trauma-focused cognitive-behavioral therapy (TF-CBT) usually emphasizes the need for youth to communicate in English and talk about the trauma they have experienced, so that cognitive and behavioral changes can occur. But many undocumented children and youth may not have command of the English language and speak another first language, such as Spanish or Chinese. Thus alternative modes of communication should be offered, so that the youth's fears and other negative emotions can be properly expressed and processed for better functioning and improved mental health. Play therapy is one of those alternative modes of communication. It is a means for children to express their feelings through the familiar and safe medium of play, in the presence of an adult who is trained to understand and help them. Because children in general are not always able to express themselves verbally, and because foreign-born children may also be confronting language barriers, they may use toys, art materials, or other aids to work through emotions and reenact the traumatic experience; this principle applies even to older children or adolescents.

Several aspects of trauma reenactment through play are important. Monahon (1993) states:

> The need to retell can appear insatiable, [and] the story may need numerous retellings for the child to experience some control over it. The retelling is generally factually accurate regarding the central events and salient details, although over time, some aspects of the young person's memory may become embellished with wishful fantasy—perhaps new details to the central story that wishfully recount the youth's heroism or efforts to foil the danger. Some individuals describe the duration of time involved in the trauma as much longer or shorter than it was in reality. These distortions appear to be related to the intensity of the experience [and/or to personal developmental issues]. (pp. 34–35)

Children and adolescents who are experiencing crises due to trauma need the opportunity to reenact that trauma in ways that will permit them to comfortably resolve some of their disturbing memories. When an undocumented youth has experienced multiple traumas, a skilled professional needs patience and culturally competent knowledge to sort through the premigration, migration, and postmigration contexts that may have contributed to the traumatic experiences. Because undocumented children and adolescents have no legal status, they have the particular burden of being forced to be invisible. They experience discrimination in not being able to obtain services or gain access to educational, financial, or social opportunities that their peers might have because of their illegal status. Many, like Julia in the case example that follows, need to figure out a personal identity that will allow them self-expression despite their undocumented status. Undocumented young people like Julia also may experience strain in their parent–child relationships when there has been separation, resulting in more mental health stressors for all family members.

THE CASE OF JULIA, AGE 12

Family Information

Julia was the eldest daughter of the Asturios Garcia family from Guatemala.

Ana: Age 32, an undocumented immigrant from Guatemala; mother of Julia; formerly a homemaker in upstate New York with her partner and their twin daughters, Adela and Inez; her current whereabouts (at the time treatment was sought for Julia) unknown.

Carlos: Age 38, also an undocumented immigrant from Guatemala; common-law spouse of Ana (they met while living in Brooklyn); former day laborer; now deported.

Adela and Inez: Age 4; twin daughters of Ana and Carlos; U.S.-born citizens; current whereabouts unknown; presumed to be living with their mother, Ana.

Julia: Age 12; Ana's daughter from a previous relationship in Guatemala; undocumented; arrived in the United States 5 years earlier to live with Ana, Carlos, and their twin daughters in upstate New York; currently in foster care; the foster parents were planning to adopt her.

Julia's bio-family thus consisted of her mother, her stepfather, and twin 4-year-old half-sisters. The bio-family had mixed immigration status: Both parents were undocumented; the twins were U.S.-born citizens; and Julia, from her mother's previous relationship, was undocumented. Although Julia had a speech disability, she could speak English. Religion (Pentecostal) was an important part of the bio-family's community life, but it was not part of Julia's current life with her foster parents. The details about Julia and her bio-family that follow in this section and the next were obtained from child protective services (CPS) records and the foster parents.

Ana's pregnancy with Julia was unplanned. Ana's health was poor at the time, and she did not have access to regular prenatal care. Julia was born at home in a house shared by Ana's mother and sister, as well as the sister's two children and husband. The family's economic situation was precarious, due in large part to the social instability, widespread corruption, and drug-related gang warfare that have negatively affected Guatemalan families for decades (see *www.worldbank.org/en/country/guatemala/overview*), especially those of lower socioeconomic status such as Ana's. The traditional social structures of family and community are disintegrating as more and more adult Guatemalans emigrate to escape violence and poverty (see *www.migrationpolicy.org/article/guatemala-economic-migrants-replace-political-refugees*).

When Julia was a year old, her mother left Guatemala and traveled to Brooklyn, New York, where she found a Guatemalan emigrant community and work. Julia was left in the care of her grandmother and aunt; Ana sent monthly remittances to Guatemala to support the family, and promised one day to send for Julia. While Ana was gone, her mother died, leaving Julia, then a year and a half old, in the care of Ana's sister. At this point, it appeared that Julia's life deteriorated quickly. Ana's sister had troubles of her own; according to Ana, her sister's husband drank heavily and would often become violent when drunk. Although little was known about the details of Julia's life while in her aunt's care, Ana began to hear rumors through former neighbors that Julia was unkempt, was often left alone, and was not well cared for. Julia remained in her aunt's care in Guatemala until she was 6 years old.

In the meantime, Julia's mother, while living in Brooklyn, met a fellow Guatemalan named Carlos, who attended the same Pentecostal church and worked as a day laborer. Carlos and Ana soon became a couple and moved into a shared apartment with other emigrant Guatemalan couples, some with children. When Ana became pregnant with the couple's twin daughters, Adela and Inez, they decided to move out of the New York City area to another Guatemalan emigrant community in upstate New York. A friend of Carlos from the church encouraged him to make this move because the cost of living was less expensive in the new community, and there was plenty of construction and renovation work in the surrounding upscale suburban communities. After the move, despite the fact that Ana was no longer working, the couple was able to save enough money to be able to pay a smuggler to bring Julia from Guatemala. When Julia was almost 7 years old, her mother traveled to a border town in Texas to meet her oldest daughter, whom she had not seen in over 6 years. Ana recalled that she wept at the sight of her: Julia was thin, haggard, and grimy, but it appeared to Ana that this was not simply the effect of the grueling 3-week journey north; rather, Julia had been severely neglected for a long time.

Ana reported that Julia's reaction to meeting her mother was muted, even strange, without any emotion. There was a perpetual half smile on Julia's vacant face, but it appeared to be unconnected to any feeling or action. Mostly Julia seemed wary of her mother, or of any adult, and when hugged she would stiffen her body and wriggle away. Julia shrieked when Ana attempted to brush her hair, yet she appeared to feel no pain when she went running barefoot across a rocky road that cut her feet. This was not the reconnection with her daughter that Ana had imagined, dreamed of, and longed for. Julia was a stranger. One incident stood out in Ana's recollection of those first months: Ana was standing in the kitchen, frying pork chops one by one in a pan. Julia stood nearby, watching her intently. A plate of raw pork chops that Ana was getting ready to prepare for frying sat on a plate next to the stove. Turning momentarily to reach for salt and spices behind her, Ana saw Julia's hand dart out to the plate of raw meat and grab a chop. Julia then turned her back and began to gnaw on it. Ana was astounded; she recalled thinking that Julia often acted "like an animal."

The longer Julia lived with Ana and Carlos, the more behavioral problems became evident. Ana described Julia's inability to sleep soundly in a bed; Julia also regularly hoarded food—hiding it under rugs, or stuffing it into her pillow, her shoes, and other places where she could access it at night when no one was watching. Moreover, Julia spoke little, which Ana at first attributed to shyness and the girl's expectable unfamiliarity with her new family. However, as time went by, Ana realized that Julia simply did not know how to speak: She had such a limited vocabulary that her inclination was to respond with either "yes" or "no" to questions, or simply to take what she wanted or needed without asking. Julia never initiated a conversation with anyone. She did however, enjoy babbling in non-word-specific "baby talk" with the twins; she also played incessantly with their baby toys, especially those that made noise. When Julia started first grade, she was initially assessed as an English language learner (ELL) and placed in an English as a second language (ESL) class; within a year, however, it was apparent that there were larger issues affecting Julia.

Julia's teacher and the school social worker tried repeatedly to reach out to Ana to discuss their concerns. Julia was markedly unprepared for school; she did not know how to hold a pencil, tried to eat crayons, would not sit still in her chair, and regularly stole lunches from the other students. She also exhibited social behaviors that some of the teachers found increasingly disturbing: Julia seemed to gravitate to adults, especially men, and would hug them obsessively. On one occasion, when Julia was in fourth grade, the assistant gym teacher alleged that Julia had groped him. The incident was reported to the principal and the school social worker, who then called Ana to come to the school. Ana, fearful that the family's immigration status would be discovered and reported, avoided the school's calls. Finally the social worker, who spoke Spanish, was able to convince Ana (through intervention with her church's pastor) to come to the school and discuss the school's concerns about her daughter.

Ana listened to the school's concerns and readily agreed to have Julia evaluated and placed in special education classes, as well as to receive counseling from the school psychologist, although she did not really understand what any of this meant. She was, however, especially perturbed about Julia's provocative, hypersexualized behaviors, as both she and Carlos had seen evidence of these at home as well. Carlos, who held rigid views about traditional gender roles and responsibilities in the family, was rarely involved in matters of the children's care or upbringing. He saw himself as the provider for the family, and upon occasion as the ultimate disciplinarian. On more than one occasion, he had resorted to harsh corporal punishment of Julia for stealing, lying, and disobedient behaviors. When Ana told Carlos that Julia had allegedly groped a male teacher, Carlos responded by repeatedly beating Julia with his belt, calling her a "whore" and a "devil's child." What struck Ana was that, despite repeated punishment, Julia never attempted to say she was sorry or to ask forgiveness for what she had done as a way to mitigate the severity of the discipline. And Julia never cried.

By the time Julia turned 11, she had failed to meet minimum state ESL academic standards in nearly every subject for the past two grade levels. She had also been in detention several times for taking other people's possessions without permission; she had once pilfered a teacher's car keys from her purse. According to the school counselor, Julia continued to come to group counseling sessions, but denied she had any issues or problems at home or in school. In fact, the counselor reported that Julia was always "happy and cheerful," but also appeared "superficial" in the group. Julia did not seem to have any significant friendships, but she did like to be around the "exciting kids" (i.e., the ones who were always creating mischief or commotion). At home, Ana had largely disengaged from Julia; she and Carlos both saw her as a "problem child" who was disruptive to their growing family.

Family Crisis

The crisis with Julia that eventually tore the family apart was precipitated by another incident of Julia's taking something that did not belong to her. One Saturday evening, while the family had a large group of friends from church over for a birthday celebration for the twins, Julia saw Carlos's new cell phone sitting on the kitchen counter. With no one watching, she took it. In the commotion surrounding the party, Carlos did not realize his cell phone was missing until the following day; then there ensued a great deal of concern and discussion within the family, and with others who had been over to the house, as to what had happened to the phone and when and where exactly it had gone missing. Carlos became increasingly upset as more time passed and the cell phone was nowhere to be found. Questioned repeatedly, Julia denied knowing anything about the missing cell phone.

Within a week, strange and disturbing things began to happen: A few teachers at school, as well as some students, began to get Facebook "friend requests" from Carlos; then friends of Carlos, especially those with male names, reported getting vague but provocative text messages from him. Ana and Carlos attributed this to his cell phone's having been stolen and the thief's using his phone and making mischief; they advised their friends that Carlos's cell phone had been stolen and that they should ignore the messages. Then a student at Julia's school received an explicitly pornographic picture, apparently from Carlos, with a text invitation to come over and see more; the student's parents went to the school, and the incident was reported to the police and to CPS. When the police arrived at the house, Carlos was arrested and charged with violating federal child pornography laws and endangering the welfare of a minor. CPS workers interviewed Ana, who was hysterical and distraught.

In the ensuing days, Ana asked the pastor of her church for help in dealing with both the police and CPS; she pleaded with him to explain to everyone that this was a terrible mistake, that Carlos was a decent man and a good provider, that his cell phone had mysteriously disappeared, and that he had never sent those messages or pictures. The emigrant community was supportive of Ana, but most community members were reluctant to step forward to vouch for Carlos publicly, as they too were afraid of drawing the authorities' attention on account of their own immigration status. The pastor did not have good news for Ana: Because Carlos had been arrested and charged with a felony, his immigration status was automatically checked. Because he was undocumented, he was subject to deportation, regardless of whether he was found innocent or guilty of the crime he was charged with committing. CPS workers in the meantime had also interviewed school personnel, who told them of their previous concerns about Julia's hypersexualized behavior and the parents' apparent lack of interest in following up with the school's concerns. Both Ana and Julia were interviewed extensively; Julia denied any sexual abuse by Carlos.

A week after Carlos's arrest, Ana was preparing lunch for Julia to take to school; when she picked up Julia's book bag, Carlos's cell phone fell out of the side pocket. Ana picked up the phone and began to scroll through it, seeing the explicit text messages and pornographic pictures that Julia had sent with Carlos's phone. Ana screamed; when Julia came into the room, Ana smacked her across the face, knocking Julia to the floor. She demanded to know how Julia had gotten hold of Carlos's cell phone. Julia responded as she always did when caught: She said she didn't know. Ana attacked Julia physically, pummeling her and shrieking that she was the "devil"; she grabbed the girl by her hair and pulled her toward the door. Ana flung Julia out of the house, screaming after her that she had destroyed the family and telling her "to go back to hell"; neighbors, hearing the disturbance, called the police. Julia was placed in foster care by CPS. When interviewed by CPS workers, Ana stated that she wanted nothing further to do with Julia. "She is not my daughter," Ana said.

Julia's Targeted Problems

At 12 years old, Julia presented as an attractive, slender preteen with obvious secondary sexual characteristics. She was menstruating, but did not appear to understand its significance; she denied any knowledge about sex education. Julia's affect was always cheery, but her speech was remarkable for its lack of expressive quality: Her vocabulary was limited, and the pattern of her speech fluctuated from rapid, jumbled sentences to stuttering and stammering. Sometimes, when she began to speak, her mouth remained wide open and she made prolonged vowel sounds before forming an actual word. Julia had previously been diagnosed with expressive–receptive language disorder with possible apraxia; she was receiving weekly speech therapy. Julia could understand and speak Spanish, but clearly preferred to use English; when spoken to in Spanish, she responded in English. Her Spanish vocabulary was even more limited than her English one. Curiously, Julia often reverted to using nonverbal "baby talk," as noted above. Previous diagnoses from psychological and cognitive evaluations requested by the school identified attention-deficit/hyperactivity disorder. Julia's IQ was assessed as being in the low average range; she had significant learning deficits in reading comprehension and logic.

Julia had been in out-of-home care for almost a year with the same foster parents, Jean and Audry, a same-sex couple with several adopted children who were now adults. They had expressed interest in adopting Julia, and at the time they brought Julia for therapy, it was anticipated that her permanency goal would be changed once Ana's parental rights were terminated. The CPS caseworker was aware that Julia's permanency plan would need to include a petition for special immigrant juvenile status, so that Julia would not "age out" of foster care with undocumented immigration status (Borelli, Earner, & Lincroft, 2008). Ana had not complied with the service plan for reunification: She had never visited Julia, attended court sessions, or met with the case manager. She had spoken only once with the counselor when contacted by telephone, repeated the problems she had had with Julia, and reiterated that she had no interest in bringing her home. According to her pastor, Ana became unable to support herself in upstate New York and moved back to Brooklyn with her twin daughters; he denied knowledge of any further contact information for Ana. Carlos, despite being cleared of all child abuse charges, was deported to Guatemala on account of immigration status violations; he was legally barred from returning to the United States for 10 years.

It was clear that Julia's childhood history of multiple losses, traumas, and severe neglect had negatively affected both her mental health and social development; her physical health was also affected. The doctor's notes from a clinic visit in the months after Julia had arrived from Guatemala indicated that Julia was significantly below normal height and weight; her head circumference was also well below normal. Barring other health factors, stunted growth is indicative of prolonged malnutrition in early childhood (*www.academia.edu/1750143/Stunted_growth_is_associated_with_physical_indicators_of_malnutrition_but_not_food_insecurity_among_rural_school_children_in_Honduras*). Chronic maltreatment and trauma in early childhood are also associated with complex posttraumatic stress disorder (PTSD), which manifests itself as significant disturbances in affective and interpersonal self-regulatory capacities. These were factors that could place Julia at risk for revictimization and negative peer influences, as well as difficulties with boundaries, trust, and control (Leenarts, Diehle, Doreleijers, Jansma & Lindauer, 2013).

Julia's foster parents initially reported that Julia was a remarkably cheerful and polite child; there were no behavioral or emotional issues, and Julia was always very eager to be helpful around the house. She had a hearty appetite. However, within a few months of the placement, Julia was once again hoarding and bingeing food, taking things that did not belong to her, and lying. She also knowingly disobeyed house rules. The foster parents were most concerned that Julia did not seem to respond to any behavioral redirection based on consequences and rewards; as one of them remarked, "She really doesn't seem attached to anything, and nothing bothers her. She just bounces along from one thing to the next and doesn't seem to learn from one incident to the other." The foster parents further reported that Julia never asked about her mother or her twin sisters; it was as if they had never existed in her life. Neither did she ever talk about Guatemala. Most recently, the foster parents stated that they felt Julia needed to be supervised around the family's cat, as she treated it more like a plush toy than a living creature; she would talk to it in "baby talk," but seemed unaware of the animal's needs. Once, when the cat scratched her in an attempt to get away from being held, she responded by trying to physically squash it headfirst into the sofa cushions to keep it from getting away.

The hypersexualized behaviors that Julia had exhibited in school at the time she stole her stepfather's cell phone appeared to have subsided. Julia denied sexual abuse by anyone. A comprehensive neuropsychological evaluation provided additional diagnoses of PTSD, generalized anxiety disorder, conduct disorder, and reactive attachment disorder. PTSD is underdiagnosed in children (Grasso et al., 2009). Both foster parents and Julia were initially included in the intervention, with the aims of addressing relationship problems, improving parent–child attachment, and changing behavior through a TF-CBT approach (Leenarts et al, 2013). However, this plan was modified because of Julia's limited verbal communication capacity; instead, play therapy was utilized to help Julia identify and express feelings, release tensions, promote social development and behavioral change.

Play Therapy Sessions

Conjoint Sessions

The counselor met with Julia and her foster parents together for three sessions over a period of 2 months. In the initial sessions, with Julia present, the foster parents discussed their concerns. Julia's affect was oddly cheerful, although she sat rigidly in a chair next to her foster parents. She seemed to listen passively. When asked how she felt or whether she had anything she wanted to say, her response was always the same: "I don't know." Some children with PTSD learn to dissociate in certain situations; as became evident, Julia often utilized this defense mechanism (Kesebir, Luszczynska, Pyszczynski, & Benight, 2011).

The first individual session took place in the fourth meeting. An incident had occurred in the home prior to this session: Jean had baked a batch of chocolate-chip cookies for a family get-together. Leaving them on top of the counter in a box, she had gone to walk the dog; Julia was alone in the house. When Jean returned, she discovered that the cookies were mostly gone; she immediately suspected Julia. Sure enough, Julia had chocolate stains in the corners of her mouth and crumbs on her t-shirt. Jean showed Julia the empty box and demanded to know what had happened to the cookies. Julia stared at the box with a puzzled air, and predictably said, "I don't know." Jean was furious and reprimanded Julia. Jean reported, "I told her this was unfair to me and to everyone else. She just stared at me like a goldfish."

First Individual Contact with Child

Content of Session	*Rationale/Analysis*
COUNSELOR: Hi, Julia, how are you doing? I am glad you came to see me.	Emphasis on Julia as an individual.
JULIA: Hi.	She is smiling with her mouth tightly closed, intently watching me but not trying to engage with me. She does not trust adult women.

COUNSELOR: The last couple of times we met, your foster parents, Jean and Audry, came too. They filled me in a little about how things are going for you at home—but, as we discussed, I thought it would be a good idea for us to meet, so you and I can talk about you. I would like to know more about what's going on with you and how you are feeling, so that I can get a better understanding of any problems that come up and we can work on them with your foster parents. Is that OK with you?

The purpose of engagement with the family was to focus on behavioral issues in the home and how these affect the entire family as well as individuals, so it is important to maintain this focus.

JULIA: (*Nods, smiles.*)

COUNSELOR: So tell me how this week is going. How are things at home? Were there any problems like the ones we talked about before, when your foster parents were here?

Body language is rigid. Mouth still tightly closed but smiling. Her use of the smile is resilient and protective behavior. She does not respond to the questions.

JULIA: (*Gets up and goes to a basket of toys, and begins to rummage around looking for a toy to play with. Picks up a blue teddy bear and begins to bounce it around on the edge of the basket, babbling to herself and keeping her back turned toward counselor.*)

Julia is taking control of the situation. She keeps her worlds separate and apart.

COUNSELOR: I see you found a toy you like. Maybe you can bring the teddy bear along with you back to the seat, and then we can talk if you feel more comfortable with the teddy bear with you. I would like it if you faced me because then we can see each other and talk.

I reinforce her need to feel safe, but push her to engage appropriately.

JULIA: Hmmm. OK. (*Sits in chair with the blue teddy bear and begins to make the bear talk in "baby talk" to counselor.*).

Julia is clearly not ready to deal with this situation. Is she even present? Where does she go when she uses "baby talk"? Dissociation?

COUNSELOR: Does the teddy bear have a name? You seem to be talking to it.	
JULIA: Alex. (*Makes the bear wave to counselor. Says in baby talk:*) My name is Alex.	Who is this? Was this anyone Julia knows? Is this person significant to her? How? Let's see if Julia can identify any kind of attachment to this person.
COUNSELOR: OK. Hi, Alex. I see you and Julia seem to be having a good time together. Can you tell me what you two like to do best when you are together?	I am engaging Julia at her level. Let's see if she feels comfortable responding if it's Alex I am talking to.
JULIA: (*Ignores the question. Continues to babble in baby talk with Alex. Is now bouncing the bear higher and higher on her knee while she twirls it by both paws. This goes on for several minutes.*)	Increasingly aggressive and agitated behavior with the toy. Tension is building up.
COUNSELOR: Julia, I am trying to understand what you are telling me. Would you rather be playing with Alex than talking with me? What's going on for you right now with Alex and me in the room with you?	Where is Julia? I am trying to push her to identify a feeling and connect it with her behavior—mirroring to her what she appears to be signaling with her body language and behavior, and normalizing it by joining with her. It's OK.
JULIA: I-I-I don't know. (*Stops bouncing the toy and clutches it to her chest on her lap, very tightly.*)	Stutters in response to identifying a feeling. Deflects. Of course she would rather play than talk! She is stuttering in response to being asked what she feels. it is difficult for her to say "I," as if being present is too vulnerable.
COUNSELOR: Well, what if I said you seem a little nervous to me, and maybe that's because you don't really know who I am, and maybe it doesn't feel safe right now for you? And that's OK if that's what you feel. I get nervous in new situations too. Are you feeling a little nervous?	

JULIA: I, I, I. *(Her mouth is wide open, and she is elongating the "I" sound.)* I think that Alex likes you.

Saying "Alex" deflects the question onto the toy. Protective.

COUNSELOR: Why does Alex like me?

JULIA: B-b-b-b-b-because you have a lot of toys. They are his friends. (*Suddenly gets up, comes over to counselor, and thrusts Alex right into counselor's face, laughing. She holds Alex there and will not stop, despite counselor's throwing up hands in an effort to signal her to stop.*)

Aggressive behavior. She wants to scare me away. When she says this, her voice is very soft and quiet. Julia is gone; her face is vacant. What happened is compartmentalized. Julia is not responsible; Alex is doing it.

COUNSELOR: Please stop and sit down! Hey, hey, what's all that about? That surprised me! Did you see that I wanted you to stop pushing the bear into my face when I put up my hands? I felt overwhelmed. What did you think I meant when I said, "Please stop"?

JULIA: I don't know.

Here she is really testing me. Can I tolerate her aggression, which she is expressing through the teddy bear?

Preliminary Assessment, and Long- and Short-Term Treatment Plans

The circumstances of Julia's early childhood had severely affected her physical, cognitive, emotional, and neuropsychological development. Although Julia was chronologically 12 years old, she was clearly not at an early adolescent stage of development—socially, emotionally, or behaviorally.

Julia's lack of insight, lack of empathy, and inability to self-regulate were profound. Recent research indicates that persistent adversity and trauma in early childhood can result in structural changes in the brain, possibly leading to lifelong learning deficits and other behavioral changes (Miskovic, Schmidt, Georgiades, Boyle, & Macmillan, 2010). The long-term goals of the treatment plan for Julia were to ensure her safety, the permanency of her placement, and her well-being by providing supportive counseling to her and her foster parents. This would include helping Julia reduce her trauma-based behavioral responses, as well as improving her insight, empathic responses, and capacity for self-regulation. The short-term goals of the treatment plan included educating Julia's foster parents about the effects of trauma on behavior, and teaching them coping skills to help manage and promote Julia's behavioral and emotional development.

The foster parents also needed to understand Julia's needs in the context of the complex trauma she had endured. Jean and Audry would need help in understanding the impact of Julia's migration journey and her early life in Guatemala when she was separated from her biological mother. To consider Julia's life in terms of Sluzki's (1979) five stages of migration, in Stage 1 apparently neither Julia nor her biological mother had been adequately prepared for their reunion when Julia was age 7 and the mother and daughter had not seen each other in 6 years. In Stage 2, during the time of migration, Julia was already showing poor attachment and hoarding behaviors, which are indicators of severe abuse and neglect. In Stage 3, there was no honeymoon period; rather, there was direct conflict between Julia and her new family members, as well as between Julia and the teachers at school. Julia was labeled a "problem child" by her biological mother and her mother's common-law spouse, Carlos.

At some point, it would be important for Julia to understand the circumstances that resulted in the disruption of her relationship with her biological mother and half-sisters. Before this possibility could be broached, further assessment would be required to determine whether Julia was emotionally and cognitively ready for such understanding. It was too early to determine whether or, if so, when she could reestablish contact with Ana, Adela, and Inez.

Progress of Treatment

Individual sessions with Julia continued twice a month over a period of 6 months. During this period, based on the assessment of Julia's PTSD as well as her cognitive and emotional needs, the foster parents also implemented a number of recommended adjustments. To minimize Julia's anxiety (De Young, Kenardy, & Cobham, 2011), her schedule at home was highly structured, with a predictable routine. In addition, she was enrolled in a special education setting with an emphasis on art and music, and with a small teacher–pupil ratio (6:1), in order to promote individual growth, self-expression, and identity formation (Bal & Perzigian, 2013; Leenarts et al., 2013). Lastly, to foster attachment and connection (Signal, Taylor, Botros, Prentice, & Lazarus, 2013), Julia began a therapeutic horseback-riding program after school several days a week. The foster parents reported that Julia appeared to be responding well to these changes and to therapy. In fact, she began to look forward to her schedule—something she had never done before.

CONCLUSION

The case of the Asturios Garcia family illustrates the central importance of culturally competent assessment and intervention in social workers' and other helping professionals' interventions. A knowledge of citizenship status issues has come to play a central role in understanding the mental health stressors affecting undocumented children, youth, and families coming to and living in the United States. Helping professionals need to be able to assess and diagnose presenting problems; however, they need to be able to place these problems in the context of migration journeys and citizenship status in order to intervene effectively. For example, in the case of the Asturios Garcia family, it was essential to understand the social conditions in the home country of Guatemala, as well as the migration journey of each family member and its potential consequences (especially for trauma). Immigrant parents, both naturalized and undocumented, may be unaware of mental health and other services that are available to assist with family problems; community-based outreach, utilizing cultural liaisons, is often necessary to reach members of at-risk immigrant communities who have well-founded fears of engagement with outsiders (Suárez-Orozco, Onaga, & de Lardemelle, 2010). School-based mental health services can be most effective in identifying and providing services to at-risk immigrant children and youth (Beehler, Birman, & Campbell, 2012; Bell, Limberg, & Robinson, 2013).

Lastly, complex trauma is often misunderstood and underdiagnosed in children; in Julia's case, early intervention might have helped the Asturios Garcia family remain intact (De Young et al., 2011; Grasso et al., 2009). Yet social services for undocumented children like Julia and her biological mother are limited because of their unauthorized status. Advocacy for more culturally competent services for naturalized and undocumented children, youth, and families is needed to serve this growing population in the United States.

STUDY QUESTIONS

1. How much knowledge and understanding does a therapist need to have about the historical and political events that have shaped the trauma a child has experienced?
2. How important was it to engage Julia's foster parents in understanding the impact of trauma on her development?
3. At the end of the session described in detail in this chapter, the therapist was wondering whether Julia had been able to link her feelings with how others (in this instance, the therapist) felt. How should the therapist have checked to see whether this link was made?
4. What should the foster parents know and understand about Julia's cultural background, and how should they use this information in promoting Julia's developmental growth?

REFERENCES

American Psychiatric Association. (2013). *Diagnostic and statistical manual of mental disorders* (5th ed.). Arlington, VA: Author.

Bal, A., & Perzigian, A. B. T. (2013). Evidence-based interventions for immigrant students experiencing behavioral and academic problems: A systematic review of the literature. *Education and Treatment of Children, 36*(4), 5–28.

Balgopal, P. (Ed.). (2000). *Social work practice with immigrants and refugees*. New York: Columbia University Press.

Beehler, S., Birman, D., & Campbell, R. (2012). The effectiveness of cultural adjustment and trauma services (CATS): Generating practice-based evidence on a comprehensive, school-based mental health intervention for immigrant youth. *American Journal of Community Psychology, 50*(1–2), 155–168.

Bell, H., Limberg, D., & Robinson, E., III. (2013). Recognizing trauma in the classroom: A practical guide for educators. *Childhood Education, 89*(3), 139–145.

Bevin, T. (1999). Multiple traumas of refugees—Near drowning and witnessing of maternal rape: Case of Sergio, age 9, and follow-up at age 16. In N. B. Webb (Ed.) *Play therapy with children in crisis* (2nd ed., pp. 164–182). New York: Guilford Press.

Borelli, K., Earner, I., & Lincroft, Y. (2008). Administrators in public child welfare: Responding to immigrant families in crisis. *Protecting Children, 22*(2), 8–19.

Canino, I., & Spurlock, J. (1994). *Culturally diverse children and adolescents: Assessment, diagnosis, and treatment*. New York: Guilford Press.

Carlson, E. (1997). *Trauma assessments: A clinician's guide*. New York: Guilford Press.

Cohen, T. (2014, July 10). After Obama's Texas trip, what now for the immigration? Retrieved from *www.cnn.com/2014/07/10/politics/immigration-seven-questions/index.html*.

Delgado, M., Jones, K., & Rohani, M. (2005). *Social work practice with refugee and immigrant youth in the United States*. Boston: Pearson Education.

Dettlaff, A., & Fong, R. (2012). *Child welfare practice with immigrant children and families*. New York: Routledge.

deVries, M. (1996). Trauma in cultural perspective. In B. A. van der Kolk, A. C. McFarlane, & L. Weisaeth (Eds.), *Traumatic stress: The effects of overwhelming experience on mind, body, and society* (pp. 398–413). New York: Guilford Press.

De Young, A. C., Kenardy, J. A., & Cobham, V. E. (2011). Trauma in early childhood: A neglected population. *Clinical Child and Family Psychology Review, 14*(3), 231–250.

Ellis, L. M., & Chen, E. C. (2013). Negotiating identity development among undocumented immigrant college students: A grounded theory study. *Journal of Counseling Psychology, 60*(2), 251–264.

Foner, N. (Ed.). (2001). *New immigrants in New York*. New York: Columbia University Press.

Fong, R. (Ed.). (2004). *Culturally competent practice with immigrant and refugee children and families*. New York: Guilford Press.

Garcia, J. A. (2012). Immigrants and suffrage: Adding to the discourse by integrating state versus national citizenship, dual domestic residency, and dual citizenship. *Harvard Journal of Hispanic Policy, 24*, 21–42.

Gilchrist, M. (2013). A personal reflection on the recent Australian discourse on asylum seekers. *Social Alternatives, 32*(3), 48–50.

Gleeson, S. (2013). Unauthorized immigration to the United States. In E. Barkan (Ed.), *Immigrants in America: Arrivals, adaptation and integration* (pp. 1539–1552). Santa Barbara, CA: ABC-CLIO.

Gleeson, S., & Gonzales, R. G. (2012). When do papers matter?: An institutional analysis of undocumented life in the United States. *International Migration, 50*(4), 1–19.

Gonzales, R. G., Suárez-Orozco, C., & Dedios-Sanguineti, M. C. (2013). No place to belong: Contextualizing concepts of mental health among undocumented immigrant youth in the United States. *American Behavioral Scientist, 57*(8), 1174–1199.

Grasso, D., Boonsiri, J., Lipschitz, D., Guyer, A., Houshyar, S., Douglas-Palumberi, H., et al. (2009). Posttraumatic stress disorder: The missed diagnosis. *Child Welfare, 88*(4), 157–176.

Grasso, D., Greene, C., & Ford, J. D. (2013). Cumulative trauma in childhood. In J. D. Ford & C. A. Courtois (Eds.), *Treating complex traumatic stress disorders in children and adolescents. Scientific foundations and therapeutic models* (pp. 79–99). New York: Guilford Press.

Henderson, S. W., & Bailey, C. D. R. (2013). Parental deportation, families, and mental health. *Journal of the American Academy of Child and Adolescent Psychiatry, 52*(5), 451–453.

Iwaniec, D. (2006). *The emotionally abused and neglected child: Identification, assessment and intervention: A practice handbook* (2nd ed.). Hoboken, NJ: Wiley.

James, D. C. S. (1997). Coping with a new society: The unique psychosocial problems of immigrant youth. *Journal of School Health, 67*(3), 98–102.

Jerome-D'Emilia, B., & Suplee, P. D. (2012). The ACA and the undocumented. *American Journal of Nursing, 112*(4), 21–27.

Kesebir, P., Luszczynska, A., Pyszczynski, T., & Benight, C. (2011). Posttraumatic stress disorder involves disrupted anxiety-buffer mechanisms. *Journal of Social and Clinical Psychology, 30*(8), 819–841.

Kliethermes, M., Schacht, M., & Drewry, K. (2014). Complex trauma. *Child and Adolescent Psychiatric Clinics of North America, 23*, 339–361.

Lee, S., & Matejkowski, J. (2012). Mental health service utilization among noncitizens in the United States: findings from the National Latino and Asian American Study. *Administration and Policy in Mental Health, 39*(5), 406–418.

Leenarts, L. E., Diehle, J., Doreleijers, T. A., Jansma, E. P., & Lindauer, R. J. (2013). Evidence-based treatments for children with trauma-related psychopathology as a result of childhood maltreatment: A systematic review. *European Child and Adolescent Psychiatry, 22*(5), 269–283.

Lynch, E., & Hanson, M. (1998). *Developing cross-cultural competence: A guide for working with children and their families*. Baltimore: Brookes.

Miskovic, V., Schmidt, L. A., Georgiades, K., Boyle, M., & Macmillan, H. L. (2010). Adolescent females exposed to child maltreatment exhibit atypical EEG coherence and psychiatric impairment: Linking early adversity, the brain, and psychopathology. *Development and Psychopathology, 22*(2), 419–432.

Monahon, C. (1993). *Children and trauma: A guide for parents and professionals*. San Francisco: Jossey-Bass.

Potocky-Tripodi, M. (2002). *Best practices for social work with refugees and immigrants.* New York: Colombia University Press.

Signal, T., Taylor, N., Botros, H., Prentice, K., & Lazarus, K. (2013). Whispering to horses: Childhood sexual abuse, depression and the efficacy of equine facilitated therapy. *Sexual Abuse in Australia and New Zealand, 5*(1), 24–32.

Sládková, J. (in press). Stratification of undocumented migrant journeys: Honduran case. *International Migration.*

Sluzki, C. (1979). Migration and family conflict. *Family Process, 18*, 379–390.

Suárez-Orozco, C., Onaga, M., & de Lardemelle, C. (2010). Promoting academic engagement among immigrant adolescents through school–family–community collaboration. *Professional School Counseling, 14*(1), 15–26.

Suárez-Orozco, C., & Suárez-Orozco, M. M. (2001). *Children of immigration.* Cambridge, MA: Harvard University Press.

Timberlake, E., & Cutler, M. (2001). *Developmental play therapy in clinical social work.* Boston: Allyn & Bacon.

U.S. Census Bureau. (2012). *The foreign-born population in the United States: 2010* (No. ACS -19). Washington, DC: U.S. Census Bureau. Retrieved from *www.census.gov/prod/2012pubs/acs-19.pdf.*

van der Kolk, B. (2005). Developmental trauma disorder: Toward a rational diagnosis for children with complex trauma histories. *Psychiatric Annals, 35*(5), 401–408.

Webb, N. B. (Ed.). (2007). *Play therapy with children in crisis: Individual, group, and family treatment* (3rd ed.). New York: Guilford Press.

Zuniga, M. (2004). Latino children and families. In R. Fong (Ed.), *Culturally competent practice with immigrant and refugee children and families* (pp. 183–201). New York: Guilford Press.

Part V

SUPPORT FOR THERAPISTS

Chapter 20

Professional Self-Care and the Prevention of Secondary Trauma among Play Therapists Working with Traumatized Youth

TINA MASCHI

My father was dying of cancer. A social worker came over to the house to talk to the family. He was such a caring, kind person—I knew right then and there that this is what I wanted to do.

—ELLIE, Practitioner

I always enjoyed helping others, listening to their problems, problem solving, and brainstorming. I thought I could make a difference one-to-one, especially with children. I'm cynical about "mankind," but I think everyone has some goodness and neediness I could tap into.

—ISABELLE, Practitioner

My father had died 8 months after I'd graduated from college with BA degrees in history/political science and Spanish. I felt like I was on a quest to learn more about human behavior, loss, and why bad things happen to good people.

—JOHN, Practitioner

Practitioners who work with children or adolescents after crises or exposures to traumatic events can experience a high level of compassion satisfaction, especially when they employ self-care strategies that foster their internal and external resources. This chapter reviews the risks and benefits for practitioners who work with children and adolescents after such events and exposures. It provides a way for practitioners to understand these risk and benefits, and a roadmap to help them foster their own resilience. First, the chapter reviews the differences between compassion satisfaction and compassion fatigue, as well as work-related adverse effects of crisis and trauma counseling. These include the effects of dealing with psychological distress, chronic bereavement, countertransference, secondary trauma/compassion fatigue, and vicarious trauma.

Then the chapter presents strategies for how practitioners can survive and thrive at the personal, interpersonal, organizational, and community levels.

As illustrated throughout this book, practitioners represent pillars of compassion and support for children/adolescents and their families after crises and traumatic exposures. As the quotations above indicate, they also are often highly motivated to help others cope and solve complex problems, and frequently experience a high level of job satisfaction by doing so. However, this level of caring does not come without a "vicarious" or "secondary" risk to practitioners. As Jennifer Freyd (1996) has so eloquently noted about humanity and the type of double vision that practitioners need to survive and thrive in their work: "If we look at the world conscious of both of our eyes, we will see peace and violence, love and hate, joy and pain, and even beauty and the beast. There is a bittersweet taste to this human reality" (p. 3). Therefore, in addition to job satisfaction, practitioners who work with children/adolescents after crises and traumatic exposures often experience work-related stressors that affect them at the personal, interpersonal, and organizational levels. This stress is confounded when they grapple with past and current traumas and stressful events in their own lives, such as the expected or unexpected death of a loved one, caregiver stress or burden, and/or direct or indirect exposure to violence.

THE CONTINUUM OF CRISIS AND TRAUMA

Practitioners working with young people after crises and exposures to traumatic events try their best to help them to cope with the immediate crises or traumas. Traumatic events are broad in scope; they have a wide range of intensity; and at times there is a dosage effect. People's experiences of trauma may range from a single childhood event to the accumulation of a series of traumatic experiences across the developmental life cycle. Examples of the latter may include physical and sexual abuse, or being a victim and/or witness to family, school, or community violence. A person's subjective response to traumatic events may be psychological, emotional, and/or physiological, and survivors may be affected in a variety of ways across the different stages of the lifespan. When the fallout from childhood or adolescent experiences is left undetected and untreated, there may be ramifications for well-being in adulthood (Maschi, Baer, Morrissey, & Moreno, 2012).

A frequent type of crisis is the unexpected or expected death of a loved one. A loss associated with death involves "any separation from someone or something whose significance is such that it impacts on our physical or emotional well-being, role, and status" (Weinstein, 2006, p. 5). Practitioners can help young people with their bereavement responses to varying types of death and losses. For example, a practitioner may work with children who have experienced the anticipated death of a significant other (e.g., a grandmother diagnosed with cancer) or with youth who have experienced an unexpected or traumatic death (e.g., witnessing the murder of a parent) (Webb, 2004; Weinstein, 2006). In particular, the unexpected and traumatic types of death—where crises, traumas, and losses intersect—create a heightened risk of indirect or secondary trauma for practitioners (Cunningham, 2004; Figley, 1995; Jenkins & Baird, 2002).

On a personal level, working with children/adolescents and their families after crises and traumatic exposures may trigger practitioners' unresolved thoughts and feelings related to their own past and current trauma, grief, loss, and separation experiences, possibly arousing feelings of low self-esteem, fear, anxiety, anger, guilt, and shame. On an interpersonal level, practitioners' use of empathy with children/adolescents after crisis and traumatic exposure may have a secondary effect on the practitioners' own worldview. For example, they may ask, "How can people do such terrible things to one another?" They also may have difficulty maintaining their own protective boundaries and remaining centered, so that they may become "empathy sponges" for others' (especially children's) pain and suffering. Too much empathy can become overwhelming! On an organizational level, practitioners may experience additional stressors, such as bureaucratic hierarchies/red tape, high caseloads, and long hours of work, which may create or exacerbate feelings of powerlessness and low professional self-esteem. All of these multilevel factors make it critical for practitioners to identify and manage their work-related trauma and stress. This includes the use of self-care strategies to sustain and reinforce the practitioners' personal well-being and sense of effectiveness in their practices.

THE BENEFITS OF CARING: COMPASSION SATISFACTION

Many practitioners, especially psychologists or social workers, are drawn to the mental health field because of a desire to help those in need. The term "compassion satisfaction" refers to the common human experience of satisfaction felt from helping other people (Radey & Figley, 2007; Stamm, 2002). The online *Merriam-Webster Dictionary* (2008) defines compassion as the "sympathetic consciousness of others' distress together with a desire to alleviate it" (p. 254). Micah, a licensed clinical social worker, noted that compassion motivates his work. He said, "I love what I do—helping children and their families to change their lives, and possibly making an impact on their lives. It was a field that was the right fit for me, as far as finding satisfaction in helping people who are disenfranchised and oppressed." It is this satisfaction with helping that drives practitioners to help others in distress (Radey & Figley, 2007). It is also this drive for compassion, which does not easily succumb to stressors, that allows practitioners to remain resilient and to thrive throughout their professional careers. One veteran practitioner noted, "After 20 years of social work, I realized that I was always a clinician in the 'trenches.' I always worked with women and children [who were] victims in their homes and in group settings. I realized I was effective [in this type of work] as a clinician."

The Empathy Conduit

Empathy is the underlying psychological and emotional experience of "being in another person's shoes" that provides the necessary fuel to move to compassionate action. Empathy is a core component of practitioners' work with people after crises and traumatic exposures. Carl Rogers (1980) eloquently described the nature of empathy as follows:

> It means entering the private perceptual world of the other and becoming thoroughly at home in it. It involves being sensitive, moment by moment, to the changing felt meanings which flow in this other person, to the fear or rage or tenderness or confusion or whatever he or she is experiencing. It means temporarily living in the other's life, moving about in it delicately without making judgments. (p. 251)

As Rogers (1980) suggested, empathy is both a cognitive skill and an affective skill: It involves seeing the cognitive and affective worlds of others from their perspectives. It does not mean that helpers lose their own perspectives, but that they temporarily suspend their own frames of reference while looking at others' worlds through their own eyes (Pearlman, 1999). It is this empathic openness that helps practitioners effectively connect with their clients to work with them to facilitate their healing process, especially after traumas or crises. However, unchecked or excessive empathy without ongoing self-care strategies also places them at risk for adverse emotional, psychological, social, and behavioral effects (Pearlman & Saakvitne, 1995a, 1995b).

THE RISKS OF CARING

The literature has documented occupational risks for practitioners working with young people and adults who have experienced crises and traumatic exposures (Cunningham, 2004; Figley, 1995; Hooyman & Kramer, 2006; Ryan & Cunningham, 2007). Practitioners are at risk for such work-related adverse effects as general psychological distress, chronic bereavement, countertransference, burnout, secondary trauma stress/compassion fatigue, and vicarious trauma.

General Psychological Distress

General psychological distress that occurs in response to listening to clients' stressful experiences is considered a minor occupational risk among practitioners. "General psychological distress" in this context refers to transitory feelings that arise after a practitioner has been exposed to a client's disturbing material, and it is a natural occurrence (Cunningham, 2004). For example, in a session in which a child details the deteriorating health of a parent, the practitioner may feel upset or helpless. However, for most practitioners, this feeling of distress is temporary and does not have an impact on their ongoing practice effectiveness.

Grief, Mourning, and Chronic Bereavement

Practitioners working with children and adolescents after crises and traumatic exposures that involve deaths and losses will be exposed to the youth's responses to those losses. Bereavement is a core human experience, and its expression varies across cultures and historical periods. In the practitioner–client dyad, grief is the interpersonal or psychological expression of the bereavement process. Practitioners who work with a caseload of children and adolescents—especially those who have experienced the death of, loss of, and/or separation from loved ones (e.g., children of incarcerated parents)—may be exposed to "chronic bereavement," which involves "multiple losses in which chronic anticipatory, unresolved grief results in the compounding effects of experiencing several episodes of grief concurrently" (Cho & Cassidy, 1994, p. 275). For example, practitioners who work in the child welfare or juvenile justice system may repeatedly hear about the multiple deaths experienced by youth in their caseloads who have lost family members and friends to drug overdoses or community violence. Practitioners' chronic exposure to these traumatized children and teens may subsequently have adverse physical, psychological, emotional, social, and spiritual impacts on them, and these feelings may challenge their foundational sense of safety, security, and personal power (Cunningham, 2004; Gamble, 2002; Meyers & Cornille, 2002; Weinstein, 2006).

Countertransference

Countertransference is another occupational risk that occurs in the context of the relationship with a client. As discussed in the psychodynamic literature, "countertransference" generally refers to unresolved personal issues that account for a practitioner's reactions to a client and/or a situation (Freud, 1912/1959; Wilson & Lindy, 1994). That is, the content of the client's narratives evokes a personal reaction based on the practitioner's own history (Ryan & Cunningham, 2007). For example, a child grieving over the death of a parent may trigger unresolved feelings related to the death of a practitioner's own parents. This infusion of the practitioner's own "unfinished business" may compromise his or her ability to be effective with the client.

Countertransference is relatively easy for practitioners to prevent or eliminate if they use strategies such as self-awareness and centeredness, and if they make it a routine to practice self-integration, anxiety management, and conceptualizing skills (Cunningham, 2004; Figley, 1999). Regular supervision can also help maintain the practitioner's objectivity and effectiveness (Webb, 2011).

Burnout

Burnout is another occupational risk for practitioners who work with children/adolescents and their families after crises and traumatic exposures. In contrast to countertransference, burnout is not contingent on the practitioner–client relationship, but rather on factors related to the workplace. "Burnout" has been described as a psychological syndrome of emotional exhaustion, depersonalization, and reduced personal accomplishment that can occur among individuals who work with other people (Maslach, 2003). An important feature is that it starts out slowly and becomes progressively worse if no intervention occurs. It may have an adverse impact on practitioners' sense of well-being, as well as on their level of effectiveness with clients and overall job performance (Maslach & Leiter, 1997).

Practitioners experiencing burnout will have increased feelings of emotional exhaustion, and may feel that they are no longer psychologically or emotionally available for others. The practitioners may experience depersonalization, often in the form of negative, cynical attitudes and feelings about their clients. Practitioners experiencing burnout may also feel a sense of reduced personal accomplishment and may view themselves and their work negatively. Factors that may contribute to burnout include high caseloads, lack of supervision at work, and a feeling of being unappreciated (Maslach, Jackson, & Leiter, 1996, 1997; Rothschild, 2006).

It is well documented in the literature that burnout may have serious consequences for clinicians, their clients, and the larger organizations in which they are employed (Lloyd & King, 2002). Studies using the Maslach Burnout Inventory (MBI) have shown that burnout (defined as emotional exhaustion, depersonalization, and decreased feelings of competence at work) among practitioners was linked to work-related problems such as low morale, absenteeism, and staff turnover, and that the condition might also create personal problems such as physical exhaustion, insomnia, substance abuse, mental health problems, and marital and family conflict (Lloyd & King, 2002; Maslach, 2003).

Secondary Trauma Stress and Compassion Fatigue

Secondary trauma stress (STS), or its more user-friendly synonym, *compassion fatigue* (CF), is another occupational risk directly related to practitioners' work with clients after crises and traumatic exposures. This is especially true, for example, when a young person's crisis was due to sudden traumatic circumstances, such as the loss of a parent in a terrorist attack or an unexpected natural disaster. In contrast to burnout, which is not necessarily linked to work with clients, STS *is* related to a worker's empathic response. STS or CF consists of the "natural consequent behaviors and emotions resulting from knowing about a traumatizing event experienced by a significant other—the stress resulting from helping or wanting to help a traumatized or suffering person" (Figley, 1995, p. 7). Rather than being directly exposed to traumatic events, in other words, practitioners are exposed secondarily through the context of their work relationships.

Paralleling the *Diagnostic and Statistical Manual of Mental Disorders*, fifth edition (DSM-5; American Psychiatric Association, 2013) criteria for posttraumatic stress disorder (PTSD), practitioners, especially first responders, may develop what Figley (1995) has called "secondary traumatic stress disorder" (STSD) by witnessing or listening to clients' trauma-related material. According to Figley's criteria, the stressor to which a practitioner is exposed must be outside the range of usual human experiences, and one that would be markedly distressing to most people. Afterward, the practitioner may continue reexperiencing the traumatic event, which may include having recollections (including dreams) of the client's traumatic experiences (Stamm, 1999, 2002).

Practitioners may have physiological and psychological reactions to their memories of clients' materials (Adams, Boscarino, & Figley, 2006). These reactions may include avoidance, numbing, and persistent arousal. Avoidance and numbing include practitioners' efforts to avoid thoughts, feelings, activities, and situations that remind them of a client or event. The practitioners also may experience adverse psychological and emotional changes as part of their avoidance and numbing strategies, such as psychogenic amnesia, diminished affect, negative thinking patterns, decreased interest in activities, and detachment from others. Persistent arousal may include somatic and emotional symptoms, such as difficulty falling or staying asleep, irritability, anger outbursts, and trouble concentrating. It may also include hypervigilance, exaggerated startle response, and physiological reactivity to cues (Bride, 2007; Bride, Radey, & Figley, 2007; Figley, 1995, 1999; Valent, 2002).

CF/STS (or STSD, in Figley's terminology) has been called "a disorder that affects those who do their work well" (Figley, 1995, p. 5). Practitioners may experience emotional, cognitive, and physical effects from assisting others (Stamm, 1999, 2002). CF/STS is also characterized by deep emotional and physical exhaustion and by a shift in helping professionals' sense of hope and optimism about the future and the value of their work. The symptoms of CF/STS are usually sudden in onset and associated with a particular event. As a result of listening to a client's material, a practitioner may feel afraid, have trouble sleeping, or have disturbing images. The level of CF/STS a practitioner experiences can ebb and flow from one day to the next. CF/STS can even affect very healthy helpers with optimal life–work balance; however, practitioners may experience higher than normal levels when they are working with a lot of traumatic content, or when they are experiencing burnout as described above (Figley, 1995; Maslach, 2003; Stamm, 2002).

Nevertheless, Radey and Figley (2007) remind us that CF/STS can have a positive and not just a negative influence. Practitioners can choose to focus on the positive fulfillment and satisfaction they get from their work, as opposed to only the negative and stressful aspects. Based on the work of Fredrickson (1998), Radey and Figley have proposed a conceptual model that includes the positive effects of this work and emphasizes the importance of utilizing internal and external resources to reduce negative symptoms.

Vicarious Trauma

Vicarious trauma (VT) is still another occupational risk of working with children and adolescents after crisis and traumatic exposure. Whereas STSD as defined by Figley (1995) is based on clinical symptoms and diagnostic criteria, its "cousin," VT, is based on theoretical constructs that are important for practitioners to understand (Pearlman, 1999; Saakvitne, Gamble, Pearlman, & Tabor Lev, 2000; Saakvitne & Pearlman, 1996). Pearlman and Saakvitne (1995a) have defined VT as

> the transformation that occurs within the trauma counselor as a result of empathic engagement with clients' trauma experiences and their sequelae. Such engagement includes listening to graphic descriptions of horrific events, bearing witness to people's cruelty to one another, and witnessing and participating in traumatic reenactments. It is an occupational hazard and reflects neither pathology in the therapist nor intentionality on the part of the traumatized client. (p. 31)

Another distinct difference between these constructs is that CF/STS can have a sudden onset as opposed to VT, which has a gradual onset in response to an accumulation of memories of clients' traumatic material that affects practitioners' perspectives on themselves, others, and the world (Figley, 1995; Pearlman, 1999).

Signs and Symptoms of VT

Practitioners who work with children and adolescents after crises and traumatic exposures are at risk for experiencing VT and thus need to be aware of the signs and symptoms of this condition. For example, the memories of practitioners affected by VT often become fragmented. That is, practitioners may be able to recall clients' trauma narratives without also recalling their own or the clients' emotional responses to it (e.g., panic or terror). They may also experience images (e.g., flashbacks) without connecting these images with the clients' trauma narratives or with their own or the clients' associated feelings.

Since VT is the "transformation of the helper's inner experience resulting from empathic engagement with the client's trauma material" (Saakvitne & Pearlman, 1996, p. 40), Saakvitne and Pearlman (1996) have noted general and specific symptoms that may have an impact on a practitioner's developing self. Practitioners suffering from VT may feel no energy, experience feeling disconnected from loved ones, become socially withdrawn, and be more sensitive to loss and trauma. They may have increasing feelings of cynicism and despair, and have ongoing nightmares. They may also experience specific intrapersonal changes, such as disruptions or impairments in frame of reference. These may include changes in such factors as self-identity, world view, spiritual beliefs, self-capacities, ego resources, and cognitive schemas. VT also may cause mental health effects such as memory and perception, intrusive imagery, dissociation, and depersonalization (Pearlman, 1999; Saakvitne et al., 2000). All these changes may result in practitioners' assuming a negative attitude about themselves and the world. This negative shift will compromise the practitioners' personal well-being and effectiveness in professional practice (Pearlman, 1999).

Factors Influencing VT

Despite the risks that VT poses for practitioners, this condition is very amenable to self-care prevention and intervention (Pearlman, 1999). The nature of social/environmental and individual-level factors may protect or place practitioners at risk for vicarious trauma (Saakvitne et al., 2000). Environmental factors such as the nature of the work, the nature of the clientele, cumulative exposure to trauma material, organizational context, and social and cultural context can influence the impact of VT on practitioners (Bell, Kulkarni, & Dalton, 2003; Catherall, 1995). Individual characteristics of practitioners that may influence the effects of VT include their personal history, personality, coping style, current life context, training and professional history, and participation in supervision or personal therapy (Crestman, 1999; Saakvitne & Pearlman, 1996).

In general, the less trauma exposure practitioners experience in their work, the more support they receive from their agencies and communities (i.e., their work environments), and the more reinforcement they receive for their personal characteristics of resilience and adaptive coping, the more likely it is that they will be able to prevent or remediate trauma-related work symptoms (Adams & Riggs, 2008; Bell, 2003; Figley, 1995, 1999; Radey & Figley, 2007). These individual and social/environmental characteristics apply to both VT and STSD. It is important for practitioners who work with children and adolescents after crises and traumatic events to conduct regular self-assessments on the impact of trauma-related content on themselves. A later section of the chapter discusses a number of assessment tools that can assist practitioners.

Constructive Self-Development Theory

Originating from constructivist psychology, constructivist self-development theory (CSDT) is the theoretical framework most commonly used to describe

VT among practitioners (Saakvitne & Pearlman, 1996). According to CSDT, VT causes "profound changes in the core aspects of the therapist's self" (Pearlman & Saakvitne, 1995b, p. 152). Because VT is a natural consequence of trauma-related work, the ongoing challenge for practitioners is to identify, address, and transform their own experiences of VT and to learn effective methods for dealing with it.

According to CSDT, practitioners are at risk for VT because their open, empathic engagement with clients involves both positive and negative material (Pearlman & Saakvitne, 1995b). As results of practitioners' persistent exposure to clients' traumatic material, they may experience cognitive disruptions that adversely affect their perceptions of themselves, others, and the world (Figley, 1995; Pearlman, 1999). In particular, the shift to a negative world view can have devastating effects on practitioners' personal and professional lives if it remains unchecked.

According to CSDT, in the face of trauma, each person will adapt and cope (Pearlman, 1999). Therefore, adaptation and coping are integral internal factors that influence what the theory refers to as the "developing self' (Saakvitne & Pearlman, 1996). Positive adaptation and coping will protect the health and well-being of a practitioner's self, whereas negative adaptation and coping will compromise that self. Internal and external factors that influence practitioners' ability to adapt and cope include environmental, interpersonal, and intrapersonal factors, such as their current life contexts, their prior histories of loss and trauma, and familial/social/cultural factors (Saakvitne et al., 2000). Parts of the developing self that are at risk when exposed to traumatic material are a practitioner's frame of reference, self-capacities, ego resources, psychological needs/cognitive schemas, and memory and perception (Pearlman & Saakvitne, 1995a; Saakvitne & Pearlman, 1996; Saakvitne et al., 2000). Figure 20.1 is a self-assessment checklist for VT that covers all these aspects.

FRAME OF REFERENCE

CSDT argues that each self has a "frame of reference" that consists of self-identity, world view, and spirituality, and that is influenced by personal and professional experiences. An individual's frame of reference shapes the person's interpretation of the self, relationships, and experiences.

SELF-CAPACITIES

The concept of "self-capacities" includes the ability to self-soothe and to achieve and maintain an inner sense of balance. On a practical level, it involves a practitioner's ability to (1) manage strong feelings, (2) feel entitled to be alive and deserving of love, and (3) have an inner awareness of others (Saakvitne et al., 2000). A practitioner's frame of reference and self-capacities may be

Use this worksheet to evaluate yourself for vicarious trauma. Rate how much you agree with each of these statements, using the following scale: 1 = strongly disagree, 2 = disagree, 3 = neutral, 4 = agree, 5 = strongly agree. Put a plus sign next to those items that are sources of strength and a check mark next to those items that are of concern.

FRAME OF REFERENCE

____ I have a strong sense of self-identity.

____ Overall, the world is a good place.

____ I am a spiritual person.

____ I am connected to my faith.

____ My life has meaning.

____ I have a purpose to fulfill.

SELF-CAPACITIES

____ I can manage my strong feelings.

____ I keep my loved ones in mind.

____ My loved ones care about me.

____ I am worthwhile.

____ I am deserving of good things.

____ I am lovable.

EGO RESOURCES

____ I use resources on my own behalf.

____ I make good decisions in my personal life.

____ I make good decision in my professional life.

____ I can protect myself.

____ I have strong personal boundaries.

____ I have strong professional boundaries.

____ I know how to use resources for self-growth.

____ I keep growing personally.

____ I keep growing professionally.

BASIC PSYCHOLOGICAL NEEDS/ COGNITIVE SCHEMAS

Safety

____ I feel reasonably safe.

____ I feel my loved ones are reasonably safe.

Self-Esteem

____ I feel proud of who I am.

____ I trust my judgment.

Trust

____ I believe I can trust others.

____ I feel I can depend on others.

Control

____ I believe I have control over my life.

____ I have the power to influence others.

Intimacy

____ I am good company for myself.

____ I feel I am close to others.

PERCEPTION AND MEMORY

____ I sleep well at night.

____ I never experience nightmares.

____ I get triggered by clients' experiences.

____ I experience stress in my body.

____ I feel nervous.

____ I feel numb.

____ I have deep insight into myself.

FIGURE 20.1. Self-assessment checklist for vicarious trauma. Adapted from Saakvitne, Gamble, Pearlman, and Tabor Lev (2000), with permission from the Sidran Institute.

disrupted by work with high levels of traumatic material; that is, this work may impair the practitioner's ability to manage his or her own emotions and personal and professional relationships.

EGO RESOURCES

An individual's ego resources may also be affected by VT. The concept of "ego resources" refers to an individual's ability to negotiate interpersonal situations, as well as to exercise good decision making and judgment (Pearlman, 1999). It consists of self-awareness (insight), the ability to take the perspective of another (empathy), the use of willpower and initiative, and a striving for personal growth. A practitioner's effective use of ego resources consists of being able to foresee consequences, make self-protective judgments, and establish healthy boundaries between the self and a client (Pearlman & Saakvitne, 1995a; Saakvitne et al., 2000). These ego resources will become compromised when practitioners are adversely influenced by VT.

PSYCHOLOGICAL NEEDS AND COGNITIVE SCHEMAS

Practitioners' psychological needs, as reflected in cognitive schemas, may be influenced by VT. The five basic psychological needs are safety, esteem, trust (or dependency), control, and intimacy. According to CSDT, these basic psychological needs are critical factors that can protect practitioners from VT or from being unduly influenced or placed in a vulnerable position by others' trauma content (Saakvitne & Pearlman, 1995a).

MEMORY AND PERCEPTION

Practitioners' memory and perception also are susceptible to adverse changes after prolonged exposure to clients' material that involves loss and trauma (Pearlman, 1999). Since memory and perception are multimodal, they involve different capacities (i.e., verbal, visual, emotional, somatic/sensory, and interpersonal), all of which can be affected (Pearlman & Saakvitne, 1995b; Saakvitne & Pearlman, 1996; Saakvitne et al., 2000). Verbal memory and perception involve the narrative of what happened before, during, and after the traumatic event; visual imagery involves the mental picture of the event; affect involves the emotions related to the event; somatic/sensory memory and perception involve the bodily experiences that represent the traumatic event; and interpersonal memory and perception involve the relational patterns and behaviors reflected in the event (particularly an abusive traumatic relationship) (Saakvitne & Pearlman, 1996). The challenge for practitioners in preventing or remediating VT effects is to maintain the integration and interconnectedness of the different parts of memory and perception, so that disconnection or dissociation does not occur.

ASSESSMENT TOOLS

There are a number of user-friendly standardized assessment tools for identifying occupational risks, such as burnout, STS/CF, and/or VT (Bride et al., 2007). These instruments include the following:

- The Professional Quality of Life Scale (ProQL-5; Stamm, 2009)
- The Secondary Traumatic Stress Scale (STSS; Bride, Robinson, Yegidis, & Figley, 2004)
- The Trauma and Attachment Beliefs Scale (TABS; Pearlman, 2003)

The ProQL-5 is a 30-item scale that measures compassion satisfaction and is available in several languages. It can be self-administered and self-scored, and is known for good psychometric properties (Bride et al., 2007; Stamm, 2009). It is available for download (*www.proqol.org/uploads/ProQOL_5_English_Self-Score_3-2012.pdf*) and can be completed and self-scored in about 10 minutes.

The STSS is a 17-item summative scale that measures the frequency of intrusion, avoidance, and arousal symptoms associated with indirect exposure to traumatic events in practice over a 7-day period. The items on the scale are consistent with the DSM-IV-TR criteria for PTSD, with subscales for intrusion, avoidance, and hyperarousal (the B, C, and D criteria). The STSS takes about 5 minutes to complete (Bride et al., 2004). A copy of this measure is available online (*http://academy.extensiondlc.net/file.php/1/resources/TMCrisis20CohenSTSScale.pdf*)

The TABS is a reliable and valid instrument that is based on CSDT. It consists of 84 items assessing practitioners' beliefs about self and others, as well as the five areas of psychological need (safety, trust, esteem, control, and intimacy), all of which may be affected by VT. The scale can be purchased from Western Psychological Services (*http://portal.wpspublish.com*).

After an assessment for trauma-related work symptoms, practitioners may engage in various self-care strategies to prevent or ameliorate their impact.

THE SELF-CARE TRIANGLE: AWARENESS, BALANCE, AND CONNECTION

It is generally agreed that practitioners' self-care prevention and intervention strategies should target the three realms of practitioners' lives: personal, professional, and organizational (Gamble, 2002; Ryan & Cunningham, 2007; Yassen, 1995). Although the pathways to work-related burnout, STS/CF, and VT may vary, practitioners often experience similar adverse physical, psychological, emotional, social, spiritual, professional, and community-related consequences. (See Figure 20.2, which is a self-care activities checklist addressing all these areas.)

Rate how frequently you do each of the following self-care activities, using the following scale: 0 = never, 1 = rarely, 2 = sometimes, 3 = frequently. Put a check mark next to those activities that you want to continue doing, and a double check mark next to self-care activities that you would like to do.

PHYSICAL SELF-CARE

____ Get enough sleep.
____ Eat three meals a day.
____ Eat healthy foods.
____ Exercise.
____ See a doctor if needed.
____ Get massages.
____ Be sexual.
____ Rest.
____ Other physical activities.

PSYCHOLOGICAL SELF-CARE

____ Make time for reflection.
____ Practice self-awareness.
____ Use guided imagery.
____ Practice relaxation.
____ Attend counseling.
____ Write in a journal.
____ Read for entertainment.
____ Make other efforts to minimize stress.

SOCIAL SELF-CARE

____ Spend quality time with family.
____ Spend quality time with friends.
____ Attend social events.
____ Participate in social action activities.
____ Ask for help when needed.

WORK SETTING

____ Take a lunch break.
____ Eat during your lunch break.
____ Participate in rewarding projects.
____ Attend work-related trainings.
____ Get regular clinical supervision.
____ Negotiate for needs (pay raise, benefits).
____ Participate in a peer support group.
____ Do some non-trauma-related work.

EMOTIONAL SELF-CARE

____ Enjoy the company of others.
____ Love yourself.
____ Allow yourself to cry when needed.
____ Laugh.
____ Engage in creative activities.
____ Express anger with social action.
____ Other emotional care activities.

SPIRITUAL SELF-CARE

____ Make time for self-reflection.
____ Spend time in nature.
____ Belong to a spiritual community.
____ Practice positive thinking.
____ Meditate.
____ Pray or chant.
____ Do yoga.
____ Read spiritual teachings.
____ Practice mindfulness.
____ Embrace hope and optimism.
____ Other spiritual activities.

PROFESSIONAL SELF-CARE

____ Maintain professional boundaries.
____ Keep to a regular work schedule.
____ Attend trainings and workshops.
____ Review agency policies.

COMMUNITY ENVIRONMENT

____ Participate in community activities.
____ Attend community groups.
____ Participate in social activism.
____ Volunteer in the community.
____ Garden at home.
____ Participate in a community garden.
____ Give donations to charity.
____ Provide community leadership.

FIGURE 20.2. Self-care activities checklist. Adapted from Saakvitne, Gamble, Pearlman, and Tabor Lev (2000), with permission from the Sidran Institute.

Thus self-care should be a critical component of all practitioners' professional activities (Pearlman, 1999; Trippany, White Kress, & Wilcoxon, 2004). Saakvitne and Pearlman (1996) have identified the three interlocking legs of a practitioner's "self-care triangle": (1) awareness, (2) balance, and (3) connection. *Awareness* is the first leg of the self-care triangle. Saavkitne and Pearlman describe awareness as practitioners' being in touch with their own needs, limits, emotions, and resources. That is, if practitioners can identify the problem, they can prepare the self-care solution. Self-care necessitates that practitioners pay careful attention to their bodies, minds, and emotions. Allowing time for quiet and reflection, and practicing mindfulness (which is an acceptance of what is in the moment without modification or judgment), are considered essential self-care strategies (Cunningham, 2004; Gamble, 2002). In particular, these practices can help facilitate the personal grief process that practitioners experience when working with children/adolescents after crisis and traumatic events, which may involve a symbolic type of "psychological death" due to an inner world influenced by clients' trauma-related content (Figley, 1995).

Balance is the second leg of the practitioner's self-care triangle. Saavkitne and Pearlman (1996) refer to balance in both inner and outer activities. Practitioners who lead balanced lives are able to balance work, play, and rest activities. Although they are active, they are also in touch with their inner resources and allow ample time for self-reflection and personal choice (Saavkitne & Pearlman, 1996).

Connection is the third leg of the practitioner's self-care triangle. Practitioners who foster connection with themselves, with others, and with something larger than themselves are practicing preventive self-care (Saakvitne & Pearlman, 1996). Being connected to self and others offers a powerful antidote to living under the shadow of despair and isolation that characterizes practitioners with untreated STS/CF and/or VT. Practitioners in tune with their inner selves can more readily recognize and respond to their changing perceptions and needs (Pearlman, 1999). Studies have shown that practitioners who foster their internal and external connections sustain hope, along with a positive outlook on themselves, others, and the world (Adams & Riggs, 2008). Connection can also serve to distract practitioners from falling into a pattern of nihilistic attitudes, despair, and isolation.

After practitioners identify symptoms of STS/CF and/or VT, these symptoms need to be addressed and transformed. The literature emphasizes self-care as an essential strategy to promote the ongoing positive development of practitioners' minds, bodies, emotions, and spirits. In addition, practitioners must actively work to transform and to release negative beliefs, feelings of despair, feelings of helplessness/hopelessness, and losses of meaning (Pearlman, 1999). See Figure 20.3 for a "self-care eco-map."

The literature suggests that the despair of STS/VT can be transformed when practitioners engage in meaning making that involves thoughts and actions. Saakvitne and Pearlman (1996) have recommended that practitioners integrate their current activities with renewed meaning. It also is important

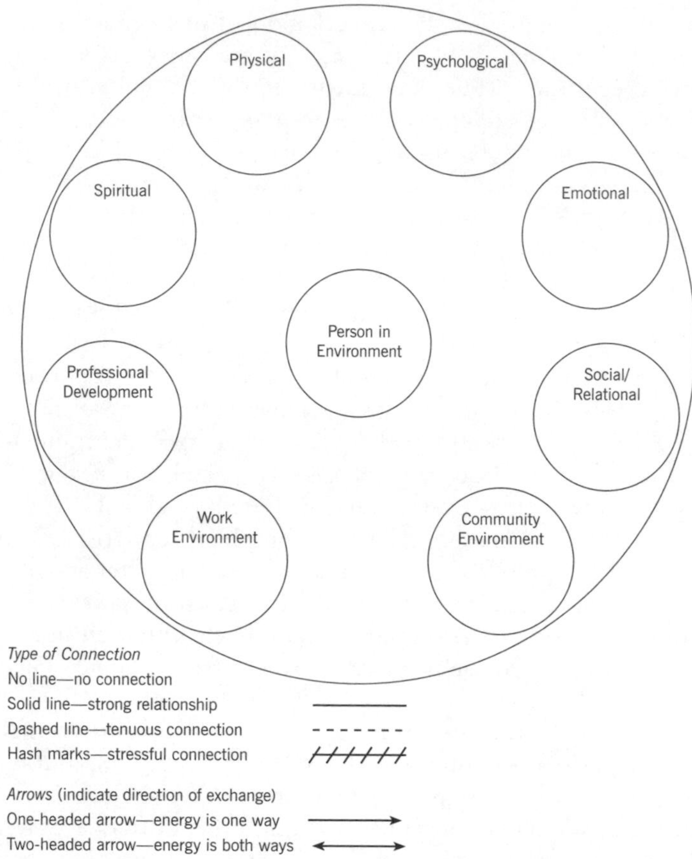

FIGURE 20.3. Self-care (inner and outer) eco-map. This visual assessment tool developed by Maschi and Brown can help practitioners identify strong and positive areas, areas of neglect, and areas of conflict (see the key code). In the center circle, the practitioner should list his or her name. Each self-care circle should list the activities, relationships, and so forth associated with the self-care area. This eco-map can also be used with clients. From Maschi and Brown (2010). Copyright 2010 by The Guilford Press. Reprinted by permission.

for practitioners to constantly challenge negative beliefs and assumptions, such as nihilism, cynicism, and despair, with positive responses (e.g., participating in community-building activities and social activism) (Yassen, 1995). Cunningham (2004) has recommended the use of mindfulness and relationship building. For example, working with other community members for a common good or goal, such as combating family and community violence, creates a community of personal and group connection and empowerment. According to Saakvitne and colleagues (2000), the processes of addressing and transforming STS/CF and VT often go hand in hand.

ECOLOGICAL MODEL FOR PREVENTION

Another useful practitioner self-care model is Yassen's (1995) ecological model for prevention (EMP). The EMP takes a multidimensional approach to preventing STS/CF, burnout, and VT, through the use of active planning that involves knowledge-building strategies and techniques. The model assumes that STS/CF and VT are normal reactions to abnormal events (e.g., violence) or unusual events (e.g., natural disasters). EMP assumes that the enduring or negative effects of trauma can be prevented from developing into psychological symptomatology, such as STSD, depression, or anxiety (Bride, 2007; Crestman, 1999). The EMP consists of the following four steps: (1) prepare, (2) plan, (3) attend, and (4) transform. For example, practitioners can develop healthier lifestyle skills that give them a solid grounding for the exposure to the ebb and flow of trauma-related experiences inherent in their work with young people affected by crises and traumatic events. These skills are described below.

Personal Self-Care

Personal self-care is aimed at self-development activities, such as self-awareness and self-care strategies in the physical, psychological, emotional, spiritual, and social domains (see the first five categories in Figure 20.2).

Self-Awareness

Similar to other self-care models, the EMP underscores the importance of self-awareness as a critical factor for prevention of STS/CF and VT. This approach, corroborated by studies, has shown that practitioners' characters and personalities may influence the level of trauma-related symptoms they experience after crisis and trauma work. It is important for practitioners to assume a nonjudgmental and compassionate attitude toward themselves and others, and to have a good understanding of their current life situations. They also should be aware of power dynamics in their lives (i.e., what they do and don't have power and control over), and especially of times when they need to ask for help. Good self-awareness skills among practitioners are critical in enabling them to recognize adverse signs of somatic, psychological, emotional, and spiritual shifts in their belief systems.

Self-Care Strategies

At the individual level, practitioners should engage in self-care strategies that target their physical, psychological, cognitive, behavioral, interpersonal, and spiritual well-being (Saakvitne et al., 2000). Adequate sleep, nutrition, and a healthy diet are vital to maintaining physical health. Other physical self-care strategies include activities that increase strength, endurance, clarity of mind, and feelings of well-being. It is important for practitioners to identify exercises that fit their specific lifestyles (Cunningham, 2004). Some physical exercises that practitioners may select include jogging, aerobics, playing on competitive sport teams, dog walking, yoga, and tai chi.

Psychological and emotional self-care strategies can also reduce practitioners' symptoms of physical arousal (Gamble, 2002; Jenkins & Baird, 2002). Practitioners should balance their work with outside interests that include a social life, personal time, and recreational activities. Daily relaxation practices, including guided imagery and breathing exercises or spending time in nature, are consistently recommended in the literature as helpful strategies that are not time-intensive (Cunningham, 2004; Gamble, 2002; Yassen, 1995). Creative activities can also help practitioners process psychological and emotional reactions, and thus prevent or remediate STS/CF and VT. Such activities include writing, poetry, drama, photography, cooking, drawing, painting, dancing, playing music, and journal writing. In addition, humor has been shown to reduce stress; release tension; and increase physical, psychological, and emotional health (Moran, 2002). Self-care strategies should also address cognitive and behavioral skills development (Yassen, 1995). Some examples of skills development activities include assertiveness training, stress management, time management, and individual and group communication skills training.

Spiritual practices, including meditation, also have been shown to be helpful self-care strategies (Ryan & Cunningham, 2007). Practitioners generally report that such practices increase their feelings of well-being (Cunningham, 2004). Meditation and other spiritual practices have been shown to offer such benefits as lowering blood pressure, improving breathing, relaxing muscles, and increasing feelings of hope and well-being among practitioners (Trippany et al., 2004).

THE CASE OF WANDA

Ever since she lost her father when she was 5 years old, Wanda wanted to grow up to be a counselor for children whose parents died. At age 35, she is doing just that. Wanda is employed as a clinical social worker at an inner-city agency's program for children ages 5–17 who have experienced exposure to crises and trauma. Of the 25 children on her caseload, 15 have lost one or more family members to community violence. After 3 years on the job, her enthusiasm for helping has given way to a feeling of emptiness. In a discussion with her team supervisor, she cannot pinpoint any one child client's story that concerns her; rather, she is experiencing a general sense of malaise and hopelessness. She is surprised by her self-deprecating thoughts. She has also stopped going out with her friends on Friday nights, and for the past 3 months, she has been having trouble sleeping and has regularly been skipping meals. She doesn't receive regular clinical supervision at work, because her team supervisor is "too busy." She has just about given up hope that anything will change in her community, and she can no longer stand the pain and suffering of so many young people. When she talks about her clients in treatment team meetings, she discusses their issues in a monotone, with flat affect.

CONCLUSION

This chapter has outlined the importance of practitioners' understanding and responding to the potential adverse affects of trauma work with children and adolescents. In order to maximize the benefits, practitioners must be mindful and practice self-care for self-protection, overall health and well-being, and professional effectiveness. Ongoing monitoring and self-care practices that promote physical, cognitive, emotional, social, and spiritual well-being are available to assist practitioners in not only surviving but thriving in the midst of their trauma-related work.

STUDY QUESTIONS

1. Think back to your decision to enter your profession. What were the reasons that led you to choose your profession? What role, if any, did compassion satisfaction (e.g., the desire to help other people) have in your decision-making process? What roles does it play for you in your current professional life?
2. Of the psychological needs and cognitive schemas described in the chapter text (i.e., safety, esteem, trust, control, and intimacy), which ones are most challenged by the types of work you do?
3. Please download and complete the ProQOL-5 (available at *www.proqol.org/uploads/ProQOL_5_English_Self-Score_3-2012.pdf*). What are your scores for compassion satisfaction and CF? Based on the results, which areas have you identified as needing intervention? (This exercise can be completed individually or in a group.)
4. Examine the self-care eco-map (Figure 20.3). What areas do you identify as personal strengths and vulnerabilities? What self-care strategies do/can you use to develop or maintain your strengths and reduce your vulnerabilities?
5. Complete the self-care activities checklist (Figure 20.1). What activities do you already do? What additional activities are you willing to incorporate into your daily life routine?
6. Based on the chapter content reading, how would you describe what Wanda is experiencing? If you were helping Wanda develop an assessment and self-care plan, what might it look like?

ACKNOWLEDGMENT

Portions of this chapter are adapted from Maschi and Brown (2010), with permission from the Guilford Press.

REFERENCES

Adams, R. E., Boscarino, J. A., & Figley, C. R. (2006). Compassion fatigue and psychological distress among social workers: A validation study. *American Journal of Orthopsychiatry, 76*(1), 103–108.

Adams, S. A., & Riggs, S. A. (2008). An exploratory study of vicarious trauma among therapist trainees. *Training and Education in Professional Psychology, 2*(1), 26–34.

American Psychiatric Association. (2013). *Diagnostic and statistical manual of mental disorders* (5th ed.). Arlington, VA: Author.

Bell, H. (2003). Strengths and secondary trauma in family violence work. *Social Work, 48*(4), 513–522.

Bell, H., Kulkarni, S., & Dalton, L. (2003). Organizational prevention of vicarious trauma. *Families in Society, 84*(4), 463–470.

Bride, B. E. (2007). Prevalence of secondary traumatic stress among social workers. *Social Work, 52*, 63–70.

Bride, B. E., Radey, M., & Figley, C. R. (2007). Measuring compassion fatigue. *Clinical Social Work Journal, 35*, 155–163.

Bride, B. E., Robinson, M. M., Yegidis, B., & Figley, C. (2004). Development and validation of the Secondary Traumatic Stress Scale. *Research on Social Work Practice, 13*, 1–16.

Catherall, D. (1995). Preventing institutional secondary traumatic stress disorder. In C. R. Figley (Ed.), *Compassion fatigue: Coping with secondary traumatic stress disorder in those who treat the traumatized* (pp. 232–248). New York: Brunner/Mazel.

Cho, C., & Cassidy, D. E. (1994). Parallel process for workers and their clients in chronic bereavement resulting from HIV. *Death Studies, 18*, 273–292.

Crestman, K. R. (1999). Secondary exposure to trauma and self-reported distress. In B. H. Stamm (Ed.), *Secondary traumatic stress: Self-care issues for clinicians, researchers, and educators* (2nd ed., pp. 29–36). Lutherville, MD: Sidran Press.

Cunningham, M. (2004). Avoiding vicarious trauma: Support, spirituality, and self-care. In N. B. Webb (Ed.), *Mass trauma and violence: Helping families and children cope* (pp. 327–343). New York: Guilford Press.

Figley, C. R. (1995). Compassion fatigues as secondary traumatic stress disorder. In C. R. Figley (Ed.), *Compassion fatigue: Coping with secondary traumatic stress disorder in those who treat the traumatized* (pp. 1–20). New York: Brunner/Mazel.

Figley, C. R. (1999). Compassion fatigue: Toward a new understanding of the costs of caring. In B. H. Stamm (Ed.), *Secondary traumatic stress: Self-care issues for clinicians, researchers, and educators* (2nd ed., pp. 3–28). Lutherville, MD: Sidran Press.

Fredrickson, B. L. (1998). What good are positive emotions? *Review of General Psychology, 2*, 300–319.

Freud, S. (1959). The dynamics of the transference. In E. Jones (Ed.) & J. Riviere

(Trans.), *Collected papers* (Vol. 2, pp. 312–322). New York: Basic Books. (Original work published 1912)

Freyd, J. J. (1996). *Betrayal trauma: The logic of forgetting childhood abuse.* Cambridge, MA: Harvard University Press.

Gamble, S. J. (2002). Self-care for bereavement counselors. In N. B. Webb (Ed.), *Helping bereaved children: A handbook for practitioners* (2nd ed., pp. 346–362). New York: Guilford Press.

Hooyman, N. R., & Kramer, B. J. (2006). *Living through loss: Interventions across the lifespan.* New York: Columbia University Press.

Jenkins, S. R., & Baird, S. (2002). Secondary traumatic stress and vicarious trauma: A validational study. *Journal of Traumatic Stress, 15,* 423–432.

Lloyd, C., & King, R. (2002). Social work, stress and burnout: A review. *Journal of Mental Health, 11,* 255–265.

Maschi, T., Baer, J. C., Morrissey, M. B., & Moreno, C. (2012). The aftermath of childhood trauma on late life mental and physical health: A review of the literature. *Traumatology, 19,* 65–72.

Maschi, T., & Brown, D. (2010). Professional self-care and prevention of secondary trauma. In N. B. Webb (Ed.), *Helping bereaved children: A handbook for practitioners* (3rd ed., pp. 345–373). New York: Guilford Press.

Maslach, C. (2003). *Burnout: The cost of caring.* Cambridge, MA: Malor Books.

Maslach, C., Jackson, S. E., & Leiter, M. P. (1996). *Maslach Burnout Inventory* (3rd ed.). Palo Alto, CA: Consulting Psychologists Press.

Maslach, C., Jackson, S. E., & Leiter, M. P. (1997). Maslach Burnout Inventory (3rd ed.). In C. P. Zalaquett & R. J. Wood (Eds.), *Evaluating stress: A book of resources* (pp. 191–218). Lanham, MD: Scarecrow Press.

Maslach, C., & Leiter, M. P. (1997). *The truth about burnout: How organizations cause personal stress and what to do about it.* San Francisco: Jossey-Bass.

Merriam-Webster. (2008). Compassion. Retrieved April 10, 2008, from *www.merriam-webster.com/dictionary/compassion*

Meyers, T. W., & Cornille, T. A. (2002). The trauma of working with traumatized children. In C. R. Figley (Ed.), *Treating compassion fatigue* (pp. 39–56). New York: Brunner-Routledge.

Moran, C. C. (2002). Humor as a moderator of compassion fatigue. In C. R. Figley (Ed.), *Treating compassion fatigue* (pp. 139–154). New York: Brunner-Routledge.

Pearlman, L. A. (1999). Self-care for trauma therapists: Ameliorating vicarious traumatization. In B. H. Stamm (Ed.), *Secondary traumatic stress: Self-care issues for clinicians, researchers, and educators* (2nd ed., pp. 51–64). Lutherville, MD: Sidran Press.

Pearlman, L. A. (2003). *Trauma and Attachment Belief Scale (TABS) manual.* Los Angeles: Western Psychological Services.

Pearlman, L. A., & Saakvitne, K. W. (1995a). *Trauma and the therapist.* New York: Norton.

Pearlman, L. A., & Saakvitne, K. W. (1995b). Treating therapists with vicarious traumatization and secondary traumatic stress disorders. In C. R. Figley (Ed.), *Compassion fatigue: Coping with secondary traumatic stress disorder in those who treat the traumatized* (pp. 150–177). New York: Brunner/Mazel.

Radey, M., & Figley, C. R. (2007). The social psychology of compassion. *Clinical Social Work Journal, 35,* 207–214.

Rogers, C. R. (1980). *A way of being.* Boston: Houghton Mifflin.

Rothschild, B. (2006). *Help for the helper: Self-care strategies for managing burnout and stress.* New York: Norton.

Ryan, K., & Cunningham, M. (2007). Helping the helpers: Guidelines to prevent vicarious traumatization of play therapist working with traumatized children. In N. B. Webb (Ed.), *Play therapy with children in crisis: Individual, group, and family treatment* (3rd ed., pp. 443–460). New York: Guilford Press.

Saakvitne, K. W., Gamble, S., Pearlman, L. A., & Tabor Lev, B. (2000). *Risking connection: A training curriculum for working with survivors of childhood abuse.* Lutherville, MD: Sidran Press.

Saakvitne, K. W., & Pearlman, L. A. (1996): *Transforming the pain: A workbook on vicarious traumatization.* New York: Norton.

Stamm, B. H. (Ed.). (1999). *Secondary traumatic stress: Self-care issues for clinicians, researchers, and educators* (2nd ed.). Lutherville, MD: Sidran Press.

Stamm, B. H. (2002). Measuring compassion satisfaction as well as fatigue: Developmental history of the Compassion Satisfaction and Fatigue Test. In C. R. Figley (Ed.), *Treating compassion fatigue* (pp. 107–122). New York: Brunner-Routledge.

Stamm, B. H. (2009). Professional Quality of Life Scale. Retrieved March 19, 2012, from *www.proqol.org/uploads/ProQOL_5_English_Self-Score_3-2012.pdf.*

Trippany, R. L., White Kress, V. E., & Wilcoxon, S. A. (2004). Preventing vicarious trauma: What counselors should know when working with trauma survivors. *Journal of Counseling Development, 82*(1), 31–37.

Valent, P. (2002). Diagnosis and treatment of helper stresses, trauma, and illnesses. In C. R. Figley (Ed.). *Treating compassion fatigue* (pp. 17–38). New York: Brunner-Routledge.

Webb, N. B. (2004). The impact of traumatic stress and loss on children and families. In N. B. Webb (Ed.), *Mass trauma and violence: Helping families and children cope* (pp. 3–22). New York: Guilford Press.

Webb, N. B. (2011). *Social work practice with children* (3rd ed.). New York: Guilford Press.

Weinstein, J. (2006). *Working with loss, death and bereavement: A guide for social workers.* Thousand Oaks, CA: Sage.

Wilson, J. P., & Lindy, J. (Eds.). (1994). *Countertransference in the treatment of PTSD.* New York: Guilford Press

Yassen, J. (1995). Preventing secondary traumatic stress disorder. In C. R. Figley (Ed.), *Compassion fatigue: Coping with secondary traumatic stress disorder in those who treat the traumatized* (pp. 178–208). New York: Brunner/Mazel.

Appendix

Play Therapy Resources

SELECTED TRAINING PROGRAMS AND CERTIFICATIONS

Play Therapy

The programs listed here represent a small selection of those available in different parts of the United States. A more comprehensive listing by state is available through the Association for Play Therapy (*www.a4pt.org*).

Boston University School of Social Work
Postgraduate Certificate Program in Assessment and Treatment of Psychological Trauma
Boston, MA 02215
www.bu.edu/ssw/professional-development/professional-education-programs-pep

California School of Professional Psychology
Alliant University
Fresno, CA 93727
www.alliant.edu/cspp

Center for Play Therapy
University of North Texas
Denton, TX 76203
http://cpt.unt.edu

Chesapeake Beach Professional Seminars
Chesapeake Beach, MD 20732
www.cbpseminars.org

Lesley University
Advanced Professional Certificate in Play Therapy
Cambridge, MA 02138
http://lesley.smartcatalogiq.com/en/2014-2015/Graduate-Catalog/Graduate-School-of-Arts-and-Social-Sciences/Division-of-Expressive-Therapies/Advanced-Professional-Certificates/Copy-of-Advanced-Professional-Certificate-in-Play-Therapy

Theraplay Institute
Evanston, IL 60201
www.theraplay.org

Play Therapy Training Institute
Monroe Township, NJ 08831
www.ptti.org

Vista Del Mar Child and Family Services
Los Angeles, CA 90034
www.vistadelmar.org

Creative Arts/Expressive Therapy

Lesley University
Advanced Professional Certificate in Expressive Therapies Studies
Cambridge, MA 02138
www.lesley.edu/certificate/expressive-therapies/advanced-professional

Expressive Arts Florida Institute
Sarasota, FL 34236
www.expressiveartsflorida.com/institute-training.html

Graduate Program in Drama Therapy
Department of Music and Performing Arts Professions
New York University
New York, NY 10012
www.steinhardt.nyu.edu/music/dramatherapy

Creative Arts and Health Certificate
The New School
New York, NY 10011
www.newschool.edu/academics

Dance/Movement Therapy
Drexel University
Philadelphia, PA 19102
www.drexel.edu/cnhp/academics/departments/Creative-Arts-Therapies

School of the Art Institute of Chicago
Chicago, IL 60603
www.artic.edu

Trauma/Crisis Mental Health Counseling

American Academy of Experts in Traumatic Stress
Ronkonkoma, NY 11779
www.aaets.org

American Association of Suicidology
Washington, DC 20015
www.suicidology.org

ChildTrauma Academy
Houston, TX 77024
www.childtrauma.org

Child Trauma Institute
Northampton, MA 01060
www.childtrauma.com

EMDR International Association
Austin, TX 78731
www.emdria.org

National Institute for Trauma and Loss in Children
Albion, MI 49224
www.starr.org/training/tlc

Grief Counseling

Association for Death Education and Counseling
Deerfield, IL 60015
www.adec.org

Certificate Program in Thanatology
Graduate School of the College of New Rochelle
New Rochelle, NY 10805
www.cnr.edu/web/graduate-school/thanatology

The Dougy Center: The National Center for Grieving Children and Families
Portland, OR 97286
www.dougy.org

Hospice Foundation of America
Washington, DC 20036
www.hospicefoundation.org

Make-A-Wish Foundation of America
Phoenix, AZ 85016
www.wish.org

National Center for Death Education
Newton, MA 02459
www.mountida.edu/academics/continuing-education/ncde

PROFESSIONAL JOURNALS ON PLAY, CREATIVE ARTS, AND TRAUMA

Anxiety, Stress and Coping (journal of the Stress and Anxiety Research Society)
www.star-society.org

Art Psychotherapy
www.elsevier.com

Art Therapy: Journal of the American Art Therapy Association
www.arttherapy.org

Brown University Child and Adolescent Behavioral Letter
www.childadolescentbehavior.com

Child Abuse and Neglect
www.elsevier.com

Child and Adolescent Group Psychotherapy
www.springerlink.com

Child and Adolescent Social Work Journal
www.springerlink.com

Child Development
www.srcd.org/publications

Child Psychiatry and Human Development
www.springerlink.com

Child Welfare Journal (formerly *Child Welfare Quarterly*)
www.cwla.org/child-welfare-journal

Children and Youth Care Forum
www.springerlink.com

Children and Youth Services Review
www.elsevier.com

Drama Therapy Review
www.nadta.org

Groupwork
www.whitingbirch.net

International Journal of Group Psychotherapy
www.guilford.com/journals

International Journal of Play Therapy
www.apa.org/journals

Journal of Abnormal Child Psychology
www.springerlink.com

Journal of Adolescence
www.elsevier.com

Journal of the American Academy of Child and Adolescent Psychiatry
www.jaacap.com

Journal of Child and Adolescent Group Therapy
www.springerlink.com

Journal of Child and Adolescent Trauma
www.springerlink.com

Journal of Child and Family Studies
www.springerlink.com

Journal of Child and Youth Care (formerly *Journal of Child Care*)
www.ucalgary.ca/ucpress

Journal of Child Psychology and Psychiatry and Allied Disciplines
www.cambridge.org

Journal of Clinical Child and Adolescent Psychology (formerly *Journal of Clinical Child Psychology*)
www.tandfonline.com

Journal of Family Violence
www.springerlink.com

Journal of Music Therapy
www.musictherapy.org

Journal of Research on Adolescence
www.onlinelibrary.wiley.com

Journal of Traumatic Stress
www.istss.org

Journal of Youth and Adolescence
www.springerlink.com

Play Therapy
www.a4pt.org

Psychoanalytic Study of the Child
yalepress.yale.edu/yupbooks

School Psychology International
www.sagepub.com/journals

Social Work with Groups
www.tandfonline.com

Trauma, Violence, and Abuse
www.sagepub.com/journals

PROFESSIONAL ORGANIZATIONS THAT SUPPORT THE USE OF PLAY/EXPRESSIVE THERAPIES

American Academy of Child and Adolescent Psychiatry
www.aacap.org

American Academy of Experts in Traumatic Stress
www.aaets.org

American Academy of Pediatrics
www.aap.org

American Art Therapy Association
www.arttherapy.org

American Association of Suicidology
www.suicidology.org

American Dance Therapy Association
www.adta.org

American Music Therapy Association
www.musictherapy.org

American Professional Society on the Abuse of Children
www.apsac.org

American Psychiatric Association
www.psych.org

American Psychological Association
www.apa.org

American Red Cross
www.redcross.org

American Society of Group Psychotherapy and Psychodrama
www.asgpp.org

Annie E. Casey Foundation
www.aecf.org

Association for Play Therapy
www.a4pt.org

Association for Traumatic Stress Specialists
www.atss.info

Association of Pediatric Oncology Social Workers
www.aposw.org

Children's Group Therapy Association
www.cgta.net

Child Welfare League of America
www.cwla.org

Child Witness to Violence Project
www.childwitnesstoviolence.org

International Expressive Arts Therapy Association
www.ieata.org

International Society for Traumatic Stress Studies
www.istss.org

National Association of Social Workers
www.naswdc.org

National Association of Perinatal Social Workers
www.napsw.org

National Child Traumatic Stress Network
www.nctsnet.org

National Coalition of Creative Arts Therapies Associations
www.nccata.org

North American Drama Therapy Association
www.nadta.org

Sandplay Therapists of America
www.sandplay.org

SUPPLIERS OF PLAY AND ASSORTED CREATIVE ARTS MATERIALS

Child Therapy Toys
www.childtherapytoys.com

Constructive Playthings
www.constructiveplaythings.com

Magic Cabin
www.magiccabin.com

Play Therapy Supply
www.playtherapysupply.com

Rose Play Therapy Toys
www.roseplaytherapy.net

School Specialty
https://schoolspecialty.com

Self Esteem Shop
www.selfesteemshop.com

Toys to Grow On
www.toystogrowon.com

U.S. Toy Company
http://ustoyco.com/constcatalogs.htm

Western Psychological Services
www.wpspublish.com

Index

Page numbers followed by *f* indicate figure, *t* indicate table

B

C

D

E

R

S

T